Polymeric Biomaterials

NATO ASI Series

Advanced Science Institutes Series

A Series presenting the results of activities sponsored by the NATO Science Committee, which aims at the dissemination of advanced scientific and technological knowledge, with a view to strengthening links between scientific communities.

The Series is published by an international board of publishers in conjunction with the NATO Scientific Affairs Division

A	Life Sciences	Plenum Publishing Corporation
B	Physics	London and New York
C	Mathematical and Physical Sciences	D. Reidel Publishing Company Dordrecht and Boston
D	Behavioural and Social Sciences	Martinus Nijhoff Publishers Dordrecht/Boston/Lancaster
E	Applied Sciences	
F	Computer and Systems Sciences	Springer-Verlag Berlin/Heidelberg/New York
G	Ecological Sciences	

Series E: Applied Sciences – No. 106

Polymeric Biomaterials

Edited by

Erhan Piskin

Hacettepe University
Chemical Engineering Department
Ankara
Turkey

Allan S. Hoffman

University of Washington
Center for Bioengineering
Seattle, Washington
USA

1986 **Martinus Nijhoff Publishers**
Dordrecht / Boston / Lancaster
Published in cooperation with NATO Scientific Affairs Division

Proceedings of the NATO Advanced Study Institute on Biopolymers, Izmir, Turkey,
August 27–September 5, 1984

Library of Congress Cataloging in Publication Data

NATO Advanced Study Institute on Biopolymers (1984 :
   Izmir, Turkey)
   Polymeric Biomaterials.

   (NATO Advanced Science Institutes series. Series E:
Applied sciences ; 106)
   "Proceedings of the NATO Advanced Study Institute on
Biopolymers, Izmir, Turkey, August 27–September 5,
1984."
   "Published in cooperation with NATO Scientific
Affairs Division."
   1. Polymers in medicine—Congresses. I. Piskin,
Erhan. II. Hoffman, Allan S. III. North Atlantic
Treaty Organization. Scientific Affairs Division.
IV. Title. V. Series: NATO ASI series. Series E,
Applied sciences ; no. 106.
R857.P6N38   1984   610'.28   86–790

ISBN-13: 978-94-010-8452-9   e-ISBN-13: 978-94-009-4390-2
DOI: 10.1007/978-94-009-4390-2

Softcover reprint of the hardcover 1st edition 1986

Distributors for the United States and Canada: Kluwer Boston, Inc., 190 Old Derby
Street, Hingham, MA 02043, USA

Distributors for the UK and Ireland: Kluwer Academic Publishers, MTP Press Ltd,
Falcon House, Queen Square, Lancaster LA1 1RN, UK

Distributors for all other countries: Kluwer Academic Publishers Group, Distribution
Center, P.O. Box 322, 3300 AH Dordrecht, The Netherlands

FOREWORD

This volume comes from manuscripts contributed by invited speakers to the NATO Advanced Study Institute on Biopolymers, which was held in Izmir, during August 27th - September 5th, 1984. Many more details have been added to the manuscripts as a result of the interchange of ideas during the symposium. This book includes 16 papers which were originally presented at the meeting by some of the world's foremost investigators.

In this volume, the existing basic knowledge across the whole field of polymeric biomaterials is reviewed. Classification, structure, composition, synthesis, modification and fabrication of these novel materials is included in detail. Fundamental phenomena involved in the interaction of polymers with the biological environment and resulting responses of blood and tissue components are discussed. Modification of polymers physically, chemically or biochemically, in order to improve their biocompatibility is included. Selected applications of polymeric biomaterials in Medicine, Dentistry, Biotechnology, Pharmacology and other related fields are also covered.

We strongly hope that this book will be a great contribution to the rapidly expanding field of biomaterials and will help to stimulate an even more exciting future for this field.

Erhan Piskin
Allan S. Hoffman

ACKNOWLEDGEMENTS

NATO Advanced Study Institute on "Biopolymers" was held in Izmir during August 27th - September 5th, 1984. I would like to express my deepest appreciation and gratitude to NATO Scientific Affairs Division, that our meeting has been accepted as a NATO ASI, and has been supported by their programmes. I wish to thank also to all the other supporting firms and organizations, especially to Hacettepe University and Turkish Scientific and Technical Research Council.

I gratefully acknowledge the kind collaboration of Prof.A.S.Hoffman in editing this book. I wish to thank also all the authors for their contributions in bringing out this volume.

I am grateful to Dr.K.Piskin, Mr.E.Erturk, Mr.A.Oncu, Mr.V.Evren, Mr.M.Mutlu, Miss M.Kiremitci, Mr.E.Marlalı for their concientious efforts in working on the organization of the meeting, and especially to Mr.V.Evren and Mr.A.Denizli for their very kind help on the preparation of this book. Lastly, I should convey our appreciation to publishers themselves for their customary efficiency in bringing out the volume.

Erhan Piskin
Director
NATO ASI on Biopolymers

CONTENTS

APPLICATIONS OF SYNTHETIC POLYMERIC BIOMATERIALS IN MEDICINE AND BIOTECHNOLOGY

A.S. Hoffman

University of Washington, Center for Bioengineering, Seattle, Washington, USA

INTRODUCTION

There is a wide variety of materials which are used in contact with biological fluids. These materials are known as biomaterials. Many different biomaterials are used clinically, as components of implants or devices for diagnosis or therapy (1,2). Other important uses are in laboratories and in industrial processes. Agricultural and marine applications to animals, birds and fish also exist. The various biomaterials include polymers (fibers, rubbers, molded plastics, emulsions, powders, coatings and fluids), metals, ceramics, carbons, reconstituted or specially treated natural tissues, and composites made from various combinations of such materials (Fig. 1).

Synthetic polymers make up by far the broadest and most diverse class of biomaterials (Figs. 2 and 3). This is mainly because synthetic polymers are available with such a wide variety of compositions, properties and forms and also because they may be fabricated readily into complex shapes and structures (Table I).

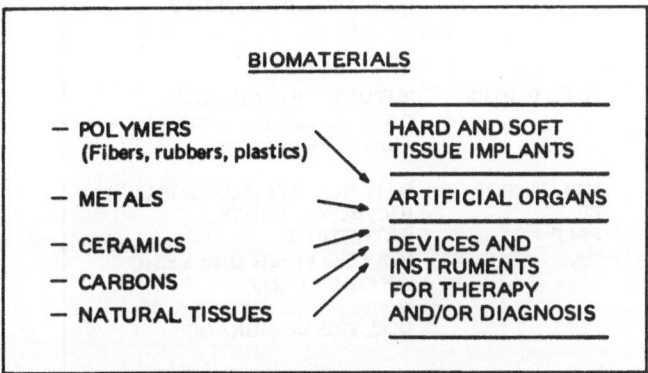

Figure 1.   Classes and General Medical Application Areas of Biomaterials.

2

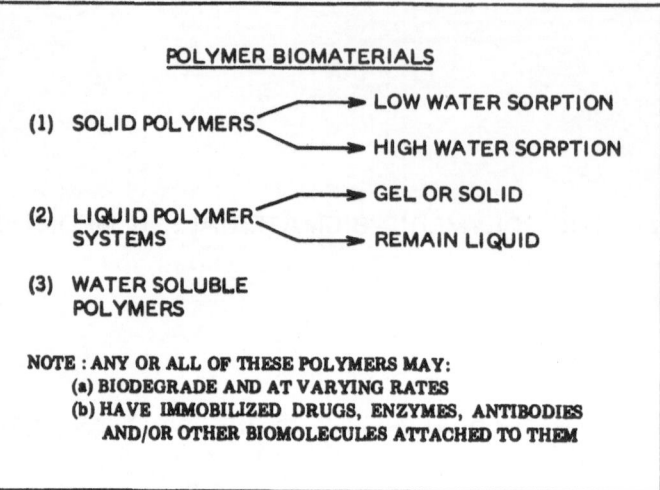

Figure 2.   Forms of Polymeric Biomaterials.

SOLID POLYMERIC BIOMATERIALS

PROPERTIES	EXAMPLES	USES
(a) SOFT (RUBBERY)		
— LOW WATER SORPTION	SR, PU, PVC	TUBES, DIAPHRAGMS, COATING, IMPLANTS, PACEMAKERS, ADHESIVES, BLOOD BAGS
— HIGH WATER SORPTION	PHEMA	CONTACT LENS, BURN DRESSING, COATING
(b) AMORPHOUS, HARD	PMMA	CONTACT LENS, IOL, DENTAL AND ORTHOPEDIC CEMENTS
(c) SEMI-CRYSTALLINE		
— LOW WATER SORPTION	PET, PP, PTFE	SUTURES, VASCULAR GRAFTS, SEWING ANCHORS, TISSUE INGROWTH
	NYLON, PGA PE PFEP CA	SUTURES, (BIODEGREDABLE) IUD, BONE, JOINTS, CATHETERS HOLLOW FIBER DIALYSER, CONTACT LENS
— MODERATE WATER SORPTION	CELL	DIALYSIS MEMBRANE.

Figure 3.   Morphology, Composition and Medical Uses of Polymeric Biomaterials.

Table I. Solid Forms of Polymeric Biomaterials (1).

1. Hollow Fibers, Tubes
2. Films, Membranes, Discs
3. Microspheres, Powders, Beads
4. Fibers, Rods
5. Molded Objects
6. All of the above as:
   a. smooth, homogeneous solids
   b. filled solids
   c. surface-rough solids
   d. porous solids
   e. water-swollen solids
   f. solid suspensions in aqueous solution
7. Coatings

Since the biologic environment is mainly composed of water, the water wettability and sorption are two important properties of biomaterials. The mechanical properties of biomaterials are also key factors in determining useful applications of such materials. These three factors are interrelated for a wide range of biomaterials in Figure 4.

MODIFIED AND BIOFUNCTIONAL BIOMATERIALS

The surfaces of polymeric biomaterials may be readily modified physically or chemically (Fig. 5) (3-6). Such surface modifications of biomaterials can significantly influence their biologic responses to blood or tissue fluids.

A wide variety of biologically active species may also be incorporated into or onto polymeric biomaterials for a wide variety of uses (Table II) (7-9). Such biofunctional polymer systems may be used in-vitro in the clinical laboratory or elsewhere for diagnostic assays, in-vivo or ex-vivo as biosensors, components of artificial organs, or for drug delivery or toxin removal from blood (Tables III and IV).

Table II. Biologically Active Species Which May be Immobilized Within or on Polymeric Biomaterials.

Enzymes	Anticancer agents
Antibodies	Drug antagonists
Antigens	Other drugs, in general
Anti-thrombogenic agents	Sugars and polysaccharides
Antibiotics	DNA or RNA sequences
Antibacterial agents	Peptide sequences
Contraceptives	Living cells

Classification of Biomaterials

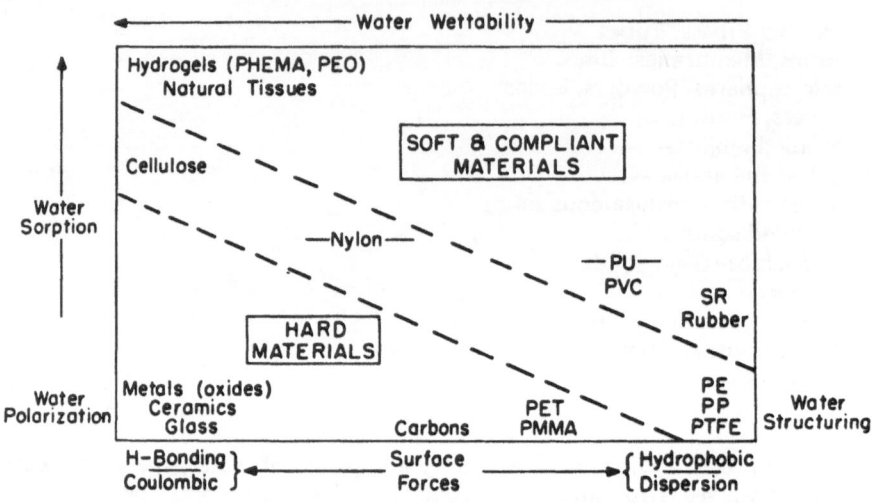

Figure 4.   Classification of Biomaterials in Terms of Water Interaction and Mechanical Properties.

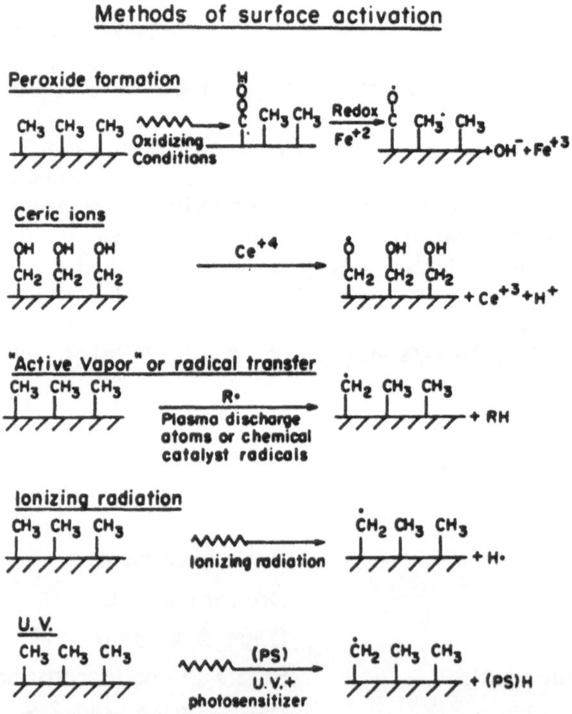

Methods of surface activation

Peroxide formation

Ceric ions

"Active Vapor" or radical transfer

Ionizing radiation

U. V.

Figure 5.   Examples of Techniques and Reactions for Generating Radicals on Surfaces (Note: The precise nature of the radical intermediates formed has not been elucidated in some cases, Representations in this figure show schematically radical species which might be formed) (6).

Table III. Some Examples of Uses of Immobilized Biomolecule-Polymer Systems.

Improved biocompatibility
Drug delivery
Toxin removal
Cell "finders" and "markers" (via antibody-antigen binding)
Diagnostic kits
Bioreactors (including artificial organs, cell and enzyme reactors)
Biomedical sensors or electrodes

Table IV. Some Specific Biomedical Applications of Immobilized Enzymes (13).

Immobilized Enzyme	Application
Brinolase, Urokinase, Streptokinase	Fibrinolytic surface
Asparaginase, Glutaminase	Leukemia treatment
Carbonic Anhydrase, Catalase	Membrane oxygenator
Urease	Artificial kidney
Glucose Oxidase	Glucose sensor (artificial pancreas component)
Microsomal enzymes	Artificial liver
Alcohol Oxidase	Blood alcohol electrode
LNase, RNase	Removal of airborn infections

In many cases the immobilized biomolecule system has particular advantages over the "free" biomolecule (Table V lists some advantages for immobilized enzymes).
One may immobilize the biologically active molecules or cells by four major techniques: (a) physical entrapment; (b) physical adsorption with or without chemical crosslinking; (c) electrostatic attraction; and (d) chemical bonding (Table VI).

Table V. Advantages of Immobilized Enzymes.

1. Enzyme more stable
2. Can reuse enzyme
3. Continuous processing possible
4. Product is enzyme-free
5. Can modify microenvironment and/or process conditions
6. Lower cost, higher quality product
7. No immunogenic response to "foreign" enzyme

Table VI. Immobilization Techniques for Biomolecules and Cells.

1. Physical Entrapment
2. Physical Adsorption with or without Chemical Crosslinking
3. Electrostatic Attraction
4. Chemical Bonding

Physical entrapment may involve sorption of the biologic species into a formed polymer, or encapsulation inside a polymeric skin via a phase separation process or polymerization of monomers ($\mp$ polymers) in solutions containing the biologic species. It is very important that either a significant pore structure exist in the final product or that it be in a finely divided form, so as to provide access for other biomolecules to reach the immobilized biomolecule, or vice versa. (The word "immobilization" refers in a temporal sense to the significantly lowered mobility of the biological species; it may never leach out or it may gradually dissolve into the surrounding medium. In either case, it is considered to have been "immobilized".)

Another immobilization technique involves nonspecific surface adsorption of biologic species sometimes followed by chemical crosslinking of the adsorbed biomolecules to themselves using bifunctional reagents as glutaraldehyde.

"Electrostatic attraction" normally signifies ion-ion or ion-dipole forces and as such may be viewed as similar to ion-exchange or affinity chromatography, when the latter is primarily based on ionic interactions. It is the basis for immobilization of polyanionic biomolecules as heparin onto cationic sites, and may control the binding of an antigen onto an already immobilized antibody, or a substrate molecule onto an immobilized enzyme. Specific biological binding requires previous immobilization of the specific binding site. Although hydrophobic binding is a special case of physical adsorption as an immobilization mechanism it may also contribute to electrostatic immobilization.

Chemical bonding involves specialized chemical reactions on specific matrix backbone groups (usually —OH or —COOH which are pre-reacted in order to activate these sites so they can form primary bonds with the species to be immobilized (usually via —NH_2 groups on such species). This is the most complex technique of all and may involve several steps. Some polymers, such as polysaccharides, already contain reactable groups, while others, as Teflon or polypropylene, are relatively unreactive. These latter polymers may be modified using radiation processing followed by chemical immobilization techniques (3-6). Radiation grafted hydrogels or radiation polymerized emulsions of HEMA or MAAc and their copolymers have been most used for subsequent immobilization of biomolecules (10-13). Soluble polymers may also be used to "immobilize" biomolocules, as exemplified with drug molecules in Figure 6 (3). Plasma discharge treatments may also be useful for surface immobilization of biomolecules (6,14). This technique is less "precise" than radiation-grafted surface immobilization in the sense that there are a larger number of poorly defined chemical groups produced on a plasma-treated surface.

APPLICATIONS OF BIOMATERIALS IN BIOTECHNOLOGY

The ability to recombine DNA in precise ways, to insert the novel plasmid into living cells and to produce new proteins with important clinical uses has led to a new and immense scientific field as well as to a modern industrial, "biotechnological" revolution (15-17). In parallel with this significant achievement, immunologists have been able to produce useful quantities of antibodies having high purity and antigenic specificity. These antibodies are called monoclonal antibodies (MAb's). These two significant developments together make up the exciting new field called biotechnology (Fig. 7).

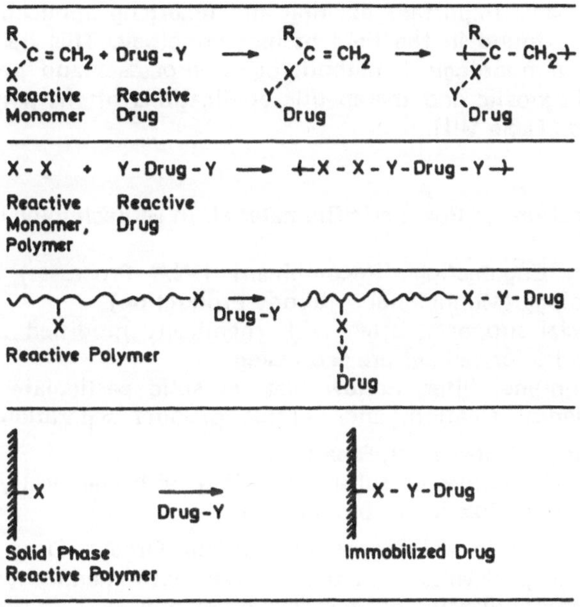

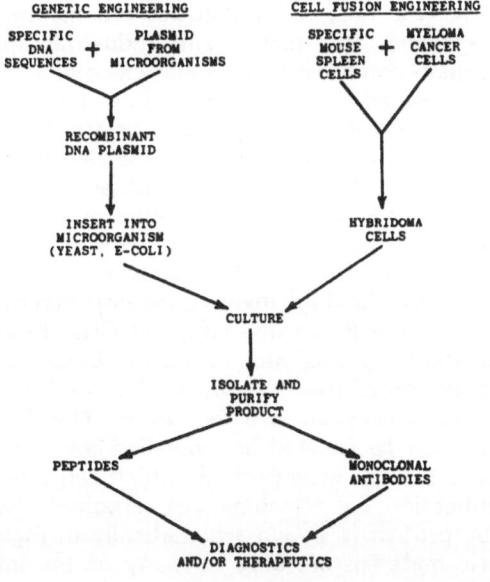

Figure 6.   Preparation Methods for Synthetic Polymer - Biomolecule Conjugates; Shown with Drugs as an Example of a Biomolecule (3).

GENETIC ENGINEERING   CELL FUSION ENGINEERING

SPECIFIC   PLASMID   SPECIFIC   MYELOMA
DNA   +   FROM   MOUSE   +   CANCER
SEQUENCES   MICROORGANISMS   SPLEEN   CELLS
                                 CELLS

RECOMBINANT
DNA PLASMID

INSERT INTO   HYBRIDOMA
MICROORGANISM   CELLS
(YEAST, E-COLI)

CULTURE

ISOLATE AND
PURIFY
PRODUCT

PEPTIDES   MONOCLONAL
                                 ANTIBODIES

DIAGNOSTICS
AND/OR THERAPEUTICS

Figure 7.   The Two Major Branches of Biotechnology Showing Applications in the Medical or Veterinary Fields. Specific Human Lymph Cells Would be Used Instead of Mouse Spleen Cells for Making Hybridomas Which Produce Antibodies for Therapeutic Uses in Humans, (20).

There are many important existing and emerging applications of polymeric biomaterials to be found in the field of biotechnology. This field involves genetic engineering and immunological methodologies, processes and products. There are also numerous diagnostic and therapeutic applications of the polypeptide products of these processes (Table VII).

Table VII. Applications of Polymeric Biomaterials in Biotechnology.

I. Genetic Engineering (Recombinant DNA Processes) and Immunologic Technology (Monoclonal Antibody Production)
   — Special supports, often with chemically modified surfaces, or microcapsules for cell culture processing
   — Membrane, filter, hollow fiber or solid particulate systems for DNA sequence isolation, and peptide product separation and purification

II. Diagnostics (Biosensors, Bioassays)
   — Special coatings or substrates, often with chemically modified surface for immobilization of biomolecules

III. Therapeutics (Novel Bioreactor/Artificial Organs, Drug Delivery Systems)
   — Exchange devices or materials, often with chemically modified surfaces for immobilization of biomolecules or cells

Recombinant DNA Biotechnology

Recombinant DNA (ReDNA) methodologies are making possible many new and revolutionary diagnostic, therapeutic and industrial applications in clinical medicine, agriculture (plants and insects), veterinary medicine, and animal husbandry. This field is commonly referred to as "genetic engineering" and more commonly as "genesplicing" technology. ReDNA processing is useful for enhancing yields over conventional tissue culture processes (e.g. for antibiotics, enzymes), for larger scale fermentation production in general or where no other practical means of synthesis is currently available (e.g. for human insulin or interferon). The full range of processes and products of ReDNA biotechnology is far from realization.

Polymers play an important role in the processing and applications of ReDNA products. Basically, ReDNA technology involves the insertion of a particular sequence of a hybrid DNA into a ring-like double stranded DNA hybrid, called a plasmid, which is then inserted into living cells, such as yeast or E. coli cells, where it is used as a template for the production of specific polypeptide products. The cells are usually cultured in dishes or in suspension, in a fermentor. The "genetically engineered" peptide products must then be isolated and purified for subsequent uses. To date, most ReDNA products are single gene proteins which can function with little or no post-translational modification, e.g. attachment of carbohydrates.

A typical ReDNA process is shown schematically in Figure 8. This figure also shows where polymeric materials are used in many of the important steps in this process. New polymers with or without special surface treatments may be developed to improve process yields, productions rates and product purity (18-22). For example, it is well known that both cell adhesion and cell motility on foreign surfaces are sensitive to surface chemistry (23-26). It is possible that replication of polypeptides

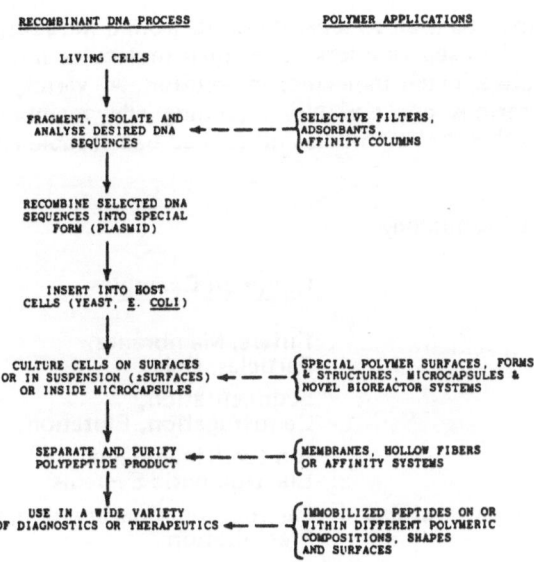

RECOMBINANT DNA PROCESS · POLYMER APPLICATIONS

LIVING CELLS

FRAGMENT, ISOLATE AND ANALYSE DESIRED DNA SEQUENCES ← − − − { SELECTIVE FILTERS, ADSORBANTS, AFFINITY COLUMNS

RECOMBINE SELECTED DNA SEQUENCES INTO SPECIAL FORM (PLASMID)

INSERT INTO HOST CELLS (YEAST, E. COLI)

CULTURE CELLS ON SURFACES OR IN SUSPENSION (±SURFACES) OR INSIDE MICROCAPSULES ← − − − { SPECIAL POLYMER SURFACES, FORMS & STRUCTURES, MICROCAPSULES & NOVEL BIOREACTOR SYSTEMS

SEPARATE AND PURIFY POLYPEPTIDE PRODUCT ← − − − { MEMBRANES, HOLLOW FIBERS OR AFFINITY SYSTEMS

USE IN A WIDE VARIETY OF DIAGNOSTICS OR THERAPEUTICS ← − − − { IMMOBILIZED PEPTIDES ON OR WITHIN DIFFERENT POLYMERIC COMPOSITIONS, SHAPES AND SURFACES

Figure 8.   Polymer Applications in ReDNA Processes, (20).

within a cell could also be sensitive to the character of the foreign surface onto which the cell is adhered. Surfaces for cell culture operations may be used in a variety of forms (Table I). Such polymer surfaces may be modified by a variety of methods as discussed above. Bioreactors or fermentors for cell culturing can incorporate synthetic polymers in different designs and operating modes (Table VIII).

Table VIII. Fermentor Designs.

Stirred Tank (Batch or Continuous)
Fluid Bed
Packed Bed
Hollow Fiber
Biological Film

Bioseparation

Separation and purification of the genetically engineered peptide product is critical to the economic viability of the process (18-19). There are many separation technologies which are commonly used or which are now emerging within the chemical, pharmaceutical and biological industries (Table IX). Classical laboratory scale chromatographic techniques (Table X) are generally useful for yielding small quantities of high purity products but are not as applicable in large scale processing. For such needs, polymeric membrane, filter or separation systems may be most useful for concentration and purification of the polypeptide products of an ReDNA process.

Microporous filters may be used to separate solids from a fluid suspension; ultrafiltration may then be used to separate large and small molecules and reverse osmosis can be used to concentrate selected molecules in solution. A variety of polymer separation device configurations are possible, including flat membrane stacks, coiled, flattened membrane tubes, hollow fibers and packed beds (Table XI).

Table IX. Separations Technology.

Basis	Common Examples
Size	Filters, Membranes, Particles, Gels
Density	Sedimentation, Centrifugation, Flotation
Charge	Ion Exchange Solids, Electrokinetic Systems
Physico-Chemical Interactions	Partitioning, Coacervation, Precipitation
Biospecific Affinity	Particles or Macromolecules with Specific Ligands
Biospecific Enzymolysis	Isomer Separation

Table X. Chromatographic Separations.

Type	Molecular Basis of Separation
Affinity	Bio-Specificity
Ion-Exchange	Change
Gel Filtration	Size
Isoelectric Focusing	Isoelectric Point
Hydrophobic Interaction	Hydrophobic Bonding

Table XI. Membrane Separations Technology.

A. Common Types:

Micro Filters	(Particles From Solution)
Ultrafilters	(Large Molecules From Small Molecules)
Permselective Membranes	(Small Molecules From Other Small Molecules)

B. Common Designs:
1) Stacked, Flat Sheets
2) Coiled Envelopes
3) Hollow Fibers

Biofunction units as immobilized cell bioreactors and immobilized enzyme reactors may also assist in product purification (18).

Monoclonal Antibody Immuno-Biotechnology

The availability of a wide range of monoclonal antibodies (MAb's) has also opened up possibilities for an immense variety of novel and revolutionary diagnostic and therapeutic applications, especially in clinical medicine (Table XII). MAb's may be prepared either (a) by fusing specialized mouse spleen or human lymph cells with long-lived ("eternal") cancer cells as myeloma cells to form MAb-producing hybridoma cells, which are then cultured, or (b) by ReDNA processing, with the information for making the MAb inserted into the cell as part of a DNA plasmid. MAb's may be made against a wide variety of clinically important antigens (20,27).

Table XII. Uses of Monoclonal Antibodies (20).

1. In-Vitro or In-Vivo Diagnostics
2. Targeting Drug or Drug Containing Systems
3. Therapeutic Agents
4. Affinity Chromatography

A major use of MAb's is in a wide variety of immunoassay diagnostic tests, (27). Included are assays for drug monitoring, viral diseases, sexually transmitted diseases, respiratory diseases, tissue typing, blood grouping, cell surface antigens and cancer. Most of these assays depend upon one of three types of signals, e.g. radioactivity as in radioimmunoassay, RIA; fluorescence as in fluorescent immunoassay, FIA; or fluorescence polarization immunoassay, FPIA; or visible color change as in enzyme immunoassay, EIA; such as enzyme-linked immunosorbant assay, ELISA; enzyme-multiplied immunoassay technique, EMIT; and enzyme-membrane immunoassay, EMIA. Typical concentration ranges of clinically important assays are shown in Table XIII.

Table XIII. Typical Concentration Range of Clinical Analystes.

	Moles / Liter
Ions	10^{-1} to 10^{-2}
Metabolites (Glucose, Urea, Cholesterol)	10^{-2} to 10^{-4}
Drugs	10^{-3} to 10^{-6}
Steroids	10^{-6} to 10^{-11}
Protein Hormones	10^{-6} to 10^{-12}
Antibodies	10^{-6} to 10^{-10}
Cellular Antigens	10^{-6} to 10^{-9}
Tumor Antigens	10^{-10} to 10^{-11}
Viral Antigens	10^{-10} to 10^{-12}

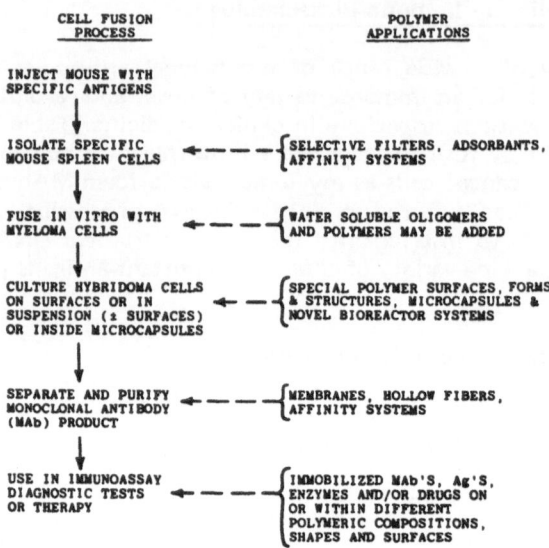

Figure 9.   Polymer Applications in the MAb Biotechnology Field, (20).

Table XIV. Possible Biosensor Signals (20).

     Optical (Visible, Fluorescent, Luminescent)
     Electrical (Potential, Current)
     Radioactive Emissions
     Chemical (pH, Redox)
     Biochemical (Aq/Ab)
     Mechanical (Swelling)
     Acoustic
     Magnetic

     MAb's may also be used therapeutically, either by themselves or as a targeting biomolecule when conjugated to a drug or to a drug containing polymeric system (as microcapsules). MAb's or antigens are immobilized to polymeric surfaces (usually by physical adsorption) in many of the immunoassay systems, as well as when they (MAb's) may be used as a targeting molecule for a drug delivery system. Specially treated or reactable polymer surfaces are also useful for these applications (6). Figure 9 summarizes the many polymer applications in the MAb biotechnology field.
     A wide range of highly specific biosensors is now possible using immobilized MAb's as the detection agent for the analyte (27,28). Some of these are miniaturized extensions of conventional assay techniques, while a number are novel fiber-optic, electronic or acoustic devices. There are important contributions to be made here by polymer scientists in collaboration with physical scientists, electrical engineers and biological scientists (Fig. 10). Table XIV lists the wide variety of biosensor signals possible. Most miniaturized devices which are intended for in vivo monitoring are still under development.

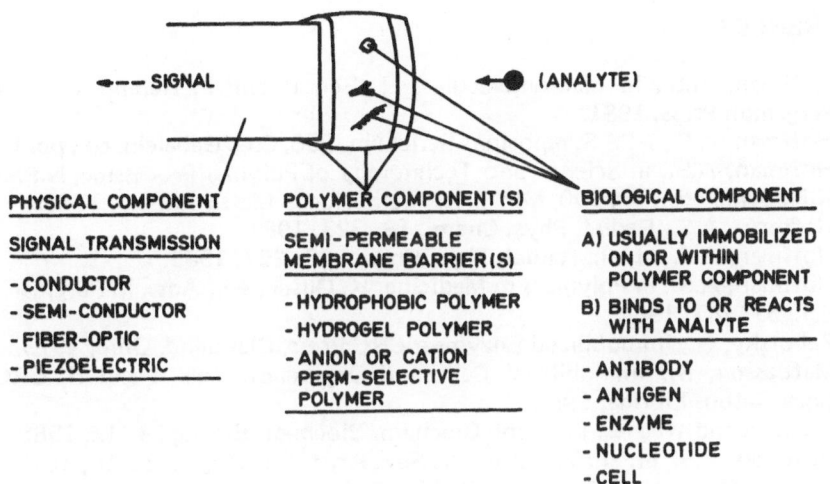

Figure 10. The Three Major Components of Biosensors, (20).

SYMBOLS

Polymers

CA	Cellulose acetate
Cell	Cellulose
PAAm	Poly (arcylamide)
PE	Polyethylene
PET	Poly (ethylene terephthalate)
PFEP	Poly (perfluoro ethylene-propylene)
PGA	Poly (glycololic acid)
PHEMA	Poly (hydroxyethyl methacrylate)
PMAAc	Polymethacrylic acid
PMMA	Poly (methyl methacrylate)
PP	Polypropylene
PTFE	Poly (tetrafluoro ethylene)
PU	Polyurethane
PVC	Poly (vinyl chloride)
SR	Silicone Rubber

Biotechnology

Ag	Antigen
MAb	Monoclonal Antibody
ReDNA	Recombinant DNA

Biomaterials

IOL	Intraocular lens
IUD	Intrauterine device

REFERENCES

1. Hoffman, A.S., in Macromolecules, H. Benoit and P. Rempp, eds., pp. 321, Pergamon Press, 1981.
2. Hoffman, A.S., ACS Symposium Series No. 256, C.G. Gebelein, ed., pp. 13, 1984.
3. Hoffman, A.S., in Science and Technology of Polymer Processing, N.P. Suh and N.H. Sung, eds., pp. 200, MIT Press, Cambridge, Massachussets, 1979.
4. Hoffman, A.S., Radiat. Phys. Chem., 18: 323, 1981.
5. Hoffman, A.S., et. al., Radiat, Phys. Chem., 22: 267, 1983.
6. Hoffman, A.S., in Polymers in Medicine, K. Dusek, ed., Adv., in Polymer Sci., 57: 141, 1984.
7. Zaborsky, O., Immobilized Enzymes, CRC Press, Cleveland, Ohio, 1973.
8. Mattiasson, B., Immobilized Cells and Organelles, Vols. I and II, CRC Press, Boca Raton, Florida, 1983.
9. Klein, J. and Wagner, F., Appl. Biochem. Biochem. Bioeng., 4: 12, 1983.
10. Hoffman, A.S., et. al., Trans. Amer. Soc. Artif. Int. Organs, 18:10, 1972.
11. Molday, R.S., et. al., Nature, 249: 81, 1974.
12. Rembaum, A., et. al., Macromol., 9: 328, 1976.
13. Ratner, B.D. and Hoffman, A.S., in Hydrogels for Medical and Related Applications, J.D. Andrade, ed., ACS Symposium Series 31, Washington D.C., 1976.
14. Yasuda, H., et. al., J. Biomed. Mater. Res., 9: 629, 1975.
15. Science, 209 (4463): 1317, 1980.
16. Scientific American, 245 (3): 66, 1981.
17. Science, 219 (4585), 1983; entire issue.
18. Michaels, A.S., Chem. Tech., 11: 36, 1981.
19. Michaels, A.S., Chem. Eng. Progress, 80 (4) 9, and 80 (6), 19, 1984.
20. Hoffman, A.S., Pure and Appl. Chem., 5b (10): 1329, 1984.
21. Albertsson, P.A., Partition of Cell Particles and Macromolecules, Wiley Interscience, 2nd Ed., 1971.
22. Brooks, D.E., Biotechnology, 1 (8): 668, 1983.
23. Baier, R.E., in Adhesion in Biological Systems, R.S. Manly, ed., pp. 15, Academic Press, New York, 1970.
24. Ratner, B.D., et. al., J. Biomed. Mater. Res., 9: 407, 1975.
25. Grinnell, F. Intl. Rev. Cytol, 53: 65, 1978.
26. van der Valk, P., et. al., J. Biomed. Mater. Res., 17: 807, 1983.
27. Sevier, E.D., et. al., Clin. Chem., 27 (11): 1797, 1981.
28. Cheung, P.W., et. al., Theory, Design and Biomedical Applications of Solid State Chemical Sensors, CRC Press, Boca Raton, Florida, 1978.

IN-VITRO AND IN-VIVO TEST METHODS FOR ASSESSING BLOOD-COMPATIBILITY

R.S. Wilson and S.L. Cooper

University of Wisconsin, Department of Chemical Engineering, Madison, Wisconsin, USA

INTRODUCTION

There has been an increased demand over the last quarter-century for materials compatible with blood. Hemodialysers, heart valves and aortic grafts, for example, are commonly used today. The recent development of the artificial heart (1) has now demonstrated that it is possible to replace entire diseased organs with artificial organs. It is clear that the number of applications for blood-contacting materials will continue to expand in the future.

Much research has been directed toward finding materials for long-term blood-contacting applications. These materials must satisfy several requirements (2). They should not cause thrombosis, destruction of the formed blood elements, alterations of plasma proteins, destruction of enzymes or depletion of electrolytes. They should not cause damage to adjacent tissue, adverse immune responses, cancer nor toxic and allergic reactions. Of these ten requirements, the requirement that a material not cause thrombosis has proved the most difficult to satisfy. Thrombus formation can lead to vessel occlusion, or thrombi may embolize from the surface and become lodged downstream, causing damage by retarding or preventing blood flow through arterioles and capillaries (3). These phenomena present serious problems to the clinical use of artificial biomaterials. Use of anticoagulants has helped to minimize the problem of thrombosis in extracorporeal devices. However, it often causes other complications, such as a hemorrhagic tendency (4).

It is generally accepted that the first event to occur when blood contacts a foreign surface is the adsorption of plasma proteins to that surface. Vroman and Adams (5) have shown that within a few seconds of contact a protein layer is formed on the surface. Dutton et al. (6) have shown, using electron microscopy, that there exists a protein layer between the surface and adhered platelets and thrombi. Thus, the interaction between blood and a foreign surface is mediated by an adsorbed protein layer. The composition of the adsorbed layer is dependent upon the material surface properties (5,7,8). Experiments with surfaces pre-coated with plasma proteins (9,10) have shown that specific proteins can affect the extent of thrombogenesis.

Albumin has been shown to passivate the surface, while proteins like fibrinogen, fibronectin, von Willebrand factor and alpha -2-macroglobulin promote the formation of thrombi. Thus, a polymer surface which preferentially adsorbs albumin over fibrinogen or alpha-2- macroglobulin would be expected to be less thrombogenic than a surface which adsorbs more fibrinogen.

Following protein adsorption, platelets adhere to the surface (6). The attached platelets undergo a series of morphological changes, from discs to spheres with extended pseudopods. They then flatten, releasing their granule contents (11). The granule contents, e.g. ADP, fibrinogen, fibronectin and thrombospondin, induce the aggregation of more platelets, forming thrombi on the surface. Under arterial flow, thrombi consist primarily of platelets and fibrin (12) and may detach, or embolize, from the surface due to shear forces (13), or by the breakdown of the thrombus by thrombolytic enzymes (14) or by a combination of these mechanisms.

Many factors affect how blood interacts with an artificial surface. These include the factors of flow rate, state of anticoagulation, surface roughness, and hematology. Many experimental systems have been developed for the examination of blood-material interactions. The Working Group on Blood-Material Interactions has defined six broad groups of tests used in the search for blood-compatible materials (15). These categories are:

1. In-vitro tests
2. Acute extracorporeal tests
3. Tests of tubular devices in/on animals
4. Tests of membrane devices using animals
5. Tests of cardiovascular devices in animals
6. Clinical tests

Most of the systems developed for the examination of blood-material interactions reported in the literature are in-vitro, where contact between blood and an artificial surface occurs separate from the body. In-vivo and ex-vivo systems involve the implantation of materials or shunts into the cardiovascular system. This paper will discuss a few of the methods currently used to examine blood-material interactions. The systems discussed are included in the first three groups above.

IN-VITRO SYSTEMS

The in-vitro test is the most common method of evaluating material biocompatibility. In-vitro experiments are often much easier, faster and less expensive to perform than those in-vivo. Test parameters are usually easier to control and the results may be more quantifiable. These advantages have resulted in the widespread use of in-vitro methods.

The types of in-vitro systems involving the contact of blood or plasma proteins with polymer surfaces can be divided into five groups

1. Static systems
2. Bead column test
3. Recirculatory systems

4. Rheological chambers
5. Protein-contacting systems

Static Systems

The static, in-vitro experiment is the simplest method of examining blood-material interactions. Blood is contacted with a test surface for a specific period of time and then removed. Both the blood and test surface may then be examined. Most of the static methods fall into two categories: the clotting time test (16,17) and the blood chamber test (18-21). The rationale behind the clotting time tests is the longer the clotting time, the less thrombogenic the material is. These tests are modifications of the Lee-White clotting test (22). A tube coated with or consisting entirely of the test material is used instead of the glass tube of the Lee-White test. For instance, Coleman et al. (17) examined the clotting times of a series of HEMA-MMA copolymers. They found that an equimolar copolymer produced the shortest clotting time, implying that this material is the most compatible of the copolymers tested.

Most static systems reported in the literature use some type of test chamber, using sheet or tubular material, in which blood sits for a period of time. These chambers are usually designed to prevent the presence of a blood-air interface. After the blood has contacted the surface for a period of time, the unclotted blood is drained from the chamber and may be examined. The most common blood tests are the partial thromboplastin time test (PTT), platelet factor 3 (PF-3) assay, prothrombin time (PT) and measurement of the platelet count. The PTT is a measure of the extent of activation of the intrinsic coagulation pathway (23), while the PT monitors the activation of the extrinsic pathway (24). The PF-3 assay is a measure of the extent of platelet activation, while platelet counts before and after contact are used to measure the retention of platelets on the surface. In addition to blood measurements, the test surface may also be examined after blood contact. Usually the degree of platelet adhesion is measured using light, phase-contrast, or scanning electron microscopy. Mason et al. (25), for example, contacted blood with tubular biomaterials. They found that their system was sensitive enough to observe dynamic interactions of blood with biomaterials and could be used to screen effects of antithrombotic agents upon the reactivity of blood with test materials.

Bead Column Tests

The bead column test is a widely used technique for evaluating the relative blood-compatibility of different materials. It has been regarded favorably because of the ease with which experiments can be performed and results obtained, and is recommended by the Working Group on Blood-Material Interactions as a primary test to screen prospective materials (15). The most common form of this test is the Salzman bead test (26). A chromatography column is packed with glass beads which have been coated with the biomaterial of interest. Anticoagulated blood or platelet-rich plasma (PRP) is pumped through the column. Measurements of platelet concentration before and after elution provide a measurement of platelet retention in the column. The degree of retention provides a relative measure of the thrombogenicity of the test material. The morphology of adhered platelets may also be examined by electron microscopy.

As an example of the research conducted with this type of system, Brier-Russell et al. (27) have used this system to examine a series of acrylate polymers in which the length of the alkane side group is varied. Their tests suggest that increasing the hydrophobic side group length increases platelet retention. These results and others (26) have suggested that the mobility of pendant groups on the polymer backbones in response to the aqueous interface has much to do with protein adsorption and platelet retention.

Recirculatory Systems

Recirculatory systems involve the flow of blood through a specially-designed chamber. Blood may contact the test surface only once or may be recirculated through the chamber. The test material may be used in the fabrication of the recirculation loop itself or may be inserted into the system in various forms, such as a heart valve, filter or flow chamber. Thus, the material may be examined in the shape it may be clinically used. Blood flow rate through this type of system can be controlled. After a period of blood-contact time the blood can be examined for hematological changes, and the material surface can be examined for adhered blood elements. Recirculation of the blood through the system may permit the amplification of alterations in blood components through repeated exposure to the material. Anticoagulants are usually used, although studies using native blood have been performed (28-30).

Platelet adhesion and changes in platelet morphology are the most common parameters measured, usually by phase-contrast or electron microscopy. Another method of measuring platelet deposition is the use of radiolabeled platelets (31,32). It is also possible to use videomicroscopy to observe the formation of platelet thrombi in real time (33-35).

One of the original recirculatory systems is the Chandler loop (28), in which a partially-filled circular loop of tubing is rotated on a tilted turntable. This system was originally used as a mechanical alternative to the conventional clotting time test, which depends largely on subjective judgment of the clotting endpoint. A modification of this system involves the removal of the blood after a period of time and the examination for alterations (36).

Most other recirculatory systems reported in the literature use a flow chamber. The annular axial flow chamber of Turitto and coworkers (30,37-39) has provided much information on the effect of wall shear rate on platelet deposition and thrombus formation. Observations of the rate of platelet deposition from citrated blood onto rabbit subendothelium have indicated that there are three experimental flow regimes (38). Below a wall shear rate of $200 \ sec^{-1}$ the rate of platelet deposition is diffusion controlled, while above $1300 \ sec^{-1}$ deposition is controlled by surface reaction kinetics. Between 200 and $1300 \ sec^{-1}$ there lies an intermediate flow regime where deposition is controlled by a combination of diffusion and reaction kinetics. Another circulatory system, the flat plate chamber of Grabowski and Didisheim (32-34,40), has been used to determine species effects on platelet adhesion to biomaterials. They have shown, for example, that rabbit and canine blood deposit three to four orders of magnitude more platelets onto Cuprophane than human, baboon, macaque, dog, calf, or sheep blood.

Rheological Chambers

In this type of system, the test surface spins in a pool of blood. As a result the flow field is usually well-defined and the shear rates or stresses at the material surface carefully controlled. Either native or anticoagulated blood may be used, depending on the design of the chamber and the purpose of the experiment. As with the recirculatory systems the measured parameter is usually the degree of platelet adhesion.

The typical configurations used are either a Couette rod (41-43) or a spinning disc (44,45). The spinning rod system provides a uniform shear rate over the test surface, while in the case of the spinning disc system, the surface shear rate varies with the radial distance from the disc center. Whicher and Brash (42) used the Couette system to demonstrate that platelet adhesion is dependent upon the material surface, the type of protein preadsorbed on the surface, and the hematocrit. Using a spinning disc system, Butruille et al. (45) demonstrated that platelets will cluster together on the surface. It was concluded that platelets cluster because their probablity of reacting with the surface is increased by the proximity of an already adhered platelet which is releasing aggregating agents.

Protein-Contacting Systems

As mentioned in the introduction, the first event of blood-material interactions is the deposition of plasma protein onto the foreign surface. All subsequent events occur following the formation of this layer, which has been found to have a great influence on the thrombogenic nature of a material (46-48). For this reason much research has been directed toward examining how specific plasma proteins interact with artificial surfaces.

Adsorption isotherms or dynamic adsorption profiles of proteins, under static or dynamic flow conditions, are typically measured. One of the more commonly used techniques to measure adsorbed protein on a surface is the radiolabeling of protein with ^{125}I (7,49,50). It has been suggested (51) that either denaturation or preferential adsorption of the labeled protein could cause serious difficulties. However, Bornzin and Miller (50) found that measured adsorption of albumin and fibrinogen onto two different surfaces was independent of the mole fraction of labeled protein, indicating no effect of radiolabeling.

In order to obtain dynamic protein adsorption profiles using radiolabeled protein, it is necessary to perform a series of experiments in which the protein solution contacts the test surface for a series of different contact-times. This procedure is time consuming and only provides discrete, scattered data points. There has been a movement recently towards real-time spectrophotometric measurements of protein adsorption, in particular by Fourier transform infrared-attenuated total reflectance (FTIR-ATR) spectroscopy (52,53). FTIR-ATR can also be used with polymer-coated ATR crystals, permitting protein studies on a variety of surfaces. This technique has the potential to collect dynamic data without dismantling the flow chamber to measure surface concentrations. Correlations with radiolabeled proteins have shown this technique to be accurate (53,54).

Bellissimo and Cooper (54) have used FTIR-ATR spectroscopy to examine fibrinogen and albumin adsorption onto germanium ATR crystals and Biomer^{R} coated crystals. The experiments were performed with a specially designed flow cell which incorporated ATR optics and nearly uniform flow characteristics. In general, the adsorption profiles obtained exhibited an initial period of rapid adsorption during which a significant fraction of the final protein layer was adsorbed. After three to five minutes, protein adsorption can be seen to continue up until about twenty-five minutes, where it appears to slow significantly.

This initial period of rapid adsorption, followed by a period of slower adsorption suggests that two modes of protein adsorption exist. The adsorption seen initially is probably associated with a layer of tightly bound protein, while that seen later on is probably indicative of protein which was loosely bound to the surface. This speculation is further supported by measurements of the protein layer before and after a protein-free rinse. After the rinse the amount of protein on the surface corresponded to the amount observed at the end of the initial period of rapid adsorption, indicating that there was a loosely bound layer of protein which was stripped from the surface during the rinse, leaving the tightly-bound layer.

IN-VIVO AND EX-VIVO SYSTEMS

The terms in-vivo and ex-vivo mean, literally, inside the body and outside the body, respectively. In-vivo experiments are defined as experiments where a material is implanted into or grafted onto the vascular system. After a period of time the material is removed and analyzed. In-vivo experiments may also include monitoring changes within the test animal, such as the rate of radiolabeled platelet consumption, changes in hematocrit, or measurements of the activation of coagulation pathways. Ex-vivo experiments involve the flow of blood from the body via a cannulated vessel through a test chamber or shunt which is examined outside the body. After flowing through the test chamber the blood may or may not be returned to the animal.

In-vivo Systems

In-vivo experiments may be separated into four categories:

1. Intravascular rings
2. Grafts
3. A-V shunts
4. Catheters

The most well-known in-vivo test is the vena cava, or Gott ring test (55,56). An intravascular ring is inserted into a dog's vena cava and is removed after two hours or two weeks. The patency of the ring is then assessed gravimetrically and visually. Gott et al. (55) used this test to demonstrate how a colloidal graphite coating would improve the compatibility of methyl methacrylate intravascular rings. They also demonstrated that a positively charged graphite-coated ring would clot shut after one hour of blood-contact, while neutral and negatively charged rings remained patent with little thrombus formation. Variations of this test include modifying the ring to change flow characteristics (57) and placing the ring in the aorta to measure the degree of embolization by the renal embolus test (58). Graft experiments differ from the intravascular ring systems primarily by the length of time of the experiment. Vascular grafts usually remain in the test subject for periods of weeks to months (59,60).

Catheter experiments involve the insertion of a catheter into the cardiovascular system of a test animal for a given period of time, usually less than three hours. Upon removal, either the degree of thrombus formation (61) or the deposition of radiolabeled blood elements (62,63) is measured. Rodvien et al. (63) demonstrated with the catheter model that platelet deposition reaches a maximum value, after which there is a very rapid decrease in the amount of platelets on the surface, indicating the occurrence of embolization. They also demonstrated that the time to reach the peak and the height of the peak are quite variable from animal to animal, although they are quite repeatable in the same animal.

Ex-vivo arterio-venous (A-V) shunt experiments are usually used to measure the extent to which platelet consumption is accelerated by the shunt material (64,65). Harker et al. (64) have shown that platelet consumption is directly related to the amount of shunt surface area and is dependent upon the shunt material (Hoffman, et al., (65)). They have also demonstrated, using a laser light scattering technique, that significant embolization of thrombi does occur from the shunt surface.

Ex-vivo Systems

In ex-vivo systems the blood flows from the test animal via a shunt and through a test chamber where the blood-material interactions are monitored. Ex-vivo systems are used primarily to examine short-term interactions. The most common measure of thrombogenicity is platelet adhesion, but many investigators also measure radiolabeled fibrinogen deposition (66-74).

There are many configurations used for ex-vivo experiments. The Dudley clotting test (36,75) is a clotting time test which involves the insertion of a tube, via a catheter, into a vein of the test animal. The time it takes for blood to stop dripping from the end of the tubing is known as the Dudley clotting time. By changing the tubing material, it is possible to compare clotting times in a manner similar to the modified Lee-White clotting test (16,17). In stagnation point experiments (76,77) the blood flows perpendicular to a transparent flat plate, which permits the direct observation of the adherence of formed blood elements with videomicroscopy. This system has been used to observe how the wall shear rate affects the sequence of events leading to thrombosis. In particular, Morton and Cumming (77) have shown that the attachment of white blood cells is shear-limited.

The rotating shaft system of Schultz and coworkers (72,73) combines some of the best features of ex-vivo systems and rheological chamber systems. The rotating shaft system imposes a Couette-type flow upon blood flowing along the shaft. In this manner, it is possible to maintain better control over the flow characteristics than is normally possible with in-vivo and ex-vivo systems. With this system they have observed (78) in some experiments that platelet and fibrinogen deposition reaches a peak value, followed by a decrease. This behavior suggests that embolization was occuring.

Flat plate chambers (74,79,80) are also frequently used. The typical procedure is to flow blood through the chamber for a period of time, flush the blood out and remove the sheet of test material for later analysis of platelet deposition. However, the process of assembling and disassembling the chamber for every blood-contact time point is time-consuming and tedious. Instead of inserting a test chamber, interactions on the surface of the A-V shunt are often examined, usually by means of radiolabeled platelets and fibrinogen (46,47,66-68).

An important modification of the A-V shunt is the insertion of a series of tubing segments of different materials. Thus, this series shunt system is able to test a number of different materials under identical blood conditions, which enables comparisons between materials to be more meaningful. Lelah et al. (81,82) have used this system to examine how the mechanical and surface properties of materials affect the processes of thrombosis and embolization in a canine model. In one set of experiments (81) the effect of Silastic tubing wall thickness on thrombus formation and embolization was examined. The various wall thicknesses provided a series of materials with identical surface chemistry but different material distensibility. It was shown that tubings possessing higher dilatation showed lower levels of platelet and fibrinogen deposition, and thrombus formation, than did the less distensible materials. The deposition behavior on the more distensible materials was also more cyclic than on the less flexible tubing. Scanning electron microscopic analysis supported the quantitative data. In addition, thrombi on the more distensible materials were smaller, less compact, and less numerous, than those observed on the less distensible materials. These results suggest that higher distensibility allows for a cyclic deposition and removal of blood components during pulsatile flow. This action may enhance blood compatibility by preventing the growth of large thrombi and their subsequent embolization.

In another set of experiments, Lelah et al. (82) examined the effect of ionically charged polyether urethanes on thrombus formation. Their results were similar to the results of Gott et al. (55). The cationic ionomer had significantly more platelet and fibrinogen deposition, and thrombus formation, than the uncharged polyether-urethane, while the anionic and zwitterionic materials had less.

ANALYSIS OF EXPERIMENTAL METHODS

This section provides a critical review of the experimental systems and methods of measurement mentioned in this paper. As mentioned previously, the most common method of investigating blood-material interactions is the in-vitro test. These experiments are usually much easier, faster and less expensive to perform than in-vivo experiments. Test parameters are usually easier to control and the results may be more quantifiable. They also have the additional advantage that human blood may be used in most systems, as opposed to in-vivo and ex-vivo experiments where animal experiments are necessary.

Two major disadvantages of in-vitro systems are that the blood is usually anti-coagulated and is often used at room temperature. Anticoagulants such as heparin and sodium citrate are used to block the activation of the coagulation pathways (83,84), but they have also been observed to affect platelet-surface interactions (40,72,85,86). It has also been observed that the experimental temperature may also affect platelet deposition (87,88). In-vitro experiments are already at a disadvantage by the fact that being separated from the body, the blood is tested under non-physiological conditions. Adding the additional factors of anticoagulants and non-physiological temperature further removes the experiment from clinical correspondence. Thus, results obtained in-vitro about the blood-compatibility of materials may not accurately describe the material's behavior under clinical conditions.

The static, in-vitro system has the advantage that anticoagulants are usually not used. Therefore, alterations in the blood are not complicated by artificial suppression of the coagulation pathways. Since there is no blood flow, however, the blood is far removed from the clinical conditions and as a result only very short-term interactions may be measured.

The bead column test is very popular. The advantages of this system are the ease of performance, low cost, ability to use human blood, and the exposure of blood to a large surface area of test material. Unfortunately, the bead column system requires the blood, usually anticoagulated, to flow under highly complex hemodynamic conditions where both platelet adhesion and aggregation occur in the column (89). In addition, the test material must be able to be cast onto beads or be fabricated in bead form. The casting, synthesis or molding process necessary to obtain the material in bead form may itself affect blood-material interactions (43,90) since differences in polymer processing modify surface properties. This is also a serious disadvantage to rheological chamber systems, where the test material usually must also be solution-cast onto the rotating section of the device (11,41,43,91).

In terms of similarity to clinical conditions, the recirculation system comes as close as any in-vitro system can. The blood is usually anticoagulated, but the test material may be inserted into the loop in exactly the shape of its intended use. Thus, the effect of material processing is not a factor in measured blood-material interactions. Flow characteristics are also usually well-characterized and controlled.

In-vivo and ex-vivo systems are naturally much more similar to clinical situations than in-vitro. The test material may also be examined in the form it will be clinically used. However, one of the principle disadvantages of in-vivo and ex-vivo systems is that non-human models must be used. Studies have shown that platelet deposition onto biomaterials is highly dependent upon animal species (40,69). Various studies (92,93) have shown that platelet aggregation characteristics are also species dependent, as is the sensitivity of red blood cells to hemolysis (94). Blood from primates is hematologically very similar to human blood (15), however the cost and shortage of primates makes their use difficult. The dog is the most commonly used animal model. Canines have a low susceptibility to cardiovascular disease and pulmonary embolism. They also have a hyperplastic vascular response to incitants and very active hemostatic and fibrinolytic systems (15). These characteristics may, however, favor the dog's use as an animal model. In some respects the canine represents a worst-case situation for comparison with human blood-material responses.

In-vivo experiments, with the exception of the two-hour vena cava ring test and the catheter experiments, only measure long-term interactions, while ex-vivo experiments generally examine the short-term (less than four hours). In addition, since the experiment is connected to a live animal, it is difficult to control many of the experimental variables involved. For example, blood flow is extremely difficult to control or characterize. Blood flow in the body, or from a cannulated vessel is pulsatile in nature due to the cyclic changes in blood pressure. Changes in blood pressure may cause the mean flow rate to change during an experiment. Some investigators (95,96) use a roller pump in the extracorporeal circuit to control the flow rate, however this use may result in increased hemolysis.

ANALYSIS OF EXPERIMENTAL MEASUREMENTS

One of the most common measurements of blood-compatibility used in in-vivo systems is the assessment of patency. A vascular graft or intravascular ring is implanted into an animal for a certain period of time or until occlusion or death. The material is removed from the animal and the degree of occlusion is determined. This is a very qualitative measurement which is greatly affected by variability between test subjects (97). Also since this type of measurement is an endpoint determination the final patency evaluation may be misleading. A ring which was removed thrombus-free may have been thrombus-free throughout blood contact, or thrombosis may have occurred, followed by a period of embolization or fibrinolysis (97).

As mentioned in previous sections, the most common method of directly assessing blood-compatibility is to measure the extent of platelet adhesion. This is obtained either through the use of photomicroscopy or by radiolabeling procedures. The primary disadvantage in counting platelets visually is that it is impossible to count the number of individual platelets within thrombi. Thus, this technique is accurate only in the regime of low surface coverage. Radiolabeled platelets do not have this limitation. However, a study comparing these two techniques at low surface concentration of platelets indicates that platelet deposition, as determined by radiolabeling, is less than the concentration observed by scanning electron microscopy by a factor of two (70).

Measurement of platelet coverage on the surface is only a partial assessment of thrombogenesis and may provide misleading results. Platelet adhesion is affected by many factors not related to the test material. As mentioned earlier in this paper, the rate of platelet deposition may be dependent upon the blood flow rate (38). Also, platelet adhesion is affected by the animal species used (40), anticoagulants (40,72,85,86), experimental temperature (87,88), and even by the amount and type of anesthetic used (98). These observations emphasize the argument that the study of blood-material interactions should include more than the measurement of platelet deposition. Platelet morphological changes may also be important in understanding the mechanism of thrombogenesis. The occurrence of embolization is an important consideration in the assessment of the blood compatibility of a material and should be monitored. Protein deposition, especially of fibrinogen, should be studied. The process of thrombosis is complex and it is necessary to study more than platelet adhesion in order to determine whether a material is compatible with blood or not.

CONCLUSION

Blood-material interactions are affected by a very complex series of reactions. Many experimental systems have been developed to measure these interactions, each with advantages and disadvantages. No one experimental system can adequately predict the clinical performance of a material. This necessitates the use of a broad approach to blood-material testing. We feel it is important to utilize a number of different in-vitro and ex-vivo test methods, and to define as many different parameters as possible in each technique. Such testing should include measurement of platelet and fibrinogen deposition, platelet morphology changes, and the activation of the coagulation pathways. A comparison of data obtained using different experimental techniques for the same materials should result in a better understanding of which materials have potential clinical value.

REFERENCES

1. Joyce, L.D., Devries, W.C., Hastings, W.L., Olsen, D.B., Jarvik, R.K., and Kolff, W.J., Trans. Am. Soc. Artif. Intern. Organs, 29:81, 1983.

2. Bruck, S.D., J. Biomed. Mater. Res., 6:173, 1972.
3. Hampton, J.R. and Mitchell, J.R.A., in Human Blood Coagulation, Haemostatis and Thrombosis, R. Biggs, ed., pp. 476, Blackwell Scientific, Oxford, 1972.
4. Cliffton, E.E., Bibl. Haematol. Basel, 29:841, 1968.
5. Vroman, L., and Adams, A.L., J. Biomed. Mater. Res. 3:43, 1969.
6. Dutton, R.C., Webber, A.J., Johnson, S.A., and Baier, R.E., J. Biomed. Mater. Res., 3:13, 1969.
7. Horbett T.A., and Weathersby, P.K., J. Biomed. Mater. Res., 15:403, 1981.
8. Noishiki, Y., J. Biomed. Mater. Res., 16:359, 1982.
9. Ihlenfeld, J.V., Mathis, T.R., Barber, T.A., Mosher, D.F., Riddle, L.M., Hart, A.P., Updike, S.J., and Cooper, S.L., Trans. Am. Soc. Artif. Intern. Organs, 24:727, 1978.
10. Young, B.R., Protein Adsorption on Polymeric Biomaterials and Its Role in Thrombogenesis, Ph. D. Thesis, University of Wisconsin, Madison, 1984.
11. Scarborough, D.E., Mason, R.G., Dalldorf, F.G., and Brinkhous, K.M., Lab. Invest., 20:164, 1969.
12. Mustard, J.F., Packham, M.A., and Kinlough-Rathbone, R.L., in Haemostasis and Thrombosis, A.L. Bloom and D.P. Thomas, eds., pp. 503, Churchill Livingston, Edinburgh, 1981.
13. Hanson, S.R., Harker, L.A., Ratner B.D., and Hoffman, A.S., J. Lab. Clin. Med., 95:289, 1980.
14. Mustard, J.F., in Thrombosis, S. Sherry, K.M. Brinkhous, E. Genton, J.M. Stengle, eds., pp. 496, Nat. Acad Sci., Washington D.C., 1969.
15. Mason, R.G. (Chairman), Guidelines for Blood-Material Interactions, NIH Publication No. 80-2185, 1980.
16. Maloney, J.V., Roher, D., Roth, E., and Latta, W.A., Surgery, 66:175, 1969.
17. Coleman, D.L., Gregonis, D.E., and Andrade, J.D., J. Biomed. Mater. Res., 16:381, 1982.
18. Nose, Y., Kambic, H.E., Kiraly, R.J., Komai, T., and Urzua, J.U., Thrombosis and Inhibitors, P.Didisheim, ed., pp. 87, F.K. Schattauer Verlag, Stuttgart, 1974.
19. Mason, R.G., and Shinoda, B.A., Biomater., Med. Devices, Artif. Organs, 3:383, 1975.
20. Lindsay, R.M., Rourke, J., Reid, B., Friesen, M., Linton, A.L., Courtney, J., and Gilschrist, T., Trans. Am. Soc. Artif. Intern. Organs, 22:292, 1976.
21. Picha, G.J., Gibbons, D.F., and Auerbach, R.A., J. Bioeng. 2:301,1978.
22. Lee, R.I., and White, P.D., Am. J. Med. Sci, 245:495, 1913.
23. Davidsohn, I., and Henry, J.B., Todd-Sanford Clinical Diagnosis by Laboratory Methods, 14 th edn., pp. 421, W. B. Saunders, Philadelphia, 1969.
24. Quick, A.J. Hemorrhagic Diseases and Thrombosis, 2nd edn., pp. 391, Lea and Febinger, Philadelphia, 1957.
25. Mason, R.G., Zucker, W.H., and Shinoda, B.A., Biomater., Med. Dev., Artif Organs, 3:57, 1975.
26. Merrill, E.W., Salzman, E.W., Sa da Costa, V., Brier-Russell, D., Wolfe, L.C., Dincer, A., Wu,J.J., Pape, P., and Lindon, J.N., Adv. Chem. Ser., 199:35, 1982.
27. Brier-Russell, D., Salzman, E.W., Lindon, J., Handin, R., Merrill, E.W., Dincer, A.K., Wu, J.S., J. Colloid Interfac. Sci. 81:311, 1981.
28. Chandler, A.B., Lab. Invest., 7:110, 1958.
29. Mason, R.G., Zucker, W.H., Shinoda, B.A., Chuang, H.Y., Kingdon H.S., and Clark, H.G., Lab. Invest., 31:143, 1974.

30. Baumgartner, H.R., Turitto, V.T., and Weiss, H.J., J. Lab. Clin. Med., 95:208, 1980.
31. Aarts, P.A.M.M., Bolhius, P.A., Sakariassen, K.S., Heethaar, R.M., and Sixma, J.J., Blood, 62:214, 1983.
32. Didisheim, P., Tirrell, M.V., Lyons, C.S., Stropp, J.Q., and Dewanjee, M.K., Trans. Am. Soc. Artif. Intern Organs, 29:169, 1983.
33. Grabowski, E.F. Herther, K.K., and Didisheim, P., Thromb. Diath. Haemorrh. Suppl., 60:127, 1974.
34. Grabowski, E.F., Adv. Exp. Med. Biol., 102:73, 1978.
35. Adams, G.A., Brown, S.J., McIntire, L.V., Eskin, S.G., and Martin, R.R., Blood, 62:69, 1983.
36. Fischer, J.P., Fughe, P., Burg, K., and Heimburger, N., Angew. Makromol. Chem., 105:131, 1982.
37. Turitto, V.T., Muggli, R., and Baumgartner, H.R., Ann. N.Y. Acad. Sci, 283:284, 1977.
38. Turitto, V.T., Weiss, H.J., and Baumgartner, H.R., J. Rheology, 23:735, 1979.
39. Turitto, V.T., Weiss, H.J., and Baumgartner, H.R., Microvasc. Res., 19:352, 1980.
40. Didisheim, P., Stropp, J.Q., Borowick, J.H., and Grabowski, E.F., ASAIO J., 2:124, 1979.
41. Feuerstein, I.A., Brophy, J.M., and Brash, J.L., Trans. Am. Soc. Artif. Intern. Organs, 21:427, 1975.
42. Whicher, S.J., and Brash, J.L., J. Biomed. Mater. Res., 12:181, 1978.
43. Whicher, S.J., and Brash, J.L., in Physicochemical Aspects of Polymer Surfaces, Vol 2, K.L. Mittal, ed., pp. 985, Plenum, New York, 1983.
44. Turitto, V.T., and Leonard, E.F., Trans. Am. Soc. Artif. Intern. Organs, 18:348, 1972.
45. Butruille, Y.A., Leonard, E.F. and Litwak, R.S., Trans. Am. Soc. Artif. Intern. Organs, 21:609, 1975.
46. Young, B.R., Lambrecht, L.K., Cooper, S.L., and Mosher, D.F., Adv. Chem. Ser., 199:317, 1982.
47. Lambrecht, L.K., Young, B.R., Stafford, R.E., Albrecht, R.M., Mosher, D.F., and Cooper, S.L., Thromb. Res., 1985. (in press)
48. Adams, G.A. and Feuerstein, I.A., ASAIO J., 4:90, 1981.
49. Baszkin, A. and Lyman, D.J., J. Biomed Mater. Res. 14:393, 1980.
50. Bornzin, G.A., and Miller, I.F., J. Colloid Interfac. Sci., 86:539, 1982.
51. Grant, W.H., Smith, L.E., and Stromberg, R.R., J. Biomed. Mater. Res., 11:33, 1977.
52. Gendreau, R.M. and Jakobsen, R.J., J. Biomed. Mater. Res. 13:893, 1979.
53. Gendreau, R.M., Leininger, R.I., Winters, S., and Jakobsen, R.J., Adv. Chem. Ser. 199:371, 1982.
54. Bellissimo, J.A. and Cooper, S.L., Trans. Am. Soc. Artif. Intern. Organs, 30:359, 1984.
55. Gott, V.L., Koepke, D.E., Dagget, R.L., Zarnstorff, W., and Young, W.P., Surgery, 50:382, 1961.
56. Ratner, B.D., Hoffman, A.S., and Whiffen, J.D., J. Bioeng, 2:313, 1978.
57. Grabowski, E.F., Derby, A.R., Koffsky, R.M., Litwak, R.S., and Leonard E.F., Ann. Biomed. Eng., 3:322, 1975.
58. Kusserow, B., Larrow, R., and Nichols, J., Trans. Am. Soc. Artif. Intern. Organs, 16:58, 1970.

59. Hiratzka, L.F., Goeken, J.A., White, R.A., and Wright, C.B., Arch. Surg., 114:698, 1979.
60. Wilson, G.J., MacGregor, D.C., Klement, P., Lee, J.M., del Nido, P.J., Worg, E.W.C., and Leidner, J., Trans. Am. Soc. Artif. Intern. Organs, 29:260, 1983.
61. Libsack, C.V., and Kollmeyer, K.R., J. Biomed. Mater. Res, 13:459, 1979.
62. Hammar, W.J., Mendelhall, H.V., Vigdahl, R.L., Ferber, R.H., and Haddad, L.C., in Proc. 2 nd Int. Conf. Chitin Chitosan, S. Hirano, and S. Tokura, eds., pp. 213, Japan Soc. Chitin Chitosan, Tottori, Japan, 1982.
63. Rodvien, R., Robinson, J., Mitchell, R.R., Litwak, R., and Price, D.C., Adv. Chem. Ser., 199:25, 1982.
64. Harker, L.A., Hanson, S.R., and Hoffman, A.S., Ann. N.Y. Acad. Sci., 283:317, 1977.
65. Hoffman, A.S., Hanson, S.R., Harker, L.A., Horbett, T.A., Ratner, B.D., and Reynolds, L.O., Adv. Chem. Ser., 199:59, 1982.
66. Barber, T.A., Mathis, T., Ihlenfeld, J.V., Cooper, S.L., and Mosher, D.F., Scanning Electron Microsc., 2:431, 1978.
67. Ihlenfeld, J.V., Mathis, T.R., Riddle, L.M., and Cooper, S.L., Thromb. Res., 14:953, 1979.
68. Baquey, C., Basse-Cathalinat, B., Masson, B., Torrielli, R., Hourdille, P., Ducassou, D., and Blanquet, P., Adv. Biomater., 1:497, 1980.
69. Lambrecht, L.K., Lelah, M.D., Jordan, C.A., Pariso, M.E., Albrecht, R.M., and Cooper, S.L., Trans. Am. Soc. Artif. Intern. Organs, 29:194, 1983.
70. Lelah, M.D., Lambrecht, L.K., and Cooper, S.L., J. Biomed. Mater. Res., 18:475 1984.
71. Lelah, M.D., Jordan, C.A., Pariso, M.E., Lambrecht, L.K., Cooper, S.L., and Albrecht, R.M., Scanning Electron Microscop., IV:1983, 1984.
72. Schultz, J.S., Goddard, J.D., Ciarkowski, A., Penner, J.A., and Lindenauer, S.M., Ann. N.Y. Acad. Sci., 283:494, 1977.
73. Schultz, J.S., Lindenauer, S.M., and Penner, J.A., Adv. Chem. Ser., 199:43, 1982.
74. Wilson, R.S., Goode, M.G., Lelah, M.D., and Cooper, S.L., Trans. Am. Soc. Artif. Intern. Organs, 28:420, 1982.
75. Dudley, B., Williams, J.L., Able and Muller, B., Trans. Am. Soc. Artif. Intern. Organs, 22:538, 1976.
76. Madras, P.N., Morton, W.A., and Petswchek, H.E., Fed. Proc., 30:1665, 1971.
77. Morton, W.A., and Cumming, R.D., Ann. N.Y. Acad. Sci., 283:477, 1977.
78. Schultz, J.S., Ciarkowski, A., Goddard, J.D., Lindenauer, S.M., and Penner, J.A., Trans. Am. Soc. Artif. Intern. Organs, 22:269, 1976.
79. Grabowski E.F., Herther, K.K., and Didisheim, P., J. Lab. Clin. Med., 88:368, 1976.
80. Friedman, L.I., Liem H., Grabowski, E.F., Leonard, E.F., and McCord, C.W., Trans. Am. Soc. Artif. Intern. Organs. 16:63, 1970.
81. Lelah, M.D., Grasel, T.G., Pierce, J.A., Lambrecht, L.K., and Cooper, S.L., Trans. Am. Soc. Artif. Intern. Organs, 30:411, 1984.
82. Lelah M.D., Pierce, J.A., Lambrecht, L.K., and Cooper S.L., J. Colloid Interfac. Sci., 104:422, 1985
83. Hermans J. and McDonagh J., Semin. Thromb. Haemostas., 8:11, 1982.
84. Rosenberg, R., Semin. Hematol., 14:427, 1977.
85. Moolten, S.E., Vroman, L., Vroman, G.M.S., and Goodman, B., Arch. Intern. Med., 84:667, 1949.

86. Bowie, E.J.W., Oven C.A., Thompson J.H., and Didisheim, P., Mayo Clin. Proc., 44:306, 1969.
87. Turitto, V.T., and Baumgartner, H.R., Haemostasis, 3:224, 1974.
88. Absolom, D.R., Policova, Z., Neumann, A.W., and Zingg, W., Trans. Am. Soc. Artif. Intern. Organs, 29:425, 1983.
89. Zucker, M.B., and McPherson, J., Ann. N.Y. Acad. Sci., 283:128, 1977.
90. Lelah, M.D., Lambrecht, L.K., Young, B.R., and Cooper, S.L., J. Biomed. Mater. Res. 17:1, 1983.
91. Mason, R.G., Scarborough, D.E., Saba, S.R., Brinkhous, K.M., Ikenberry, L.D., Kearney, J.J., and Clark, H.G., J. Biomed. Mater. Res., 3:615, 1969.
92. Sinakos, Z., and Caen, J.P., Thromb. Diath. Haemorrh., 17:99, 1967.
93. Wurzinger, L.J., and Schmid-Schonbein, H., ASAIO J., 4:149, 1981.
94. Wennberg, A., and Hensten Pettersen, A., J. Biomed. Mater. Res. 15:433, 1981.
95. Olijslager, J., The Development of Test Devices for the Study of Blood Material Interaction Ph. D. Thesis, Delft University. The Netherlands, 1982.
96. Baumgartner, H.R., and Haudenschild, C., Ann N.Y. Acad. Sci., 201:22, 1972.
97. Litwak, R.S., Silvay, G., Shiang, H., and Leonard, E.F., Ann. N.Y. Acad. Sci., 283:542, 1977.
98. Joist, J.H., Cazenave, J.P., and Mustard, J.F., Thromb. Diath. Haemorrh., 30:315, 1973.

IN VIVO BIOCOMPATIBILITY STUDIES: PERSPECTIVES ON THE EVALUATION OF BIOMEDICAL POLYMER BIOCOMPATIBILITY

J.M. Anderson

Case Western Reserve University, Department of Pathology, Cleveland, Ohio, USA

INTRODUCTION

The term "Biocompatibility" is commonly used to provide an indication of the host and material responses which occur in the specific application of a given material. Biocompatibility has recently been addressed from the issue of biocompatibility is that a given material performs satisfactorily in the biological application under consideration (1). The following definitions have been suggested by Black and provide a basis for our discussion of the biocompatibility of biomedical polymers. Biocompatibility is the biological performance of a given polymer in a specific application that is judged suitable to that situation. Biological performance is the interaction between a polymer and a living system. The two aspects of this performance are the host response which is the local and systemic response, other than the intended therapeutic response, of living systems to the polymer, and the material response which is the response of the polymer to living systems. The level of host (or polymer) response is the nature of the host (or polymer) response in a standard test with respect to the response obtained with a reference polymer. A polymer that, by standard test, has been determined to elicit a reproducible, quantifiable host or polymer response can be considered to be a reference or control polymer.

It should be noted that a clear, specific and absolute definition of biocompatibility does not exist at this time. This is not surprising considering the numerous and interdisciplinary factors which must be used to describe the biocompatibility of a given polymer in a given application for a given duration. In general, the biocompatibility of a given polymer is dependent on the polymer/host or tissue interactions which occur over the anticipated duration of the use of the material under appropriate service conditions. Table I contains interrelated factors which can influence the biocompatibility of polymers.

The purpose of this manuscript is to provide an overview of issues important to determining the biocompatibility of polymers. We have directed our efforts to appreciating issues of tissue compatibility, that is, extravascular interactions between polymers and tissues. The blood compatibility of polymers is, in many respects, an entirely different area and will not be addressed here.

Table I. Factors Influencing the Biocompatibility of Polymers.

Type and Form of the Polymer
Surface and Bulk Composition of the Polymer
Chemical, Physical and Mechanical Properties of the Polymer
Influence of Service Conditions on the Properties of the Polymer

Animal Model
Implant Site: Tissue and/or Organ
Anticipated Duration of Implant
Infuence of Service Conditions on the Tissues of the Implant Site

GENERAL ISSUES OF BIOMEDICAL POLYMER BIOCOMPATIBILITY

In determining the biocompatibility of a polymer, a series of tests and studies is undertaken to investigate the interaction which occurs between the polymer and the tissue. This series of tests is usually initiated with tests and studies in-vitro and in animals. In general, these tests are nonfunctional and emphasis is placed on determining the direct interaction between the polymer and the chemical and biological species of the implant environment. In-vitro tests involve the use of cell cultures and are designed to provide information on one or more specific aspects of the tissue/polymer interaction. Following these tests and studies, the polymer is then examined in functional or "in-use" tests in animals. These tests are usually carried out on polymers which are in their final design on "in-use" configuration and the implant site is that which is to be utilized in humans. Following successful completion of "in-use" tests in animals, clinical trials in humans are undertaken.

It should be noted that the initial tests and studies are usually directed towards appreciating the acute interactions which occur between the polymer and the tissue. These involve a variety of implant sites which include subcutaneous, intramuscular, and intraperitoneal sites. Long-term implant studies to investigate the effects of the systemic physiology on the material and host responses can also be carried out.

In considering the in-vitro tests and the implant sites to be utilized in the initial determination of the biocompatibility of a material, it is important to consider the tissue interface and the expected duration of the implant or device. Obviously, a material which will be used for only a short period of time (minutes, hours, days) may not exhibit and/or require the same biocompatibility characteristics that a material must exhibit if its intended use is for longer periods of time (weeks, months, years). This is an extremely important issue in the consideration of the biocompatibility of a given polymer. For example, Table II provides a partial classification of devices by usage. Nylon 6 and Nylon 6,6 are used clinically as suture materials and their biocompatibility characteristics are appropriate in suture applications. However, in applications where long-term stability and maintenance of strength is a requirement, these polymers may fail. The long-term degradation of nylons in vascular graft applications has been shown. This illustrates how the biocompatibility characteristics of a polymer, i.e., nylon, can dictate the applications in which the polymer can be used. A polymer considered to be biocompatible in short-term applications or usage may not be biocompatible in long-term usage. Table II provides a partial classification of polymeric devices by usage.

Table II. Classification of Devices According to Usage.

1. Internal Devices
   Short-term devices are introduced into the body (actually penetrate the surface of the body or penetrate the wall of a passage leading to the exterior of the body) for a period of 30 days or less, e.g., intravenous catheters, drainage tubes,etc. Long-term devices are introduced into the body and are left in situ for a period longer than 30 days, e.g., vascular prostheses, heart valves, orthopedic prostheses, etc.

2. Topical Devices
   Devices that contact the skin, e.g., gloves, orthopedic casts, dressings, tapes, etc. Devices that contact mucous membranes, e.g., urinary catheters, endotracheal tubes and cuffs, intravaginal devices, etc.

3. Indirect Devices
   Devices that are not introduced into the body or contact the body, but serve as a means of delivering medication, collecting body fluids, administering blood or blood constituents, or dialyzing and oxygenating blood, e.g., infusion and transfusion assemblies, oxygenators, dialyzers, etc.

4. Nonpatient Contact Devices
   Devices that do not touch the body, but physically come in contact with those devices that do contact the body, e.g., mayo stand covers, dressing trays, operating room back table covers, etc.

ACUTE AND CHRONIC TISSUE RESPONSES TO IMPLANTED POLYMERS

Several types of tissue responses may occur acutely or chronically following the implantation of a polymer (Table III). The local tissue response is considered to be an acute response and the result of the inflammatory response to the surgical trauma and the initial host response to the implanted material. The systemic toxic effect may occur acutely or chronically and usually is the result of the diffusion of a small molecular weight material which was absorbed or formed in the material during its synthesis, fabrication, or sterilization. Chronic toxicity effects may be seen as these small molecular weight materials are released over a period of time or the material undergoes biodegradation with the release of toxic materials. Allergic responses to biomedical polymers are extremely rare. They may be developed by similar mechanisms to that seen for systemic toxic effects. Carcinogenic, teratogenic and mutagenic responses are considered to be chronic. Carcinogenesis may occur through the presence of a carcinogenic agent in the material, the generation of a carcinogenic agent through degradation of the material, or carcinogenesis through physical effects. Important considerations in the determination of carcinogenic effects include the form of the material and the animal species used in the determination of the biocompatibility of the material. Adaptive responses are considered to be chronic or long-term and include the effects of mechanical forces on the tissue/polymer interaction.

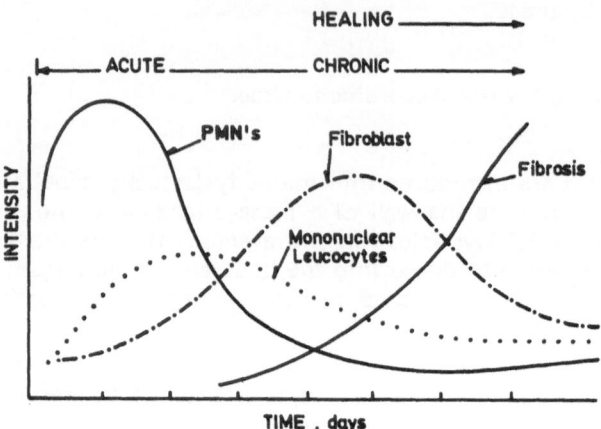

Figure 1. The Wound Healing Response to an Implanted Material. The Intensity and Duration of the Response Will be Determined by the Size and Nature of the Implanted Material and by Host Factors.

Table III. In Vivo Tissue Responses.

    Local Tissue Responses
    Systemic Toxic Effects
    Allergic Responses
    Carcinogenic, Teratogenic and Mutagenic Responses
    Adaptive Responses

All polymers undergo a local tissue response when implanted. In general, the implantation of any synthetic material initiates a wound healing mechanism that is characterized by the inflammatory response. However, the inflammatory response itself involves complex and highly regulated interactions between specific cells and various molecular mediators.

Inflammation is the host's response to injury or the presence of injurious agents. The surgery of implantation induces the initial reactions which include a series of interdependent events that begin with hemodynamic changes, followed by alterations in vascular permeability. The increased permeability of the adjacent microvasculature promotes the transport of protein-rich inflammatory fluid or exudate into the extra-vascular tissues and wound site. Simultaneously, circulating leukocytes interact with stimulatory factors, adhere to the blood vessel endothelium and subsequently pass through the vessel wall and into the extravascular tissue around the implant. Figure 1 illustrates the wound healing response during an inflammatory reaction to an implanted material. The intensity and duration of the response is controlled by a variety of mediators and determined by the size and nature of the implanted material, the site of implantation and the reactive capability of the host. A brief cellular response of low intensity would be indicative of tissue compatibility.

The acute phase of inflammation is characterized by the preferential migration of the neutrophil (a polymorphonuclear leukocyte (PMN)). The peak migration usually occurs within the first 72 hours following injury. Mononuclear leukocytes (macrophages and lymphocytes) predominate at later stages of the inflammatory process. Macrophages are derived from blood monocytes. Once monocytes leave the circulation and enter the tissue they undergo a transformation in response to various stimulate and differentiate into macrophages. It is now accepted that PMNs, monocytes and, to a lesser extent, lymphocytes are drawn from the vasculature to the site of injury by locally generated chemotactic factors.

In the presence of a polymer implant, activation of the inflammatory cells is considered to occur following the adhesion of the cells to the polymer surface or through a nonadhesive mechanism where phagocytes in the exudate are activated through cell-cell interactions or cell-mediator interactions. (2). For macrophages, cellular activation by adhesive and non-adhesive events can lead to the presence of extracellular lysosomal enzymes through non-cytolytic release by an exocytosis mechanisms or as a result of necrosis with lytic release. For PMNs, however, the importance of cell-surface adhesion with respect to the exocytosis mechanism has been shown by Gallin (3) and Henson (4). The studies of Wright and Gallin (3) have shown that the extracellular release of the contents of specific granules in PMNs were significantly augmented when the cells actively adhered to polymeric surfaces.

A polymeric implant generally represents a particle which PMNs and macrophages are unable to completely engulf. This can lead to the incomplete fusion of the phagolysosomes with the plasma membrane and thus to the extracellular relase of enzymes by exocytosis. This process has been referred to by Henson (4) as frustrated phagocytosis. Henson suggested that the specific mode of cell activation in the inflammatory response is dependent on the size of the implant and that a material in powder or particulate from which is suitable for phagocytosis may provoke a different degree of inflammation than the same material in a nonphagocytosable form such as a film, where frustrated phagocytosis and exocytosis probably will prevail.

The macrophage is probably the most highly regulatory cell associated with the inflammatory response, because of its de novo synthesis abilities and the fact that it remains available and active for a long period. The multiple macrophage functions have broad effects. In addition to complement associated regulation of the inflammatory response, the macrophage, through the secretion of mediators, regulates inflammatory cells like PMNs and fibroblasts, which, in turn, will generate soluble products that affect the macrophage. Consequently, the fate of the macrophages fllowing surface interactions with a biomaterial will strongly influence the level of inflammation and thus, the degree of tissue compatibility of a polymer (5).

Under favorable circumstances, an acute inflammatory reaction is followed within a few days by histological evidence that healing is taking place. Large numbers of capillaries will be observed in the granulation tissue of the wound area. The capillary branches grow into the wound with its disorganized mass of fibrin, leukocytes and injured tissue. Macrophages present at the wound site release interleukin 1 which stimulates the proliferation of fibroblasts. Fibroblasts are responsible for the synthesis of tropocollagen which subsequently aggregates to form collagen fibers, which are usually laid down through a proteoglycan matrix. Over a period of time, the healing wound will show a decrease in leukocytes, capillaries, proteoglycans and water, and an increase in the amount of collagen (i.e., fibrosis). At still later time points the wound area will contain mostly collagen with perhaps a few leukocytes. The wound is now in the final stages of healing.

The most favorable result of an inflammatory response is the complete return to the normal structure and function of the injured tissue. Unfortunately, with polymer implants this rarely occurs and the result most commonly seen is that of reorganization where repair is through fibrosis. In addition, the presence of the polymer will almost inevitably lead to a period of chronic inflammation, the intensity of which will depend on the size of the area involved and the consequences of the previous leukocyte/material interactions.

A chronic inflammatory response implies the continued presence of the injurious agent which may be represented even by a relatively inert polymer. Other factors which can provoke chronic inflammation include: the persistent release of cytotoxic agents from the implant, an implant which causes physical irritation to neighboring tissues, extensive surgical injury, bacterial infection or host factors such as poor blood supply or nutrition. Chronic inflammation is characterized by the predominance of mononuclear leukocytes, particularly macrophages. One also may observe signs of acute inflammation (i.e., PMNs) at foci within a chronic inflammatory lesion as well as foreign body giant cells.

If the biomaterial is either too large to be phagocytized or quickly degraded, fibrous tissue begins to form about the mass of leukocytes and encapsulates the foreign body in a dense capsule of connective tissue. This sequence of events is known as the foreign body reaction and tends to isolate the implant from the rest of the body. A foreign body granuloma is composed of the foreign body surrounded by giant cells, macrophages, lymphocytes and a few PMNs encapsulated by fibrous tissue. Accumulation of blood pigments, lipids or calcium salts are sometimes observed within the granuloma and is indicative of a continuing chronic inflammatory reaction.

Multinucleated foreign body giant cells are commonly observed around polymer implants and are believed to be derived from the cytoplasmic fusion of macrophages after they have simultaneously attempted to phagocytize the same particle (6,7). It appears inevitable therefore that giant cells will eventually form on the surface of a large polymer, providing that the macrophages are able to adhere to the surface.

The biocompatibility of an implanted polymer is a dynamic and two-way process that involves the time dependent effects of the tissue on the polymer and the polymer on the tissue. Time dependent effects of tissues on polymers may involve absorption phenomena or degradation and failure of the polymer.

The physiological environment may alter the functional characteristics of a material through absorption processes and these processes are usually considered to be chronic or long-term effects. This tpe of effect has illustrated the need for comprehensive and in-depth biocompatibility testing of materials prior to clinical use in humans. In the 1960's, reports appeared in the clinical literature on the gradual deterioration of prosthetic heart valve poppets and the physical changes observed included discoloration, swelling and cracking. Subsequent investigations showed the selective absorption of lipids from the blood. Chemical and physical changes were made in the poppet materials and further evaluation of these materials showed a minimum of changes due to absorbed processes.

Absorption of blood and tissue components may lead to a plasticizing effect with a decrease in the elastic modulus and an increase in the yield stress of a material. Changes in these and other mechanical properties of a material may lead to its inability to function appropriately in the physiological environment.

It is appropriate to mention here the effect of leaching induced by the physiologic environment. Leaching of small molecular weight components of a material such as a polymeric plasticizer may lead to an increase in the elastic modulus with a concomitant decrease in the yield strength. In general, the usual effect of exposure to physiological fluids is to decrease the effective elastic modulus but in determining the biocompatibility of a material both absorption and leaching processes must be considered.

The implantation of a polymer into the physiological environment can lead to chemical, physical or mechanical alterations in the material which may eventually lead to acute or chronic failure. Degradation and failure can occur through a number of mechanisms which are dependent on the properties of the polymer.

Wear between two components of a prostheses may lead to the ultimate failure of the prostheses. Clinical examples include wear which occurs on polyethylene surfaces in hip and knee prostheses. The majority of hip and knee prostheses involve the articulation of a metallic surface with a polyethylene surface and the mismatch in the properties of these two materials can lead to wear on the polymeric component. Wear has been noted also between components of prosthetic heart valves where the poppet or occluder, usually a silicone rubber or Teflon, comes in contact with the metallic struts of the cage and results in wear on the polymer. Extensive wear of the poppet or occluder of a prosthetic heart valve can lead to embolization of this component resulting in cardiac valve insufficiency.

Polymers may undergo degradation through a variety of mechanism which include absorption, leaching, hydration, oxidation, chain scission, and hydrolysis. In general, polymer degradation in-vivo can occur in four stages: bond cleavage, strength loss, mass integrity loss and mass loss or solubilization. The potential for bond cleavage to occur is of special importance to condensation polymers. This group of polymers contains hydrolyzable bonds in their polymeric backbone or main chain and cleavage of these bonds may rapidly lead to a loss in strength. Examples of materials in this class include polyamides (nylons), polyesters and polyurethanes.

Mechanical forces also may lead to the failure of biomaterials. Bone immediately adjacent to polymethylmethacrylate bone cement in hip prostheses and especially in knee prostheses may undergo remodelling changes to the extent that the bone at long implant periods is much stronger than the polymethylmethacrylate bone cement with which it interdigitates in fixation. This may lead to fracture of the bone cement with subsequent loss of stress transfer capabilities at the interface and development of an inflammatory response. Another example of the mismatch in mechanical properties which can develop between tissue and a polymer is the site of anastomoses of vascular grafts with natural arteries. Natural arteries are compliant and exhibit viscoelasticity. When a noncompliant vascular graft material is implanted, hemodynamic alterations may take place which result in tissue proliferation with a decrease in graft patency. This is a commonly recognized mechanism of failure of vascular grafts and points out the importance of the tissue/polymer interaction.

STANDARD TESTS FOR BIOCOMPATIBILITY

A standard test is a well-defined, repeatable test. It is generally accepted that a standard test also be accurate, significant, specific and economical. These criteria coupled with the multi- and interdisciplinary factors which control biocompatibility illustrate the task which the biomedical material scientist faces in determining the biocompatibility of a given polymer in a given application for a given implant time. The interpretation of tests or studies to determine tissue/polymer are complicated by the lack of standard tests and guidelines for polymer characterization, in particular, polymer surface characterization. In determining the tissue biocompatibility of a polymer, the limitations of the test methodology must be considered. This is an extremely important consideration as there is a tendency to extrapolate results from a static test to the dynamic situation, and the compatibility under non-functional conditions to that of functional conditions.

Tests and procedures exist for determining the tissue/material interaction from the point of view of biocompatibility. These include primary acute toxicity screening on material and material extracts as described by Autian and coworkers (8) and in-vivo implantation studies on materials in the powder form as described by Gourlay et al (9). Acute toxicity screening and in-vivo implantation represent the minimum initial studies which should be carried out on a candidate material for the determination of its biocompatibility. Table IV describes the tests used by Autian et al. in their primary acute toxicity screening and the rationale and time period for each individual test. It should be noted that the Acute Toxicity Screen is a short-term test, maximum time of 7 days, and is principally designed to determine the toxic effects of leachables. Gourlay et al. have described a test system utilizing the in-vivo implantation of polymer powders. This is shown in Table V with the indicators of toxicity and the mean standard toxicity scores relative to the behavior of known polymers. This test is for longer periods, weeks, and is based on determining the extent and degree of the induced inflammatory reaction. This system utilizes powders, not films, and it must be recognized that the biocompatibility of a material may be different in the film or sheet form.

Table IV. Primary Acute Toxicity Screening Material and Material Extracts (8).

1. Tissue Culture-Agar Overlay Responses for the Material and Extracts: detects the response of monolayer cell culture to readily diffusible components from materials, 1 day.

2. Intramuscular Rabbit Implant Test - Gross Observation and Histopathology Evaluation: detects the response of tissue to leachable components from materials, 7 days.

3. Rabbit Blood Hemolysis Test: detects the ability of the material to lyse red blood cells, 1 hour.

4. Intracutaneous Test in Rabbits on Extracts: detects the irritant response elicited by extracts, 3 days.

5. Systemic Toxicity in Mice on Extracts: measures the systemic toxicity of extracts, 7 days.

6. Inhibition of Cell Growth Test on Aqueous Extracts: measures the ability of distilled water extracts to inhibit cell growth in culture, 3 days.

We have developed an in-vivo method for determining the biocompatibility of polymers in the film or tube form. This system is called the "Cage Implant System" and involves the subcutaneous implantation of stainless steel mesh cages in rats.

Table V. Biocompatibility Testing : In-Vivo Implantation Studies on Polymer powders (9).

1. Indicators of Toxicity
    Degree of Muscle Cell Damage
    Thickness of Tissue Response
    Overall Cell Density
    Number of Polymorphonuclear Leukocytes and Erythrocytes
    Number of Eosinophils, Lymphocytes and Foreign-Body Giant Cells

2. Mean Standard Toxicity Scores (MSTS)
    Nontoxic: Polymers with MSTS's equal to or significantly greater than that for poly (glycolic acid), but significantly less than that of poly (isobutyl-2-cyanoacrylate).
    Moderately Toxic: Polymers with MSTS's not significantly different than that of poly (isobutyl-2-cyanoacrylate).
    Toxic: Polymers with MSTS's significantly greater than that of poly (isobutyl-2-cyanoacrylate) and equal to or greater than the value of poly (methyl 2-cyanoacrylate).

Table VI. The Cage Implant System: Analysis of the In-Vivo Inflammatory Reaction and Materials.

COMPONENT	ANALYSIS	METHOD
Inflammatory Exudate	Quantitative and Differential Leukocyte Counts	Hemacytometer Wright's and NSE Staining
	Intracellular Lysosomal Enzymes	NSE Staining
	Cell Viability	Trypan Blue Exclusion
Extracellular Fraction of Inflammatory	Extracellular Lysosomal Enzymes	Colorimetry
Exudate	Quantitative and Differential Protein Analysis	Electrophoresis Immunoelectrophoresis
	Complement Activation	Aggregometry
		Radioimmunoassays
Material	Adherent Leukocytes and Foreign Body Giant Cells	LM, SEM, and TEM of Thin Films
	Protein Adsorption	ATR-FTIR, SEM, ESCA, Contact Angle
	Material Surface Changes Material Bulk Changes	Tensile testing, X-Ray, DSC, GPC, Mechanical Relaxation.
Fibrous Capsule	Tissue Reaction Collagen and GAG Quantification and Identification	Histopathology Electropherosesis

The cages contain films of the polymer under investigation and empty cages are used as controls. The Cage Implant System is based on monitoring the time-dependent variation in the inflammatory reaction which is interacting with the polymer within the cage. The cages permit the withdrawal of small volumes of the inflammatory exudate for analysis without sacrificing the animal. This system allows the evaluation of selected aspects of the biocompatibility of a polymer. The influence of cells and enzymes on the material and the influence of the polymer on cells and enzymes in the inflammatory response can be measured in a time-dependent fashion.

The Cage Implant System offers a wide variety of methods and techniques for investigating the in-vivo behavior of polymers. The methods and techniques conveniently used for analysis of the inflammatory exudate and material in the cage implant system are found in Table VI. We have utilized this system to measure the biocompatibility of a wide variety of materials which include a biodegradable hydrogel (2), Biomer[R] (10-12), a cytotoxic PVC (13), and several drug-releasing polymers (14,15). In addition, we have carried out investigations on cellular interactions with materials in the cage system.

We have examined the in-vivo biocompatibility of a biodegradable hydrogel, poly(2-hydroxyethyl-L-glutamine) (2). Stress-strain measurements on the implanted biodegradable hydrogel samples showed that significant in-vivo degradation had occurred during the acute inflammatory phase of the response. This was indicated by a decrease in tensile strength. Several studies have been carried out on the segmented polyether polyurethane, Biomer[R] (10-12). These studies indicate that cellular adhesion does occur within the cage system and that cells may be activated during this adhesive process (16). Studies with the cytotoxic PVC indicate that the cytotoxic agent is released from the PVC during the period of time in the cage and this results in an acute inflammatory response of prolonged duration. We have used drug-releasing polymers in the cage system and in a study with gentamicin-silicone rubber system, it appears that the decreased biocompatibility of this system is due to the high concentrations of the gentamicin which are released, not the silicone rubber polymer.

SUMMARY

Any test system utilized to determine the tissue compatibility of the material must consider the end point of evaluation, the site of the implant, the animal species used, and the shape of the implant as these factors influence the behavior of the material in the physiological environment. The cage implant system has been presented as a test method for the simultaneous evaluation of tissue biocompatibility and material changes which may occur in-vivo.

REFERENCES

1. Black, J., Biological Performance of Materials Fundamentals of Biocompatibility, Marcel Dekker, New York, 1981.
2. Marchant, R.E., Hiltner, A., Hamlin, C., Rabinovitch, A., Slobodkin, R. and Anderson, J.M., J. Biomed. Mater. Res., 17:301, 1983.
3. Wright, D.G. and Gallin, J.I., J. Immunol., 123:285, 1979.
4. Henson P.M., Am. J. Pathol., 101:494, 1980.
5. Anderson, J.M. and Miller, K.M., Biomaterials, 5:51, 1984.

6. Chambers, T.J., J. Pathol., 122:71, 1977.
7. Murch, A.R., Grounds, M.D., Marshall, C.A. and Papadimitriou, J.M., J. Pathol., 137:177, 1982.
8. Autian, J., Artif. Organs, 1:53, 1977.
9. Gourlay, B.J., Rice, R.M., Hegyeli, A.F., Wade, C.W.R., Dillon, J.G., Jaffe, H. and Kulkarni, R.K., J. Biomed. Mater. Res., 12:219, 1978.
10. Marchant, R.E., Phua, K., Hiltner, A and Anderson, J.M., J. Biomed. Mater. Res., 18:309, 1984.
11. Anderson, J.M., Marchant, R.E., Suzuki, S., Hamlin, C., Rabinovitch, A. and Hiltner, A., in Polyurethanes in Medicine, H. Plenck, ed., Elsevier Publishing Co., The Netheriands, 1984.
12. Marchant, R.E., Miller, K.M. and Anderson, J.M., J. Biomed. Mater. Res., 18: 1169, 1984.
13. Marchant, R.E. and Anderson, J.M., unpublished results.
14. Anderson, J.M., Marchant, R. and McClurken, M., in Long-Acting Contraceptive Delivery Systems, G.I. Zatuchni., A. Goldsmith., J.D. Shelton, and J.J. Sciarra., eds., Harper and Row, New York, 1984.
15. Spilizewski, K., Marchant, R.E. and Anderson, J.M., unpublished results.
16. Marchant, R.E., Miller, K.M., Hiltner, A. and Anderson, J.M., in Polymers as Biomaterials, S. Shalaby., A. Hoffman., T. Horbett, and B. Ratner., eds., Plenum Press, New York, 1984.

PHYSICOCHEMICAL CHARACTERISTICS OF BIOPOLYMERS

N. Lotan

Technion—Israel Institute of Technology, Biomedical Engineering Department, Haifa, Israel

INTRODUCTION

In recent years, chemists, biochemists and biologists have developed a growing concern for understanding the pathways along which metals are involved in biological systems (1-3). The "no man's land" between inorganic chemistry and biological sciences has thus developed into a discipline by itself, the inorganic biochemistry.

Living organisms utilize a variety of metal ions, some in trace amounts, some others in larger quantities. The tasks assigned to these ions are diverse: from support electrolytes to charge carriers, from Lewis acid to redox catalysts, from biopolymer structure stabilizers to enzyme activators. Last but not least, metal ions perform as key agents in some regulatory devices of the living cell function, much in the same way as hormones, drugs and allosteric affectors do. This diversity of functions is expressed-among others-by a wide variation in the ion content of the various systems. Such a situation prevails at various levels of biological organization, and a few examples are set forth in Table I (for a more detailed account see Ref.4). It can be seen that the concentration of a given ion differs from one system to another or-for a given system-on the two sides of the membrane separating various compartments of it; also, these differences vary from one ion to another. Moreover, for various ions in a given system, even opposite concentration gradients are observed. In order for such an apparently unequilibrated distribution of ions to be preserved, a sine qua non condition is, obviously, to prevent their diffusion. This is achieved, among others, by the membrane, itself, the structure of which represents a hydrophobic barrier for the free movement of the hydrophilic ions. In this case, however, one can legitimately ask: How then is such a distribution generated? The answer to this question is to be related to the process of active transport across biological membranes and, in 1967, Pressman suggested the generic name of "ionophores" for the compounds that bind metal ions and carry them across the lipid membranes in the form of a lipidsoluble complex (5). It is obvious that, in order to perform properly, the ionophores must be ion specific, and the complexes they form in the lipophilic medium must dissociate in contact with water, thus releasing the ion. Such properties are, indeed, exhibited by the natural ionophores, and the behaviour of these compounds in complex biological systems has been dealt with in numerous investigations. For a summary of them the reader is referred to recent review articles (6-12). We have concerned ourselves with some of the physico-chemical aspects of cation binding by a natural ionophore and by synthetic polymers and, in the following, the results of part of our in vitro studies are presented.

Table I. Distribution of Cations in Biological Systems.

	Na^+	K^+	Mg^{++}	Ca^{++}
B. subtilis (dried), mmoles/kg				
whole bacteria		1260	124	2.5
spores		231	206	400
B. cereus (dried), mmoles/kg				
whole bacteria		1180	450	7.5
spores		51	124	475
Tolypella intricata (algal cell), mM				
chloroplasts	36	340		
vacuole	7	100		
outside	1	0.4		
Human red cell	11	92	2.5	0.1
Whole blood	85	44	1.6	
Squid nerve, mM				
inside	49	410		
outside	440	22		
Crab leg nerve, mM				
inside	52	410		
outside	510	12		

IONOPHORE A—23187

There are very many compounds which, under the definition of Pressman (5), may in principle qualify as ionophores. And, although not all of them have established themselves as such after being actually tested in defined biological systems, their ability to complex with cations in non-aqueous solutions has nevertheless been well proven. Some of these compounds are natural, others are synthetic. Of the latter class, polyethers have been extensively investigated; macrocyclic polyethers (the "crown ethers") were first obtained already twenty years ago (13-16), but it was only about ten years later that the complexing power of these compounds was discovered (17). Since then, a vast literature that covers this and connected topics has appeared (for reviews see Refs. 18-21) and, among the structurally related compounds, the cryptates (polycyclic derivatives) (22,23) and a multi-chain polyethylene oxide ("octopus molecule") (24) are to be mentioned. The syntheses and some ion binding properties of amino acid-containing compounds have also been reported (25-29).

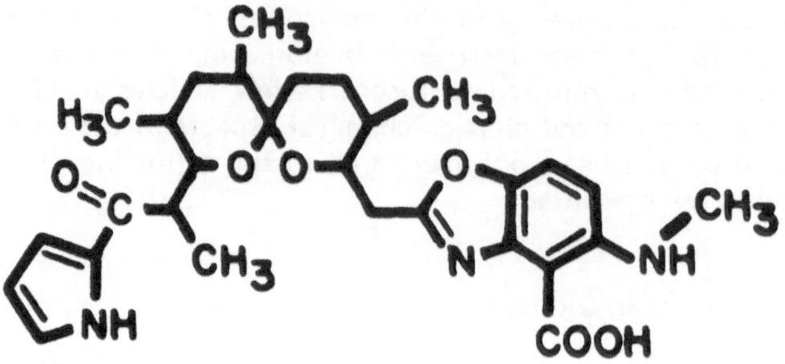

42

Figure 1. Chemical Structure of Ionophore A-23187.

For the biologists, however, by far the most appealing group of ionophores are the natural ones. Using the basic chemical structure the criterion, these compounds can be classified as polypeptides and related amino acid derivatives (e.g. gramicidin, alamethicin, antamanide, enterochelin), depsipeptides (e.g. valinomycin, beauvericin, eniantin), or macrotetralides (e.g. monactin). The compound A-23187 (30-32) belongs to a different group of natural ionophores, together with nigericin (33), monensin (34), X-537A (35), and salinomycin (36): these are monocarboxylic polyethers, which form-with the cations-electrically neutral complexes (37-39).

The structure of A-23187 (Fig. 1) has only recently been elucidated (40): the molecule contains a pyrrole and a benzoxazole ring, connected by a spiroketal bridge. Some spectral characteristics of the ionophore and of its metal complexes have been investigated, using electronic absorption and fluorescence spectroscopy (41-43) as well as electron paramagnetic resonance (EPR) (44) and nuclear magnetic resonance (NMR) techniques (40,45). It was concluded that A-23187 is highly specific for di-valent cations (38,43,44). However, under appropriate conditions the ionophore binds -although weakly-monovalent cations too, and it was reasoned that all these com-plexes most probably assume a similar structure (43). In order to further investigate the correlation between ion specificity and the structure of the complexes, we have studied the circular dichroic (CD) properties of A-23187 and of its adducts with various cations. Some representative spectra are presented in Figure 2. It can be seen that addition of Li^+ or Ca^{++} affects the CD spectrum of the ligand, indicating that complexation is associated with changes in the conformation of the latter. A some-what more detailed information as to the origin of these changes can be gained by considering the difference spectra, i.e. the differences between the spectra of the complexes and that of the free ligand, and these are shown in Figure 3. Some simi-larity can now be noticed between these two spectra, suggesting a similarity in the structure of the corresponding complexes, particularly in those parts of the molecule that express themselves in the 240-320 nm region of the spectrum. This is even more clearly seen in the normalized difference spectra, which are shown in Figure 4. From our data one can conclude that the lithium and calcium complexes of A-23187 indeed have some common structural features, as it had already been suggested earlier (43); these complexes, however, also exhibit some structural differences, and these are to be related to the large difference in the corresponding stability constants (43).

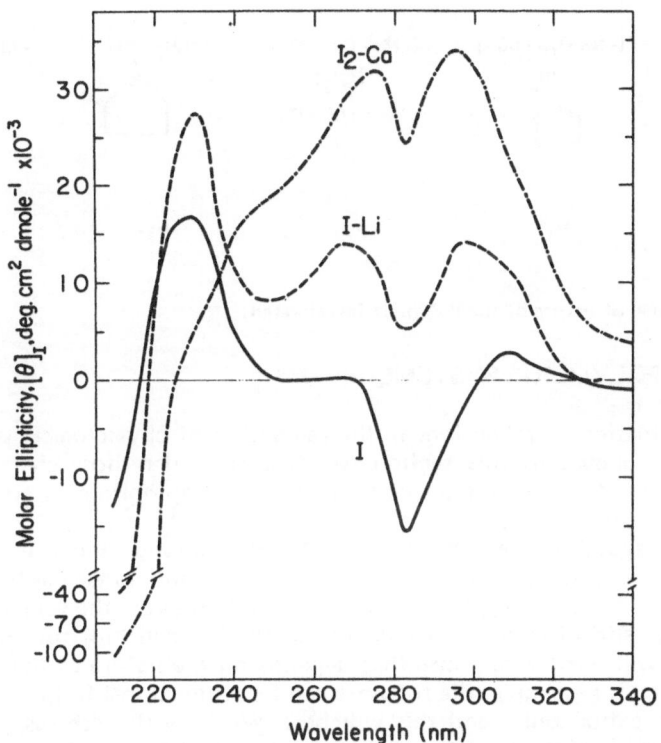

Figure 2. Circular Dichroism Spectra of Ionophore A-23187 of Its Complexes in Methanol: Chloroform (9:1 v/v); (——), no Salt Added; (— —) Complex with Li$^+$, (—·—), Complex with Ca^{++}.

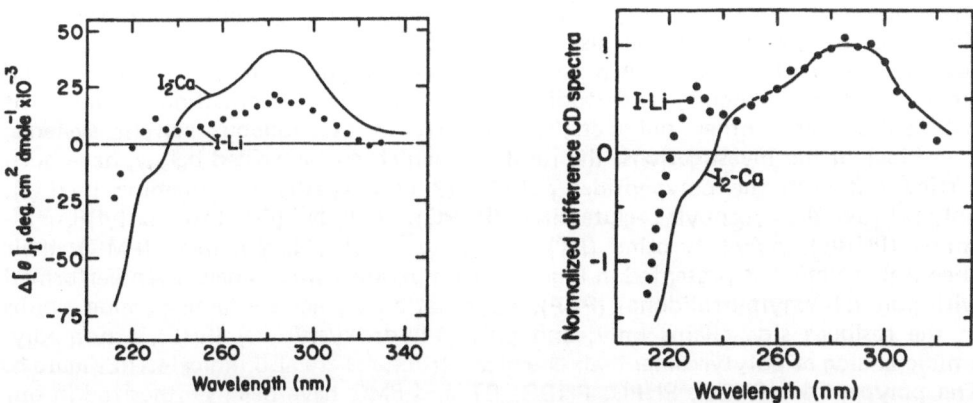

Figure 3. Difference CD Spectra of the Calcium-Ionophore (——) and of the Lithium-Ionophore (···) Complexes. The Difference Spectra were Calculated from the Data in Figure 2, by Substracting the Spectrum of the Ionophore from that of the Complex.

Figure 4. Difference Spectra of Figure 3, Normalized at 290 nm.

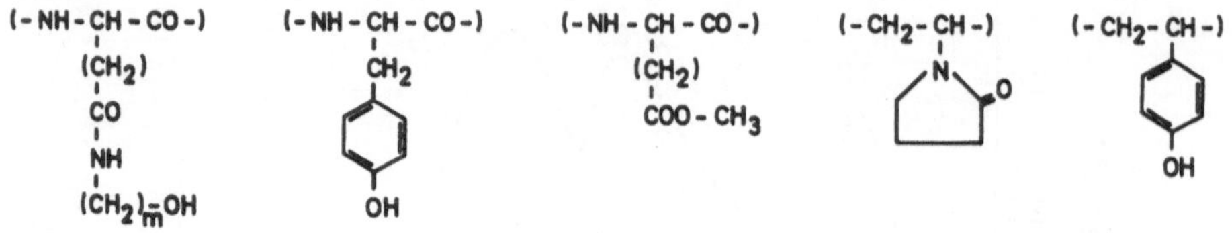

Figure 5. Chemical Structure of the Polymers Investigated.

ION BINDING POLYMERIC SYSTEMS

The participation of metal ions in the regulation of physiological processes has been mentioned above. In this section we shall consider those characteristics of synthetic polymers that, in this respect, make them appropriate as study systems, analogues to the natural ones.

Biological regulatory devices are characterized, among others, by the average level of affector at which the system is expected to respond, as well as by its range of allowed variation. It has been pointed out that ionophores are the vehicles that bring the ions at their site of action. Once arrived at the locus-in this case the regulation system-the ion will elicit a response that depends on the nature of the receptor-ion interaction. Thus, for example, the response can be proportional to the concentration of the affecting cation only, and this will be a relatively sluggish response. On the other hand, an interaction involving both the cation and the accompanying anion is obviously more complex, allowing also for a wider choice of the affectors. However, an even more advanced control system can be envisaged by having a receptor that, as a result of its interaction with the affector, will undergo a cooperative transformation. This process is characterized by a sigmoidal response i.e. a large response is produced when the level of the affector changes in a relatively small range. Such receptors are the proteins, due to their ability to undergo highly cooperative conformational transitions. Similar transitions have also been observed with synthetic polyamino acids (46-56), and the latter are thus most appropriate as model systems. We have pursued along this line of inquiry and studied the ion-induced conformational changes of polypeptides and other polymers, particularly in non-aqueous solvent systems.

Most of the investigations, the results of which are described below, have been carried out with the polypeptides poly-N^5-(2-hydroxyethyl)-L-glutamine (PHEG), poly-N^5-(3-hydroxypropyl)-L-glutamine (PHPG), poly-N^5-(4-hydroxybutyl)-L-glutamine (PHBG), poly-L-tyrosine (PT), and poly-γ-methyl-L-glutamate (PMG); their chemical structure is presented in Figure 5. Comparative studies have been performed with poly-(N- vinylpyrrolidone) (PVP), a synthetic polymer containing amide groups in the residues side chains only, and poly-(4-hydroxystyrene) (PHS), a non-poly-amidic analog of polytyrosine; their chemical structures are also indicated in Figure 5. The polypeptides PHEG, PHPG, PHBG, PT and PMG have been synthesized in our laboratory. The PVP sample used was a commercial preparation (pharmaceutical grade, Polyciences, Inc., Warrington, Pa., USA). PHS was a gift from Dr. M. Fridkin of the Weizmann Institute of Science in Rehovot.

The approach that we have used involved optical rotatory dispersion (ORD), circular dichroism (CD), hydrodynamic and nuclear magnetic resonance (NMR)

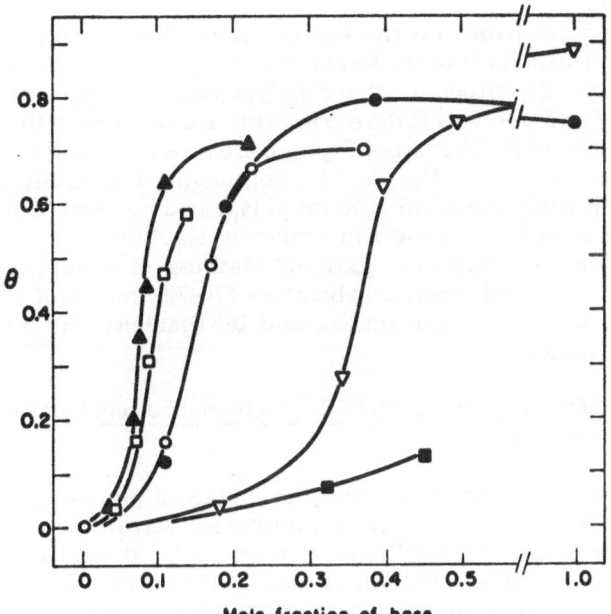

Figure 6.   Helicity, θ, of PHPG in Solutions of Formic Acid Containing: (▲) Ammonium Formate, (□) Sodium Formate, (0) Urea, (●), Formamide, (V) Acetic Acid, and (■) Chloroform as Additives.

measurements. For polyamino acids, we have interpreted our results in terms of structural interconversions between the disordered form(s) of the polymeric chain and regular entities such as the α-helix (57) and an extended but yet undefined form (58,59) of the chain. Such correlations have been extensively used in the past, and proved themselves most appropriate for such studies (53,60-63).

Polypeptides in Formic Acid Containing Solvent Systems

The interaction of protons with polypeptides has been investigated by following-by ORD measurements-the conformational changes of PHEG, PHPG and PHBG in formic acid containing solutions (64). In pure formic acid the three polymers assume a disordered conformation, as indicated by a value of zero for the Moffitt-Yang parameter b_0 (65). Obviously, formic acid strongly interacts with the polymer, not allowing it to arrange itself into the intramolecularly hydrogen bonded α-helical structure. Addition of chloroform, acetic acid, formamide, urea, sodium formate or ammonium formate to these solutions produces an increase in the α-helix content of the polymers, and the results obtained with PHPG are summarized in Figure 6. It can be seen that merely diluting the strong acid with a neutral solvent (e.g. chloroform) has only a limited effect on the conformation of the polypeptide; formamide, sodium and ammonium formate, on the other hand, are most efficient.

Of particular interest is the observation that urea affects the conformation of PHPG in various ways, depending on the solvent used. Thus, in water, it disrupts the α-helical structure of the polymer (66); in formic acid, however, at concentrations up to 10 M, urea confers stability to the α-helical form, thus belonging to the same class of additives as formamide and the formate salts. A common characteristic of these additives is their basicity towards formic acid and one can thus infer that, in the presence of the latter, the structure of the polypeptide is largely dictated by the overall acidity of the medium. This feature is even more evident from the presentation in Figure 7, where some of the data from Figure 6 are now compared not on the basis of the molar fraction of the additive, but by considering the acidity of the corresponding solvents, this being expressed in terms of H_o, acid Hammett acidity function (67). Related effects of salts in formic acid containing solutions have previously been reported by Schaefgen and Trivisonno (68) and Mattiussi et al. (69) for polycaprolactam, by Selegny, Vert and their collaborators (70-72) for poly(-) 1,2-diaminopropane sebacamide and related polyamides, and by Bradbury and Yuan (73) and by Saunders (74) for nylon.

Polymers in LiCl-Methanol and LiCl-Trifluoroethanol Solvent Systems. Formation of Pseudopolyelectrolytes

Lithium seem to be involved in a variety of biological processes, particularly in brain biochemistry. These ions are actively transported across membranes (75-77), and effectively discriminated by the "sodium pump" (78); they affect brain cortex respiration (79), glucose uptake (80), and various fundamental processes in the nerve cells (81), as well as the concentration level of neurotransmitters such as norepinephrine, acetyl choline, γ-aminobutyric acid, glutamic acid, and glutamine (82-86).

Lithium salts have been found to be remarkably effective and highly specific psychiatric drugs, particularly in the treatment of the manic depression (85) and of some states of aggression (87,88), as well as in reducing the "high" feelings associated with the intake of alcohol, marijuana and other stimulants (89). As to the mode of action of Li^+ at the molecular level it has been shown that it affects or even strongly inhibits adenyl cyclase and succinate dehydrogenase (85,90), and DNA polymerase (91), a group of enzymes which all catalyze processes involving energy-rich bonds.

The denaturing effect of certain inorganic lithium salts on proteins, in aqueous solutions, is well established (92,93); the process requires high concentration of these compounds, and it is assumed to be the result of direct ion-macromolecule interactions. Investigations of the conductivity of LiCl in non-aqueous solvents (94) have suggested that, in some of these systems, a high thermodynamic activity of Li^+ can be attained, and these results prompted us to use LiCl in organic solvents as possible affector of the tridimensional structure of polypeptides.

We have investigated the conformational changes of PHBG in the LiCl-methanol solvent system, using ORD and hydrodynamic techniques (58,59). The results are summarized in Figure 8. The changes in the b_o parameter indicate that the polymer-which is α-helical in methanol undergoes a helix-coil transformation as the LiCl content increases; the transition is complete at 4 M salt. Further increase of the LiCl concentration up to 6 M has no additional effect on the b_o parameter. Intrinsic viscosity measurements, on the other hand, reveal a more complex behavior of the system. In the range 2-4 M LiCl, the viscosity decreases, as expected for the rod-like to disordered chain transformation suggested by the ORD data. In the range of 4-6 M salt, however, one observes an increase in the viscosity, i.e. a change in the opposite direction. The changes described above for b_o and $[\eta]$ are not specific to PHBG, as we have obtained similar results with the related polypeptides PHEG and PHPG, as well as with poly-L-tyrosine (see below). Such changes are usually encountered with polyelectrolytes upon varying their degree of ionization in aqueous solutions (95-98).

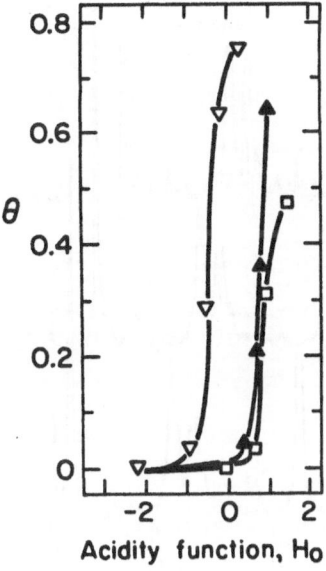

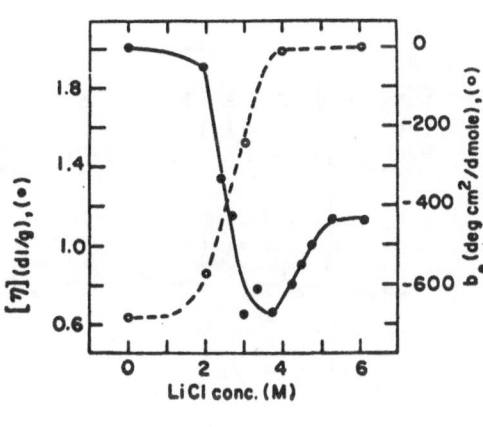

Figure 7.   Helicity, θ, of PHPG in Solutions of Formic Acid Containing Ammonium Formate (▲) Sodium Formate (□),or Acetic Acid (V), as a Function of the Acidity of the Solvent.

Figure 8.   Conformational Changes of PHBG in the LiCl-Methanol Solvent System, as Followed by (0) ORD, and (●) Viscosity.

We have therefore interpreted our results to say that, at high LiCl concentrations, the polypeptides bind Li^+ ions thus acquiring a pseudopolyelectrolyte character, while Cl^- ions are preferentially involved in a complex formation with methanol. These conclusions imply that, at the elevated LiCl concentration used, the flexibility of the polymeric chain is reduced. That this is indeed the case is suggested also by the results of our NMR measurements, and Figure 9 shows some representative spectra that have been obtained with PHPG. It can be seen that, as the salt concentration is raised, extreme broadening of the resonance lines takes place and, above 6 M, the peaks can hardly be discerned. (*),(**) We have related these changes to alterations in the mobility of the polymeric main chain and of the amino acid side chains, and not to a non-specific solvent perturbation. These considerations find support in the results of a parallel study on N-(2-hydroxyethyl)-acetamide, a low molecular weight compound modelling the side chains of the residues in the polyamino acid studied (Fig. 10): In this case the increase of salt concentration alters the splitting pattern of the protons in the methylene groups, but the resonance lines still remain relatively sharp.

(*) In these spectra a sharp peak is observed at about 3.2 ppm. It is due to traces of CHD_2-OD present in the deuterated methanol that we have used, and it has been observed in all the spectra of methanol-containing solutions, as well as in the spectrum of the solvent itself.

(**) In the spectrum obtained at 6.6 M LiCl separate resonance peaks are seen for CD_3-OH and HOD. The phenomenon is related to the strong interaction between salt and methanol.

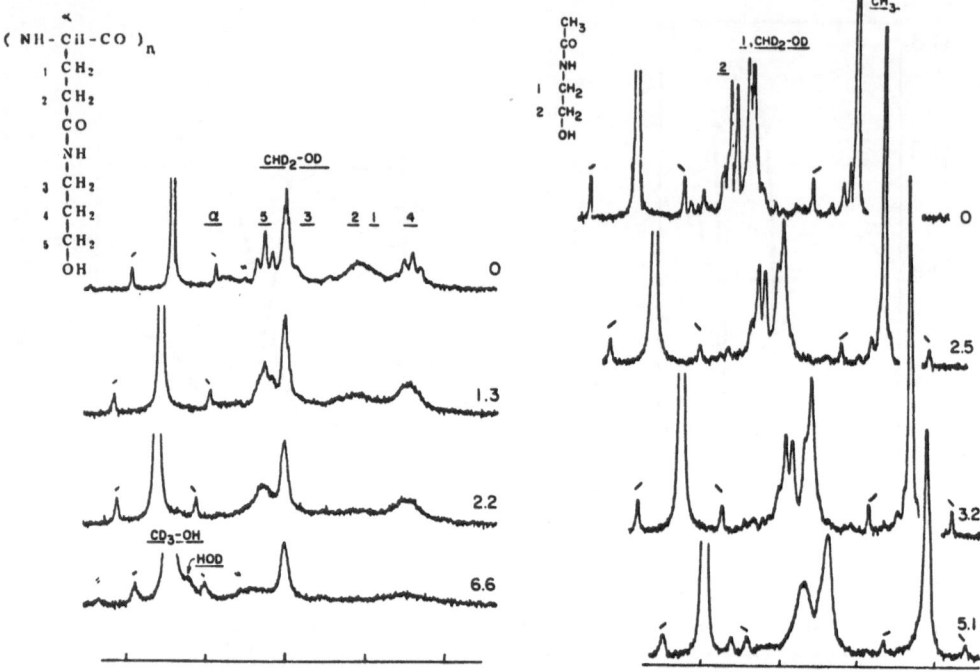

Figure 9.   NMR Spectra of PHPG in the LiCl-Methanol Solvent System. The Numbers Identifying the Spectra Indicate the LiCl Molarity in the Solvent. The Spectra are Arbitrarily Aligned on the Resonance Line of CHD$_2$-OD. In This Subsequent Figures Presenting NMR Spectra, the Scale at the Bottom of the Figure was Marked in ppm Units, and the Peaks Identified by / and // are Spinning Side Bands, the Slashes Pointing Towards the Parent Resonance Line.

Figure 10.   NMR Spectra of N- (2-hydroxyethyl)- Acetamide in the LiCl- Methanol Solvent System. The Numbers Identifying the Spectra Indicate the LiCl Molarity in the Solvent.

The polymers described above are all polypeptides. For a more general assessment for the pseudopolyelectrolyte effect in the LiCl-methanol system, we have investigated the behavior of poly-(N-vinylpyrrolidone), a polymer bearing the amide groups only in the side chains of its monomeric residues (see Figure 5). The results are summarized in the Figures 11 and 12. In methanol the PVP chain has a disordered conformation and, accordingly, its viscosity is low. Upon addition of LiCl, the intrinsic viscosity of the polymer increases (Fig. 11) and the NMR spectrum broadens (Fig. 12); these changes suggest that a more expanded and rigid macromolecular structure is formed, thus indicating that, in this respect, PVP and the polyamino acids behave alike.

We have subsequently extended our studies to include polymers containing not only the amide moiety, but other functional groups too. Poly-L-tyrosine, like the other polyamino acids mentioned above, is α-helical in methanol (99,100). The properties of polytyrosine in LiCl-methanol solutions have previously been investigated and, based on UV and IR absorption, as well as ORD and CD measurements it was concluded that, at a salt concentration of about 3 M, the polymer undergoes an α-helix-to-random coil transformation (99). In view of our results obtained with other polypeptides in this solvent system (see above), we have reconsidered the study

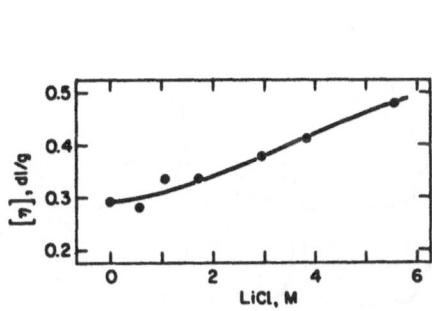

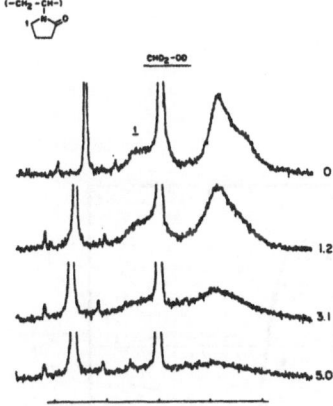

Figure 11. Intrinsic Viscosity of PVP in the LiCl-Methanol Solvent System.

Figure 12. NMR Spectra of PVP in the LiCl-Methanol Solvent System. The numbers Identifying the Spectra Indicate the LiCl Molarity in the Solvent.

of Shiraki and Imahori (99), focusing our attention on the hydrodynamic and NMR properties of the polymer.

Viscosity measurements have shown that, at LiCl concentrations below 1 M, polytyrosine behaves as expected for an electroneutral polymer, i.e. its reduced viscosity [η_{red}] decreased with decreasing polymer concentration (c_p). At higher salt concentrations (1 to 6 M), however, an opposite dependence is observed, i.e. the reduced viscosity increases with decreasing c_p. In all cases, in the polymer concentration range investigated (3 to 10 mg/ml), η_{red} shows a linear dependence on c_p, and our results, expressed in terms of the Huggins constant k', are presented in Figure 13. Furthermore, the intrinsic viscosity of the polymer, as obtained by the normal extrapolation to c_p=0, exhibits a salt concentration dependence that resembles the one of PHBG (see Fig. 8), i.e. it decreases then increases with increasing the LiCl concentration, the minimum being at about 2.5 M.

NMR spectra of poly-L-tyrosine in the LiCl-methanol solvent system are presented in Figure 14. In methanol, the resonance lines of α-CH and β-CH$_2$ protons are broad, as normally encountered with α-helical polypeptides (60,101-104). In the region of the aromatic protons the peaks are fairly well developed, but their splitting pattern is recognized with difficulty. A similar spectrum has been previously reported for poly-L-tyrosine in other helix-supporting solvents (105). Addition of LiCl has drastic effects on the spectrum: the resonance lines broaden and then are no more discernible, the α-CH and β-CH$_2$ first, the aromatic CH last. The behavior closely resembles that of poly-(4-hydroxystyrene), the non-polypeptidic analog of poly-L-tyrosine (see Fig. 15A).

The effects of LiCl on polytyrosine-as expressed in the hydrodynamic and NMR properties-most probably originate in a strong interaction between salt and the biopolymer. The changes in the NMR spectrum of the aromatic protons (see Fig. 14) suggest that this interaction involves the phenolic moieties. We believe, however, that one is not faced merely with the formation of phenolate species: a comparison of the spectra of the polymer in aqueous 0.3 N NaOD (a solvent in which all the phenolic groups are ionized) and in methanolic 5.7 M LiCl (see Fig. 16) clearly indicates that there is a large difference between the status of the polymer in the two solvents.

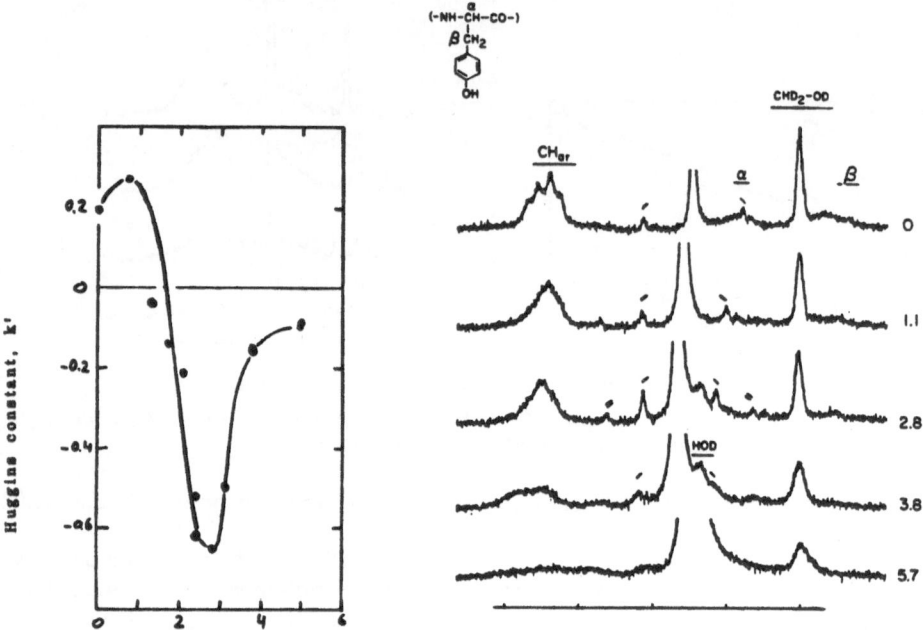

Figure 13. Salt Concentration Dependence of the Huggins Constant, k , for Poly-L-tyrosine in the LiCl-Methanol Solvent System. For Details, See Text.

Figure 14. NMR Spectra of poly-L-tyrosine in the LiCl-Methanol Solvent System. The Numbers Identifying the Spectra Indicate the LiCl Molarity in the Solvent.

A similar situation is also encountered with poly-(hydroxystyrene) (see Fig. 15). Furthermore, in aqueous alkali, the spectrum of the aromatic protons of polytyrosine (Fig. 16) closely resembles the corresponding spectrum of p-cresol (not shown), the model compound for the phenolic side chain of the tyrosine residue.

The complexity of the interaction between Li^+ and phenolic moieties is also illustrated in Figure 17, where presented are the NMR spectra of cresol and of its homologue, catechol. Addition of LiCl to the methanolic solutions produces the coalescence of the aromatic protons peaks of the former compound, while for the latter an opposite effect is observed.

It has been shown above that, in the lithium chloride-methanol solvent system, a variety of polymers exhibit the pseudopolyelectrolyte effect at very high salt concentration; we have suggested that this effect is the expression of Li^+ binding by the polymer, a process favorized by the preferential solvation of Cl^- by methanol. It was therefore expected that, if this mechanism is indeed operative, then LiCl will be more effective in solvents which, compared to methanol, are stronger solvators for the anion and/or weaker ones for the cation. Fluorinated alcohols indeed exhibit such properties (94), and we have therefore searched for the pseudopolyelectrolyte effect in trifluoroethanol (TFE). The results obtained by CD measurements of PHEG are shown in Figure 18. The spectrum in TFE is characteristic for the right-handed

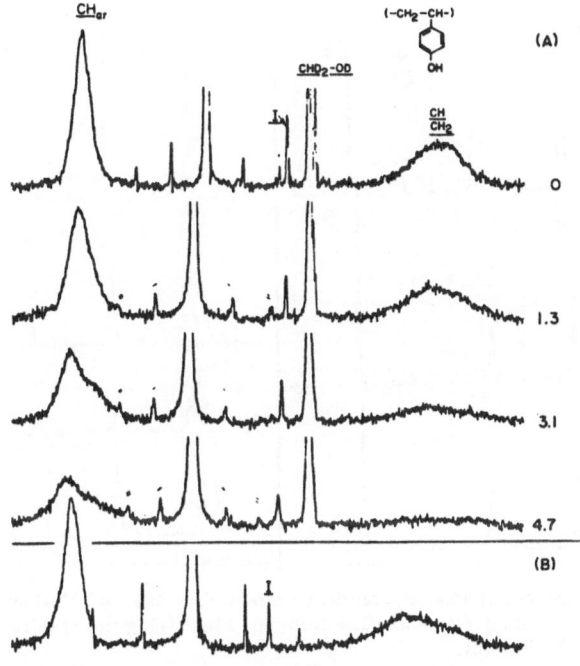

Figure 15. NMR Spectra of Poly (4-hydroxystyrene): Part A, in the LiCl-Methanol System, the Numbers Identifying the Spectra Indicating the LiCl Molarity in the Solvent: Part B, in 1 M NaOD in D_2O. In the Spectra, the Peak Marked I is Due to an Unidentified Impurity Present in the Polymer Sample.

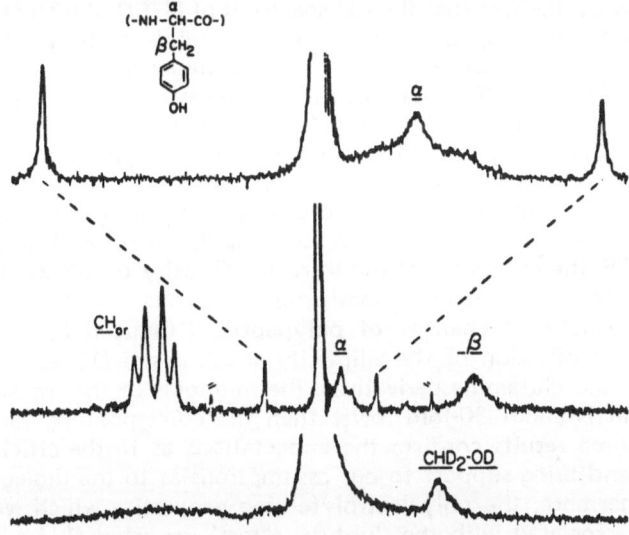

Figure 16. NMR Spectra of Poly-L-Tyrosine. Lower Tracing: in 5.7 M LiCl in Methanol (Taken from Figure 14): Middle Tracing: in 0.3 M NaOD in D_2O: Upper Tracing: Part of the Spectrum in Aqueous Alkali, Enlarged for a Convenient Identification of the α-CH Resonance Line.

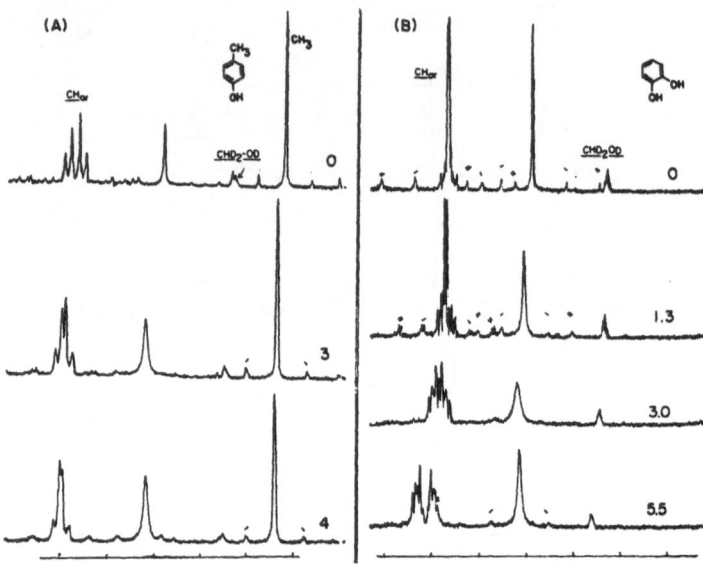

Figure 17. NMR Spectra of Phenolic Model Compounds in the LiCl-Methanol Solvent System. Part A Cresol. Part B: Catechol. The Numbers Identifying the Spectra Indicate the LiCl Molarity in the Solvent.

α-helical form of polypeptides (53,61,106). This structure is disrupted upon addition of small amounts of LiCl, and the transition is complete at about 0.2 M salt (107).

The conformational change described above and expressed in the CD properties of PHEG (see Fig. 18) does not lead to the disordered form of the polymeric chain; this is indicated by the fact that the CD spectrum of PHEG at high salt concentration in TFE (thereafter type S) differs from the one exhibited by the same polymer in water (see Fig. 18), a solvent in which this macromolecule assumes the random coil structure (101,108-112). CD spectra of the S-type have also been measured for PHBG and PMG in LiCl-containing TFE (107), and for PHEG, PHPG and PHBG at high concentration (above 4 M) of LiCl in methanol (113). In parallel to the CD studies, we have also carried out measurements on the viscosity of the polymers in the LiCl-TFE system. The results (107) show the same general features as observed with PHGB in methanol-containing solvents (see Fig. 8), with the difference that in the presence of TFE the minimum of the intrinsic viscosity occurs at about 0.2 M salt, rather than at 4 M, as observed with methanolic solutions.

The conformational changes of polypeptides, induced by LiCl in TFE and measured by the variation of the ellipticity at 222.5 nm (107), are summarized in Figure 19. For the glutamine derivatives, the midpoint of the transition is at about 0.1 M salt, that is about 30-fold lower than the corresponding value in methanol (see Fig. 8). These results confirm the expectations as to the efficiency of TFE in such systems, and bring support to our assumptions as to the molecular mechanism involved. Furthermore, the polyelectrolyte-type properties which we have observed are not to be associated with the "upturn effect" reported (114,115) for the non-Newtonian viscosity of polymer solutions, since our results have been obtained in methanol- and TFE-containing solutions of widely different viscosity (see also Fig. 23). We therefore associate the S-type CD spectra of polypeptides with their pseudopolyelectrolyte form, the latter being revealed by the hydrodynamic and NMR

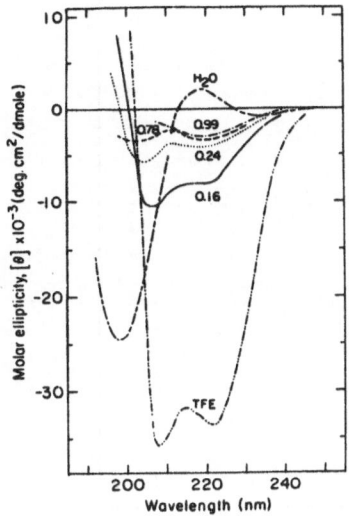
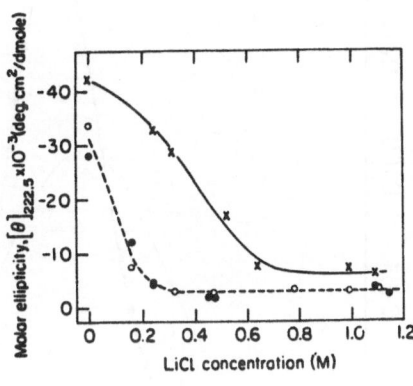

Figure 18. CD Spectra of PHEG in the LiCl-TFE Solvent System. The Numbers Identifying the Spectra Indicate the LiCl Molarity in the Solvent. For Comparison, the Spectrum of the Same Polymer in Water is Also Included.

Figure 19. Conformational Transitions of Polypeptides in the LiCl-TFE Solvent System: (x) PMLG, (0), PHEG, and (●). PHBG.

measurements. Our results are in line with previously reported cases of neutral polymers which, in the presence of salts, acquire polyelectrolyte character in non-aqueous solutions. These include, for example, poly(ethylene oxide) (116-118), poly(vinyl crown ethers) (119), poly(N-vinylpyrrolidone) (120), nylon 66 (121,122), poly(-) 1,2-diaminopropane sebacamide (70), and poly(hexamethylphosphamide (123,124). Related phenomena have also been observed in aqueous solutions (124-129).

Recently, additional evidence for the validity of our interpretation of the pseudopolyelectrolyte effect has been forwarded by Haas et al. (130,131). These investigators have carried out a systematic study on a series of hydroxyethyl-L-glutamine oligopeptides of well-defined length, each containing at its ends a donor and an acceptor of electronic excitation energy. Measurements of the kinetics of the fluorescence decay of the donor moiety of these compounds in TFE-glycerol mixtures containing various amounts of LiCl (up to 3 M) have been performed and, from the results obtained, the distribution of distances between the chromophores at the two ends of the molecules, F(R), was evaluated according to Grinvald et al. (132). The results obtained with the pentapeptide (131) are brought, for exemplification, in Figure 20. It can be seen that, for the 2.8 M LiCl containing system, the F(R) function is characterized by a mean distance which is larger and by a variance which is smaller than the corresponding values calculated for the system lacking the salt. These results indicate that the conformation of the oligopeptide is more stretched in the presence of LiCl than in its absence.

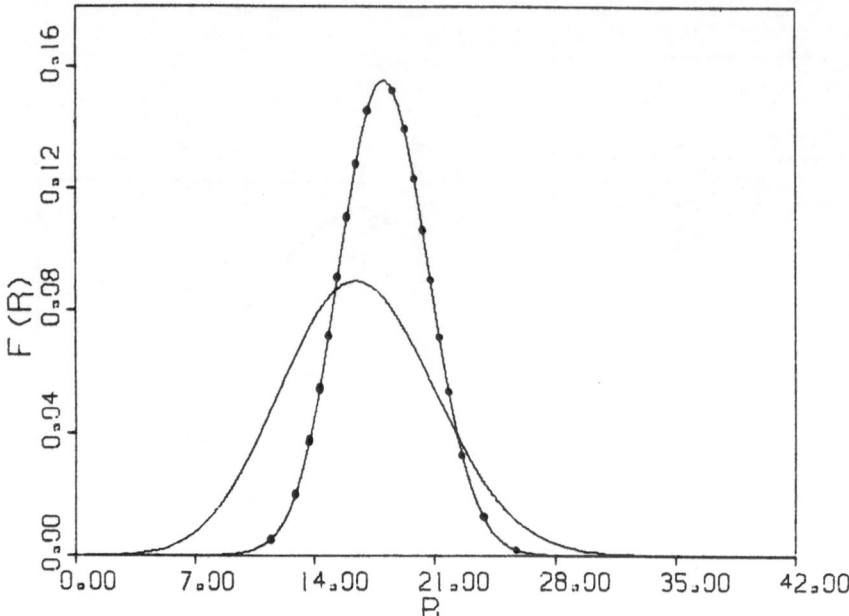

Figure 20. Distribution of the End-to-End Distances for a Modified PHEG (Degree of Polymerization 5) in TFE-Glycerol (3:7 wt/wt): (—●—), in the Presence of 2.7 m LiCl: (——), no Salt Added. The Data are Reproduced from Ref. 131, with Permission.

Effect of Water on Ion Binding by Polymers in Organic Solvents

It has been pointed out above that in order for an ion chelator to perform as ionophore, it should not only bind ions in a non-aqueous environment, but it should also release them in the presence of water. We have considered this aspect, too, in our studies on ion binding polymers, and a summary of the results obtained is presented below.

In formic acid, all our polyglutamine derivatives assume a disordered conformation (64). In water, this is also the conformation of PHEG (101,108-112), while the helix content, Θ, of the propyl and butyl derivatives in this solvent is 15% and 65% respectively (108). In formic acid-water mixtures the dependence of Θ on solvent composition takes an apparently peculiar course, and the experimental data are presented in Figure 21-A. Such a behavior can, however, be understood under the considerations that follow. In non-interacting solvent, polypeptides assume the intramolecularly hydrogen bonded α-helical conformation. In interacting solvents, on the other hand, the disordered structure prevails, and this is the case for formic acid containing solutions. Water resembles formic acid with respect to PHEG, but less so for the two higher homologues (108). On addition of water to formic acid containing solutions a complex is formed between the two solvents (133-135) and, consequently, the polymer releases the protons bound in the absence of water. This transfer also allows the polymer to regain its ordered, α-helical structure. Based on this approach, theoretical curves have been calculated (64), using the Bixon-Lifson formalism (136) for solvent-induced conformational transitions and assuming differ-

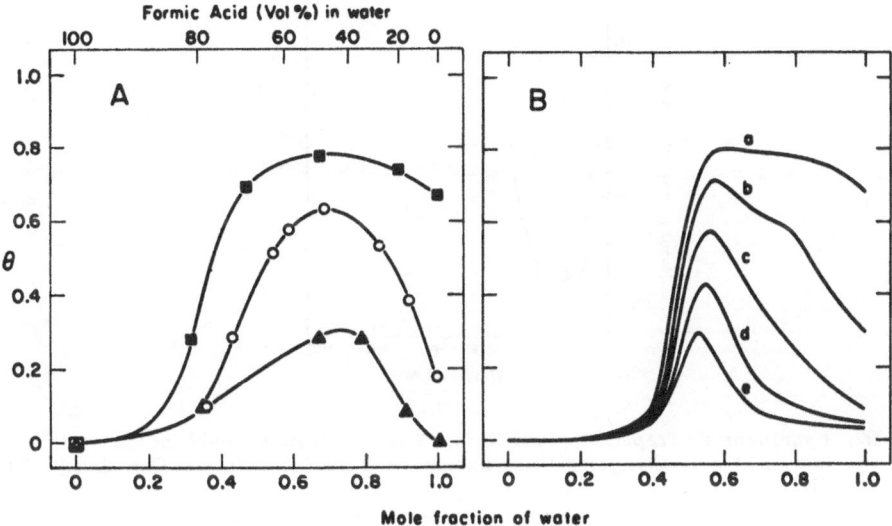

Figure 21. Part A: Helicity of (▲) PHEG, (0) PHPG, and (■) PHBG in Formic Acid-Water Mixtures. Part B: Theoretical Transition Curves for a Polyamino Acid. The Curves a-e were Obtained by Assuming Increasing Values for the Binding Constant of Water to the Polymer. For More Details, See Ref. 64.

ent values for the parameters involved. Some of the calculated curves are presented in Figure 21-B; their resemblance to the experimentally determined ones is obvious, thus providing support for the mechanism assumed. Experimental evidence for the occurrence of coil-to-helix conformational transitions, induced by addition of water to solutions of polypeptides in strong acids, have also been reported previously (137-141).

The disruptive effect of water on the ion binding ability of polymers-which has been described above for the case of protons in formic acid-has also been observed with regard to Li^+ in methanolic solutions, particularly at high salt concentrations. This was expressed by changes in the CD as well as in the hydrodynamic properties of the polymers. Representative results are shown in Figure 22, where the viscosity characteristics of PHEG in methanol-water mixtures-in the presence of 5.7 M LiCl-are expressed in terms of the Huggins constant, k'. A minimum in the k' values is observed at a water content of about 10%, i.e. at a concentration that is equimolar to that of LiCl. At higher water content, the pseudopolyelectrolyte effect is progressively abolished. Related effects of water have also been observed in studies dealing with the contractility of collagen fibers in acetone solutions in the presence of LiBr (142,143), for poly(-)1,2-diaminopropane sebacamide in the $CaCl_2$-methanol system (144), for poly(ethylene oxide) in KI-methanol (118), and for Co^{2+} complexes of poly(hexamethylphosphamide) in nitromethane (124).

56

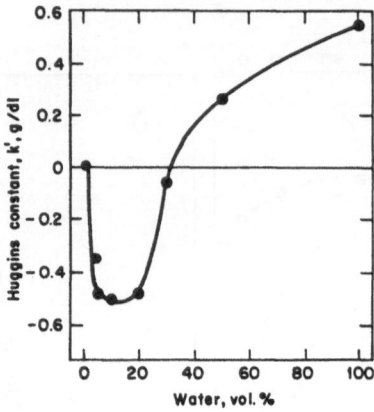

Figure 22. Hydrodynamic Properties of PHEG in 5.7 M LiCl in Methanol-Water Mixtures. The Values of k' were Calculated Using Experimental Data on Solutions Containing 4-10 mg PHEG/ml.

CONCLUDING REMARKS

Cation binding by ionophores and by polymeric ionophore models is associated with alterations in the conformation and conformational mobility of the ligand. A large body of experimental evidence has accumulated to indicate that monovalent ions - Li^+ in particular - interact with amide containing compounds yielding stable complexes (see Refs. 59, 145-147, and references quotes therein). Theoretical analyses - using semi-empirical potential functions (148,149) as well as the molecular orbital formalisms (see Ref. 148 and references quoted therein) - have been carried out for these complexes; and, although the numerical values calculated for the corresponding stabilization energy (tens of kcal per mole) are certainly not definite, they nevertheless indicate that very strong interactions are involved.

It has been pointed out (150) that binding of ions to polymers is a process not necessarily associated with polyelectrolytes; our results amply confirm this view, and the pseudopolyelectrolytes described are most suitable for studying this process in non-aqueous systems.

ACKNOWLEDGEMENTS

This research was supported by a grant from the United States-Israel Binational Science Foundation (BSF), Jerusalem, Israel.

The author also acknowledges Dr. R.L. Hamill of the Eli Lilly Co. for a gift of the A23187 ionophore, Dr. M. Fridkin of the Weizmann Institute for the gift of a poly-(4-hydroxystyrene) sample, and Mrs. R. August and B. Romano for their technical assistance.

REFERENCES

1. Sigel, H., Ed., Metal Ions in Biological Systems, Dekker, New York, 1974.
2. Eichorn, G.L., Ed., Inorganic Biochemistry, Elsevier, New York, 1973.
3. Hughes, M.N., The Inorganic Chemistry of Biological Processes, Wiley, New York, 1975.
4. Kruhoffer, P., Thaysen, J.H., and Thorn, N.A., in: Handbuch der Experimentellen Pharmakologie, pp. 196, Springer-Verlag, Berlin, 1960.
5. Pressman, B.C., Harris, E.J., Jagger, W.S., and Johnson, J.H., Proc. Natl. Acad. Sci. U.S., 58:1949, 1967.
6. Lauf, P.K., Biochim. Biophys. Acta, 415:173, 1975.
7. Ovchinnikov, Y.A., Ivanov, V.T., and Shkrob, A.M., Biochim. Biophys. Acta Library, 12:11, 1974.
8. Ulbricht, W., Biophys. Struct. Mechanism, 1:1, 1974.
9. Lardy, H.A., and Ferguson, S.M.F., Ann. Rev. Biochem., 38:991, 1969.
10. Henderson, P.J.F., Ann. Rev. Microbiol., 25:393, 1971.
11. Grell, E., Funck, Th., and Eggers, F., in: Molecular mechanisms of Antibiotic Action on Protein Biosynthesis and Membranes, E. Munoz, et al., eds., pp. 646, Elsevier, Amsterdam, 1972.
12. Dulbecco, R., and Elkington, J., Proc. Natl. Acad. Sci. U.S., 72:1584, 1975.
13. Ackman, R.G., Brown, W.H., and Wright, G.F., J.Org. Chem., 20:1147, 1955.
14. Luttringhaus, A., and Sichert-Modrow, I., Makromol. Chem., 18-19:511, 1956.
15. Stewart, D.G., Waddan, D.Y., and Borrows, E.T., Brit. Pat., 785 229, 1957.
16. Down, J.L., Lewis, J., Moore, B., and Wilkinson, G.W., Proc. Chem. Soc., 209, 1957.
17. Pedersen, C.J., J. Am. Chem. Soc., 89:2495, 1967.
18. Pedersen, C.J., and Frensdorff, H.K., Angew. Chem., 11:16, 1972.
19. Christensen, J.J., Eatough, D.J., and Izatt, R.M., Chem. Rev., 74:351, 1974.
20. Cram, D.J., and Cram, J.M., Science, 183:803, 1974.
21. Lehn, J.M., Simon, J., and Wagner, J., Angew. Chem., 12:579, 1973.
22. Simmons, H.E., and Park, C.H., J. Am. Chem. Soc., 90:2428, 1968.
23. Dietrich, B., Lehn, J.M., and Sauvage, J.P., Tetrahedron Lett., 2885, 1969.
24. Vogtle, F. and Weber, E., Angew Chem., Int. Ed., 13:814, 1974.
25. Schwyzer, R., Tum-Kyi, A., Caviezel, M., and Moser, P., Helv. Chim. Acta, 53:15, 1970.
26. Wudl, F., J. Chem. Soc., Chem. Commun., 1229, 1972.
27. Deber, C.M., Torchia, D.A., Wong, S.C.K., and Blout, E.R., Proc. Natl. Acad. Sci. U.S., 69:1825, 1972.
28. Blout, E.R., Deber, C.M., and Pease, L.G., in: Peptides, Polypeptides and Proteins., E.R. Blout, F.A. Bovey, M.Goodman, and N.Lotan, eds., pp.266, Wiley, New York, 1974.
29. Davis, D.G., Gisin, B.F., and Tosteson, D.C., Biochemistry, 15:768, 1976.
30. Hamill, R.L., Gorman, M., Gale, R.M., Higgens, C.E., and Hoehn, M.M., Intersci. Conf. Antimicrobial Agents and Chemotherapy (12th), Abstr., 65, 1972.
31. Reed, P.W., Fed. Proc., 31:1208, 1972.
32. Wong, D.T., Wilkinson, J.R., Hamill, R.L., and Horng, J.S., Arch. Biochem. Biophys., 156:578, 1973.
33. Steinrauf, L.K., Pinkerton, M., and Chamberlin, J.W., Biochem. Biophys. Res. Commun., 33:29, 1968.

34. Agtarap, A., Chamberlin, J.W., Pinkerton, M., and Steinrauf, L.K., J. Amer. Chem. Soc., 89:5737, 1967.
35. Johnson, S.M., Herrin, J., Lin, S.J., and Paul, I.S., Chem. Commun., 72, 1970.
36. Kinashi, H., Otake, N., and Yonehara, H., Tetrahedron. Lett., 49:4955, 1973.
37. Ashton, R. and Steinrauf, L.K., J. Mol. Biol., 49:547, 1970.
38. Reed, P.W. and Lardy, H.A., J. Biol. Chem., 247:6970, 1972.
39. Pressman, B.C., Fed. Proc., 32:1698, 1973.
40. Chaney, M.O., Demarco, P.V., Jones, N.D., and Occolowitz, J.L., J. Amer. Chem. Soc., 96:1932, 1974.
41. Caswell, A.H. and Pressman, B.C., Biochem. Biophys. Res. Commun., 49:292, 1972.
42. Case, G.D., Vanderkooi, J.M., and Scarpa, A., Arch. Biochem. Biophys., 162:174, 1974.
43. Preiffer, D.R., Reed, P.W., and Lardy, H.A., Biochemistry, 13:4007, 1974.
44. Puskin, J.S. and Gunter, T.E., Biochemistry, 14:187, 1975.
45. Deber, C.M. and Pfeiffer, D.R., Biochemistry, 15:132, 1976.
46. Birshtein, T.M. and Ptitsyn, O.B., Conformation of Macromolecules,Interscience, New York, 1966.
47. Fasman, G.D., in Poly-∝-Amino Acids, G.D. Fasman., ed., pp. 499, Dekker, New York, 1967.
48. Flory, P.J., Statistical Mechanism of Chain Molecules, Interscience, New York, 1969.
49. Goodman, M., Verdini, A.S., Choi, N.S., and Masuda, Y., Top. Stereochem., 5:69, 1970.
50. Poland, D. and Scheraga, H.A., in: Theory of Helix-Coil Transition in Biopolymers, Academic Press, New York, 1970.
51. Engel, J. and Schwarz, G., Angew. Chem., Int. Ed., 9:389, 1970.
52. Scheraga, H.A., Chem. Rev., 71:195, 1971.
53. Lotan, N., Berger, A., and Katchalski, E., Ann. Rev. Biochem. 41:869, 1972.
54. Lifson, S. and Lotan, N., Isr. J. Chem., 12:201, 1974.
55. Blout, E.R., Bovey, F.A., Goodman, M., and Lotan, N., Eds., Peptides, Polypeptides and Proteins, Wiley, New York, 1974.
56. Schellman, J.A., Biopolymers, 14:999, 1975.
57. Pauling, L., Corey, R.B., and Branson, H.R., Proc. Nat. Acad. Sci. U.S., 37:205, 1951.
58. Lotan, N., Bull. Isr. Phys. Soc., 14, 1973.
59. Lotan, N., J.Phys. Chem., 77:242, 1973.
60. Bovey, F.A., Polymer Conformation and Configuration, Academic Press, New York, 1969.
61. Bayley, P.M., in: Progress in Biophysics and Moleculer Biology, A.J.V. Butler and D.Noble, eds., Vol. 27, pp.1, Pergamon Press, Oxford, 1973.
62. Yang, J.T., Adv. Protein Chem., 16:323, 1961.
63. Bradbury, J.H., in: Physical Principles and Techniques of Protein Chemistry, Part B, S.J. Leach, ed., pp.99, Academic Press, New York, 1970.
64. Lotan, N., Bixon, M., and Berger, A., Biopolymers, 5:69, 1967.
65. Moffitt, W. and Yang, J.T., Proc. Nat. Acad. Sci. U.S., 42:596, 1956.
66. Lotan, N., Yaron, A., Berger, A., and Sela, M., Biopolymers, 3:625, 1965.
67. Hammett, L.P., and Deyrup, A.J., J. Amer. Chem. Soc., 54:2712, 1932.
68. Schaefgen, J.R., and Trivisonno, C.F., J.Amer. Chem. Soc., 73:4580, 1951.

69. Mattiussi, A., Gechele, G.B., and Francesconi, R., J. Polymer. Sci., Part A-2, 7:411, 1969.
70. Selegny, E., Vert, M., and Hamoud, M.R., Tetrahedron. Lett., 4:235, 1969.
71. Hamoud, M.R., Ph. D. Thesis, University of Paris, 1971.
72. Vert, M., in: Polyelectrolytes, E. Selegny, ed., pp.347, Reidel Publ. Co., Dordrecht, Holland, 1974.
73. Bradbury, J.H. and Yuan., H.H.H., Biopolymers, 11:661, 1972.
74. Saunders, P.R., J. Polymer Sci., Part A, 2:3765, 1964.
75. Bystrov, G.S., Komanenko, G.I., Nikolayev, N.I., Grigoreva, G.A., and Ataman-chuk, L., Biofizika, 17:623, 1972.
76. Brinkman, A.J., Diss. Abstr., B, 33:6040, 1973.
77. Reinach, P.S., Candia, O.A., and Siegel, G.J., J. Membrane Biol., 25:75, 1975.
78. Shaw, D.M., Brit. Med. J., 2:262, 1966.
79. Fieve, R.D., Int. J. Psychiat., 375, 1969.
80. Plenge, P., Mellerup, E.T., and Rafaelson, O.J., J. Psychiat. Res., 8:29, 1970.
81. Giacobini, E., Acta Psychiatrica Scand., Suppl. 207, 1969.
82. Davis, J.M., Fann, W.E., Ann. Rev. Pharmacol., 11:285, 1971.
83. Aghajanian, G.K., Ann. Rev. Pharmacol., 12:157, 1972.
84. Osborne, N.N., Maier, M., and Neuhoff, V., Biochem. Soc. Trans., 1:118, 1973.
85. Samuel, D., and Gottesfeld, Z., Endeavour, 32:122, 1973.
86. Pandey, G.N., Dorus, E.B., Dekirmenjian, H., and Davis, J.M., Fed. Proc., 34: 778, 1975.
87. Sheard, M.H., Nature, 230:113, 1971.
88. Eichelman, B., Thoa, N.B., and Perez-Cruet, J., Pharmac. Behav., 1:121, 1973.
89. Judd, L.L., Symposium of the Intra-Science Research, Biochemistry of Mental Disorders, Santa Monica, Calif., USA, 1975.
90. Moore, W.V. and Wolff, J., J. Biol. Chem., 249:6255, 1974.
91. Bishop, Jr., C.C., and Gill, J.E., Biochem. Biophys. Acta, 227:97, 1971.
92. von Hippel, P.H., and Schleich, T., Accts. Chem. Res., 2:257, 1969.
93. von Hippel, P.H., and Hamabata, A., J. Mechanochem. Cell Motility, 2:127, 1973.
94. Fennel-Evans, D., Nadas, J.A., and Matesich, M.A., J. Phys. Chem., 75:1708, 1971.
95. Fuoss, R.M., and Strauss, U.P., J. Polymer Sci., 3:602, 1948.
96. Doty, P., Wada., Yang, J.T., and Blout, E.R., J. Polymer Sci., 23:851, 1957.
97. Applequist, J. and Doty, P., in: Polyamino Acids, Polypeptides and Proteins, M.A. Stahman, ed., pp.161, University of Wisconsin Press, Madison, Wisconsin, 1962.
98. Rice, S.A., and Nagasawa, M., Polyelectrolyte Solutions, Academic Press, New York, 1961.
99. Shiraki, M., and Imahori, K., Sci. Pap., Coll. Gen. Educ., Univ. Tokyo, 16:215, 1966.
100. Chen, A.K., and Woody, R.W., J. Amer. Chem. Soc., 93:29, 1971.
101. Joubert, F.J., Lotan, N., and Scherage, H.A., Biochemistry, 9:2197, 1970.
102. Jardetzky, O., and Wade-Jardetzky, N.G., Ann. Rev. Biochem., 40:605, 1971.
103. Bradbury, E.M., Cary, P.D., Crane-Robinson, C., and Hartman, P.G., Pure Appl. Chem., 36:53, 1973.
104. Bovey, F.A., Macromolecular Reviews, 9:1, 1974.
105. Bradbury, E.M., Crane-Robinson, C., Giancotti, V., and Stephens, R.M., Polymer, 13:33, 1972.

106. Beychok, S., in: Poly-α-Amino Acids, G.D. Fasman, ed., pp.293, Dekker, New York, 1967.
107. Lotan, N., in: Peptides, Polypeptides and Proteins, E.R. Blout, F.A. Bovey, M. Goodman, and N. Lotan, eds., pp.157, Wiley, New York, 1974.
108. Lotan, N., Yaron, A., and Berger, A., Biopolymers, 4:365, 1966.
109. Adler, A.J., Howing, R., Potter, J., Wells, M., and Fasman, G.D., J. Amer. Chem. Soc., 90:4736, 1968.
110. Mattice, W.L., Lo, J.-T., and Mandelkern, L., Macromolecules, 5:729, 1972.
111. Mattice, W.L., and Lo, J.-T., Macromolecules, 5:734, 1972.
112. Lotan, N., Chen, K., and Roche, R.S., Isr. J. Chem., 12:207, 1974.
113. Lotan, N., unpublished results.
114. Burow, S.P., Peterlin, A., and Turner, D.T., Polymer, 6:35, 1965.
115. Bianchi, U. and Peterlin, A., J. Polymer Sci., A-2, 6:1011, 1968.
116. Liu, K.-J., Macromolecules, 1:308, 1968.
117. Liu, K.-J., and Anderson, J.E., Macromolecules, 2:235, 1969.
118. Liu, K.-J., in: Polyelectrolytes, E. Selegny, M. Mandel and U.P. Strauss, eds., pp.391, Reidel, Dordrecht, 1974.
119. Kopolow, S., Hogen-Esch, T.E., and Smid, J., Macromolecules, 6:133, 1973.
120. Yamazaki, N., Hirao, A., and Nakahama, S., Polymer J., 7:402, 1975.
121. Ford, R.A. and Marshall, H.S.B., J. Polymer Sci., 22:350, 1956.
122. Nakajima, A. and Tanaami, K., Polymer J., 5:248, 1973.
123. Bello, A., Bracke, W., Grodzinski, J.J., Sackmana, G., and Szwarc, M., Macromolecules, 3:98, 1970.
124. Ozari, Y., Ph. D. Thesis, Weizmann Institute of Science, Rehovot, Israel, 1975.
125. Erlander, S.R., J. Colloid Interface Sci., 34:53, 1970.
126. Murai, N., Makino, S., and Sugai, S., J. Colloid Interface Sci., 41:399, 1972.
127. Breuer, M.M. and Robb, I.D., Chem. Ind., 530, 1972.
128. Shchori, E. and Jagur-Grodzinski, J.,J. Appl. Polymer Sci. (in press)
129. Schulz, R.C. and Trisnadi, J.A., Macromolekulare Chemie. (in press)
130. Haas, E., Wilchek, M., Katchalski-Katzir, E., and Steinberg, I.Z., Proc. Nat. Acad. Sci., U.S., 72:1807, 1975.
131. Haas, E., Ph. D. Thesis, Weizman Institute of Science, Rehovot, Israel, 1976.
132. Grinvald, A., Haas, E., and Steinberg, I.Z., Proc. Nat. Acad. Sci. U.S., 69:2273, 1972.
133. Campbell, A.N. and Campbell, A.J.R., Trans. Faraday Soc., 30:1109, 1934.
134. Melnikov, N.P. and Tsirlin, A. Yu., Zh. Fiz. Khim., 30:2290, 1956.
135. Rivenq, F., Bull. Soc. Chim. France, 1505, 1960.
136. Bixon, M. and Lifson, S., Biopolymers, 4:815, 1966.
137. Steigman, J., Peggion, E., and Cosani, A., J. Amer. Chem. Soc., 91:1822, 1969.
138. Steigman, J., Verdini, A.S., Montagner, C., and Strasorier, L., J. Amer. Chem. Soc., 91:1829, 1969.
139. Peggion, E., Strasorier, L., and Cosani, A., Chem. Commun., 97, 1969.
140. Zezin, A.B., Bakeiov, N.F., Gourevitch, V.M., and Kozlov, P.V., Vysokomol. Soed., A, 13:99, 1971.
141. Puett, D. and Ciferri, A., Biopolymers, 10:547, 1971.
142. Sherebrin, M.H. and Oplatka, A., Biopolymers, 6:1169, 1968.
143. Katchalsky, A. and Oplatka, A., in: Principles of Receptor Physiology, W.R. Loewenstein, ed., pp.1, Springer-Verlag, Berlin, 1971.
144. Le Bris, J., Vert, M., and Selegny, E., J. Polymer Sci., Part C. (in press)

145. Adams, M.J., Baddiel, C.B., Jones, R.G., and Matheson, A.J., J. Chem. Soc., Faraday Trans. II, 70:1114, 1974.
146. Rao, C.N.R., Gurudath-Rao, K., and Balasubramanian, D., FEBS Lett., 46:192, 1974.
147. Balasubramanian, D. and Misra, B.C., Biopolymers, 14:1019, 1975.
148. Saluja, P.P.S., and Scheraga, H.A., J. Phys. Chem., 77:2736, 1973.
149. Talekar, S.V., Biochem. Biophys. Acta, 375:157, 1975.
150. Gregor, H.P., in: Polyelectrolytes, E. Selegny, M. Mandel and U.P. Strauss, eds., pp.87, Reidel, Dordrecht, 1974.

62

BIODEGRADABLE POLYMERS FOR MEDICAL PURPOSES

J. Feijen

Twente University of Technology, Department of Chemical Technology, Enschede, The Netherlands

INTRODUCTION

In this course the development and application of biodegradable polymers for medical purposes will be discussed. It has been argued by Williams (1) that the degradation effects normally found with materials in the physiological environment cannot be considered as 'true' biodegradation unless they involve some specific vital activity of that environment. Thus by this definition any degradation mechanism in polymers that is completely reproducible in an equivalent nonvital medium is not biodegradation. The ability of enzymes and bacteria to influence the degradation of implanted polymers was used as an example of 'true' biodegradation.

Other authors have used a broader definition of biodegradation, which includes all the processes leading to the degradation of implanted polymers. These include both enzymatically catalyzed processes, acid or base catalyzed hydrolysis, oxidation and other processes.

There is no reason to use the limited definition because even the simple acid or base catalyzed hydrolysis could be influenced by adsorption of biological compounds in the living organism and in principle enzymatically catalyzed processes can be simulated in vitro.

As mentioned by Gilding (2) biodegradable polymers have three major applications in medicine : (a) The temporary scaffold; (b) the temporary barrier; and (c) the drug delivery matrix.

The temporary scaffold is meant to restore the natural situation after surgical removal of parts of the living body like a blood vessel, ureter, bladder, heart valve or tympanic membrane or as an artificial support after surgical trauma. The latter application includes suture materials and bone plates. In principle also composites of biodegradable and non biodegradable materials can be considered for these purposes.

A temporary barrier is of major importance for the prevention of adhesions and later fibrosis between sliding surfaces of the tendon or between the surface of the cardiac wall and the pericardiac sac.

Biodegradable matrices for the delivery of drugs have received increasing attention during the last decade. We can distinguish between matrices where the drug is physically incorporated and those and where the drug is covalently bound. In the first case the release of the drug may be governed by diffusion and after complete release of the drug the matrix will degrade. Alternatively the release may also be controlled by the gradual degradation of the matrix (bioerodible systems). In the case of covalently coupled systems we can further distinguish between water soluble polymers meant to be taken up by specific cells, to degrade and to release the bioactive agent in the cell, and non-soluble polymers which after implantation first have to release the drug by a chemical process and then either dissolve or further degrade into soluble decomposition products. Recent reviews have been given by Kim et al. (3) and Langer et al. (4).

The requirements for biodegradable materials are directly related to their applications.

The elastic modulus of the materials has to meet the requirements for the particular application and the materials should be strong enough to stand the maximal stress and strain.

Changing mechanical properties as a consequence of biodegradation should be in phase with the healing processes in the body. Degradation products should be nontoxic and should not cause any adverse tissue reaction. The implant itself during degradation also should not cause adverse tissue reactions nor cause carcinogenesis.

In the following we will first concentrate on the use of natural occurring polymers for biomedical purposes. Then the development and application of synthetic biodegradable polymers will be discussed. Finally we will emphasize some examples of chemically-controlled release systems for bioactive agents.

NATURAL POLYMERS

Natural polymers have been used for biomedical purposes since ancient times. The main application was for sutures. Materials include gut, linen and silk. The degradation of silk being a proteinaceous material is very slow, whereas catgut is known to degrade within weeks.

Major problems encountered with natural polymers are the removal of compounds with antigenic or other adverse properties and the variation of mechanical and biodegradation properties of the materials with the site of origin, species, age and sex of the animal.

For this reason a lot of effort has been put into the development of methods to obtain purified collagen which has predictable biodegradation properties after implantation. Also various methods have been applied to substantially reduce the rate of biodegradation.

The application of collagen as a biomaterial has been reviewed by several authors (5,6). In order to understand the behaviour of collagen after implantation some information about the biochemical and biophysical properties is required. The chemistry and molecular biology of collagen have been extensively reviewed (see f.i. ref. 7,8).

In tissue, collagen fibers (2μ) form fiber bundles $(10-50\mu)$. The fibers are composed of bundles of fibrils $(0.1-0.2\mu)$ which are in turn built up from filaments $(0.01-0.02\mu)$. These filaments are the basic subunits of collagen called tropocollagen, which are rigid rods with a molecular weight of 300,000 a length of 2800 Å and a width of 15 Å.

The rod-like molecules are aligned in such a way that each molecule overlaps its neighbor for approximately one-fourth of its length.

Electron microscopy reveals a characteristic band pattern with a repeat of 690 Å (one-fourth the length of the entire molecule). 'Holes' or areas of decreased molecular density are formed because the repeat is not entirely one-fourth. The holes are sites for prosthetic groups like glycoproteins and are important for bone repair and calcification. Tropocollagen in turn is composed of three polypeptide chains with molecular weights of about 100 000 which are called α - chains. These chains constitute the triple, righ handed super helix of tropocollagen (tertiary structure) whereas the peptide chains are left-handed helices (secondary structure). The tertiary structure is stabilized by hydrogen bonding between adjacent chains.

Individual polypeptide chains might have differing amino acid sequences (α_1 and α_2). A combination of two α_1 chains and one α_2 chain is common. The characteristic structure of both chains is a repeating unit of three amino acids, Gly-X-Y, where X and Y can be a variety of amino acids. The X position is frequently occupied by proline and the Y position by hydroxyproline. The latter two amino acids account for about 22 % of the total number of amino acids, whereas glycine comprises about one third (9). Polar and apolar regions are formed when appropriate amino acids are substituted in X and Y. The amino acid sequences of a variety of animal collagens have been studied by using cyanogen bromide (CNB) cleavage of peptide chains followed by separation of the peptides on ion-exchange columns. CNB cleaves at methionine sites in the chains.

Only 2-3 % of native collagen can be solubilized in dilute acid solution. Most of the insoluble collagen (95%) can be solubilized with proteolytic enzymes without destroying the triple-helical structure (10,11). Proteolytic enzymes other than collagenase such as pepsin, trypsin, pronase and proctase digest peptides present in the non helical regions of collagen (telopeptides).

After denaturation so called α collagen (one peptide chain) is obtained, whereas after denaturation of dilute acid solubilized collagen, α collagen as well as β and γ collagens are released which have two and three chains respectively still covalently connected. A schematic representation of the collagen structure at different levels of organization is given in Figure 1. (taken from Stenzel et al. (5)).

Enzyme solubilized collagen can be purified by repeated precipitation, washing and resolubilization. The precipitation can be achieved by raising the pH or ionic strength. Aggregation of atelocollagen (collagen which is poor in telopeptides) still takes place under appropriate conditions and in this way collagen may be reconstituted. The procedure also removes contaminating connective tissue proteins.

Hydrogen bond disruption can be caused by heating tropocollagen in dilute acid at 38-40°C or by using reagents such as KSCN. The polypeptide chains assume a random coil configuration and the material obtained is gelatinous.

Collagenases are capable to cleave the peptide bonds of collagen within the triple-helix structure. The reaction takes place at physiological pH and temperature. Two types of collagenases have to be distinguished. Human collagenase severs the tropocollagen across the polypeptide strands into two segments (TCA and TCB), which still retain their helical conformation (12). Bacterial collagenase attacks the collagen molecule at both ends producing fragments of different lengths (13).

Several mechanisms have been proposed for the remodelling of mature connective tissue. Milson et al. (14) proposed a depolymerase first cleaving small fragments of the collagen, which could then be phagocytosed and degraded intracellularly. Steven et al. (15) and Etherington (16) detected that first the telopeptides were cleaved.

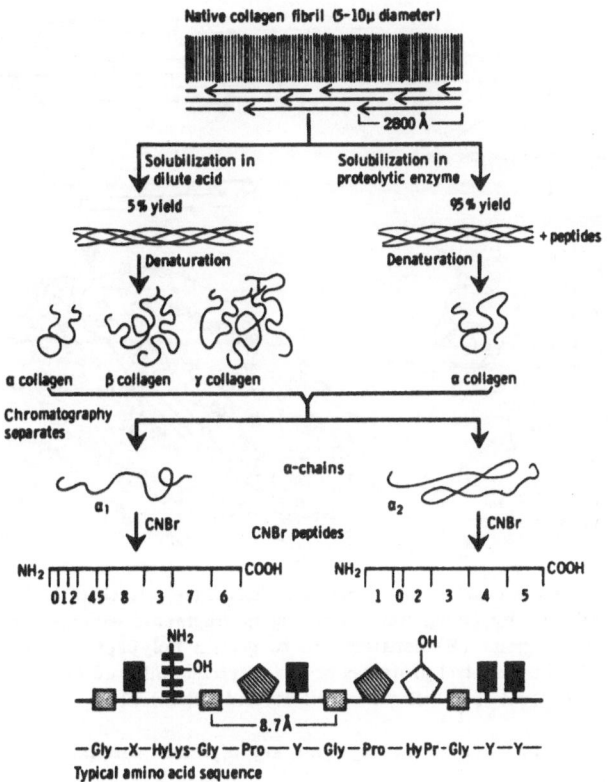

Figure 1.   Collagen at different levels of organization (from K.H. Stenzel et al) (5).

Harris and Krane (17) summarized the pathways as follows (Figs. 2 and 3 from Harris and Krane modified) : (a) Release of collagenase in the extracellular space, (b) cleavage in TCA and TCB fragments, (c) denaturation at the temperature > 32°C, and (d) digestion by proteases in the extracellular space or by intracellular degradation by lysosomal enzymes after phagocytosis. Rapid degradation might occur by uptake of small fragments of intact fibrils by phagocytes followed by digestion by phagolysosomes.

Osteoclasts, fibroblasts, foreign body giant cells, macrophages and endothelial cells are involved in the phagocytosis of collagen. The enzymes involved are cathepsins and especially cathepsin B1 which is active at a pH of 3.4-3.5. When this enzyme is released into the extracellular space it will loose its activity. The initial degradation product consists of α-chains whose telopeptides are missing. The α-chains are then rapidly degraded to peptides of low molecular weight (18).

Salthouse et al. (19,20) showed that gut and collagen sutures degrade by sequential attack of lysosomal enzymes depending on the implantation site. After implantation in muscle, acid phosphatase is acting during the period where the major loss of strength is occurring and leucine amino peptidase activity is observed during the absorption phase. In the eye, alkaline phosphatase was causing the initial hydrolysis.

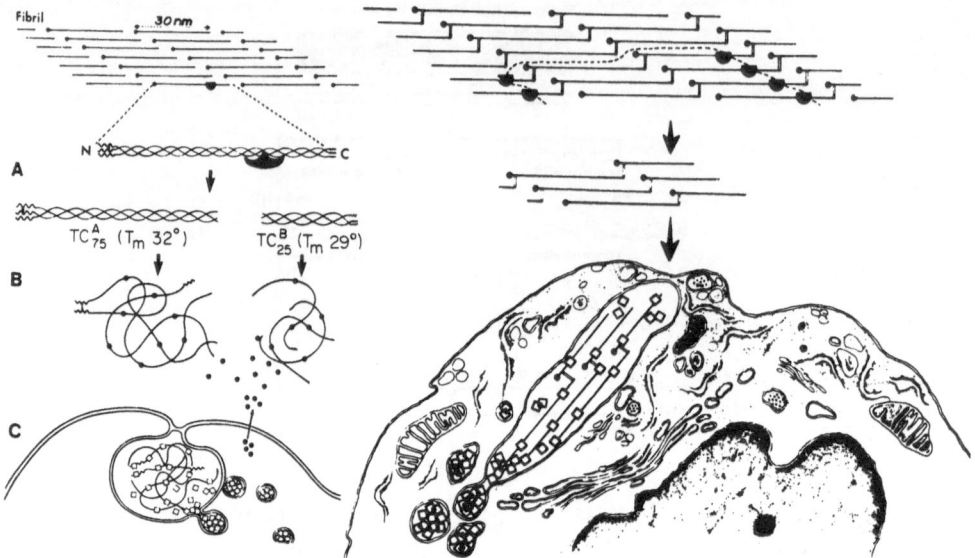

Figure 2. Pathway for the breakdown of collagen fibrils. (A) attack of helical portion of the collagen molecule by collagenase, resulting in fragments which are released by attack of telopeptide regions. (B) denaturation to gelatin polypeptides, (C) digestion of gelatin polypeptides by neutral proteases or phagocytosis followed by intracellular digestion by lysosomal enzymes (modified from Harris and Krane) (17).

Figure 3. Phagocytosis of inact fibril compounds and digestion with phagolysosomes (from Harris and Krane) (17).

Medical Applications

Collagen type materials have been used for a variety of medical applications. Basically two types of approaches can be distinguished.

In the first approach biological structures are treated to remove non-collagenous material and the remaining structure is often strengthened by crosslinking. In the other approach collagen is solubilized, purified and the material is reformed and crosslinked in the desired shape.

Drawbacks of the first approach are that we have to deal with predetermined configurations, but an advantage is that the three dimensional structure of collagen is retained. The second approach is often limited by the final strength which can be obtained.

Application in the first group include collagen heterografts like vascular prostheses (21) and heart valve prostheses (22). In these applications it is essential that the original structure is retained for longer times. The heterografts are often first treated with a protease, like ficin and then crosslinked under different conditions using formaldehyde, glutaraldehyde, dialdehyde starch or chromic oxide.

Collagen sutures comprise surgical gut (catgut) which is derived from submucosal fibrous tissue of sheep intestine or the serosal connective tissue layer of bovine intestine and sutures derived from reconstituted collagen. In both cases the tanning process using formaldehyde, alum or chromium salts is very important to obtain the desired strength and degradation times. The biocompatibility of sutures has been described by Salthouse (23).

Reconstituted collagen has been applied for hemodialysis, skin substitutes, burn dressings, heart valves, blood vessels, replacement of dura, repair of nerves, vitreous replacements, drug delivery systems, bone healing and aids for hemostasis (review 5).

Degradation is reduced by the use of specific metal ions and aldehydes as cross-linking agents or polyelectrolyte complexes with sulfated polysaccharides. Other natural materials for medical purposes, which can be absorbed in the body include crosslinked gelatins (2,24), fibrin (25) and chitin (26).

SYNTHETIC MATERIALS

Contrary to the use of natural materials, synthetic biodegradable materials can be optimized in terms of mechanical properties and rate of degradation.

We will concentrate on the development of biodegradable polyesters. An important example in the literature was the introduction of poly(glycolic acid) (PGA) by Schmitt and Polistina (27) which was applied as the suture material Dexon[R]. PGA is synthesized by the ring opening polymerization of glycolide at 220°C using a tin catalyst.

PGA is a crystalline (up to 50%) tough, inelastic material with a T_m of 230°C and T_g 36°C. The tensile strength of the oriented suture is typically 4.5-5 g/denier (28). The in-vitro and in-vivo degradation behaviour were studied by Reed and Gilding (2,29). The in-vitro tensile data at pH 7 and 37°C for different types of Dexon[R] sutures are given in Figure 4 (29). No effect of suture gauge (i.e. 0 vs 3-0) or filament denier (2-6 denier) was observed. About 80 % of the suture strength is retained for two weeks but after four weeks most of the strength is lost. From stress/strain curves it turns out that elongation decreases simultaneously with tensile strength indicating that the material is becoming more brittle. The mass loss data of two sutures exposed at the same conditions are given in Figure 5 (29). There is no effect of filament denier size. Mass loss begins in the fourth week and is completed by ten to twelve weeks when no agitation is applied.

From these data it can be concluded that the degradation mechanism might be quite complex. The MWD plots for 0,1,2 and 3 weeks degradation periods show a steady decrease in the MW of the peak of the distribution, with the high MW tail of the distribution being reduced (Fig. 6). The low MW tail increases up to 3 weeks then begins to decrease, which implies that mass loss is taking place. From these data which are representative for the hydrolytic degradation of a partially crystalline material, it can be concluded that the degradation is taking place in the amorphous regions and the material remains highly crystalline over the initial 6 week period.

In the pH range 5-9 there is no change in degradation characteristics, which was explained by the authors in terms of combined effects of crystallinity and hydrophobicity. However, the temperature has a very pronounced effect on the loss of initial strength (Fig. 7) (29).

Above the glass transition temperature the percent of initial strength loss per week increases more rapidly with temperature than below the glass transition temperature, which indicates that above T_g, water diffusion and hydrolysis is more facile. The in-vivo degradation behaviour compares quite well with the in-vitro results. However, the influence of certain enzymes cannot be completely excluded.

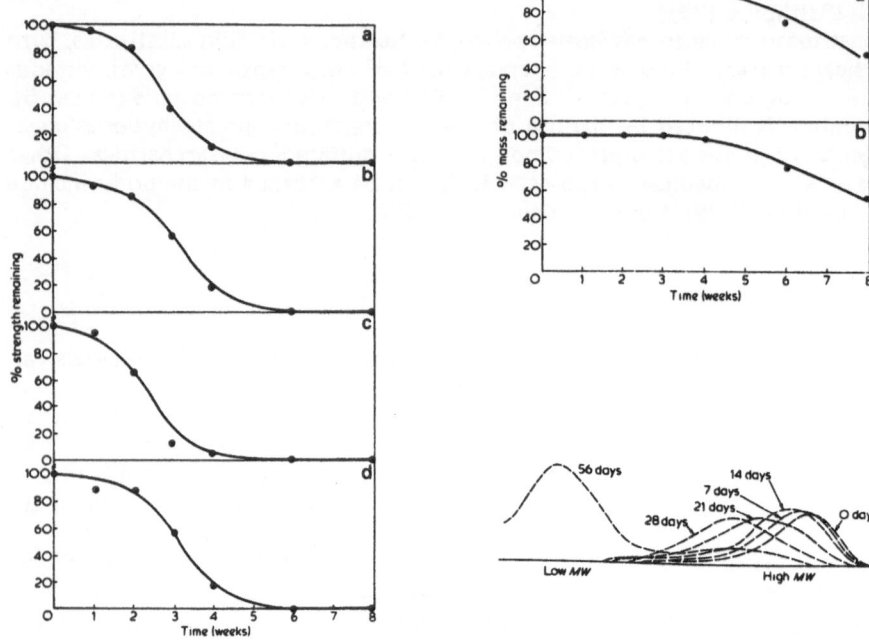

Figure 4.   Tensile strength data of Dexon[R], PGA sutures as a function of exposure time to a buffer solution (pH 7, 37°C). (a) 'O' Dexon; (b) 'O' Dexon[R] 's'; (c) '30' Dexon[R]; (d) Dexon[R] 's' (from A.M. Reed and D.K. Gilding) (29).

Figure 5.   Mass loss data of Dexon[R], PGA sutures as a function of exposure time to a buffer solution (pH 7, 37°C) (a) 'O' Dexon[R]; (b) 'O' Dexon[R] 's' (from A.M. Reed and D.K. Gilding) (29).

Figure 6.   Change in molecular weight distributions for Dexon[R] ('O'), PGA sutures as a function of time after exposure to buffer with a pH of 7 at 37°C (from A.M. Reed and D.K. Gilding) (29).

In the case of poly(lactic acid) first evaluated by Kulkarni et al. (36,37), we have to differentiate between poly(L-lactic acid) (PLA) which is a crystalline, tough inelastic material with a T_m of 180°C and a T_g of 67°C and poly(D,L-lactic acid), (PDLA), which is amorphous, tough inelastic and has a T_g of 57°C. The presence of the methyl groups makes the polymers more hydrophobic and also increases the T_g.

The in-vitro mass and molecular weight loss for PLA which has a crystallinity of 37 % show that over a 16 week period only 10-15 % of the mass of a 0.5 mm thick disc is lost and MW is reduced to ~50 % of its initial value (29). Furthermore, relatively small changes in mechanical properties over a 26 week period were observed. As expected the hydrolysis of the amorphous PDLA is more rapid than that of PLA (31-33).

An in-vitro degradation study of PDLA in acetone/water mixtures (10:1 v/v) at 60-70°C revealed that in time smaller molecular weight distributions were obtained (34) than expected on the basis of a random chain scission process (35).

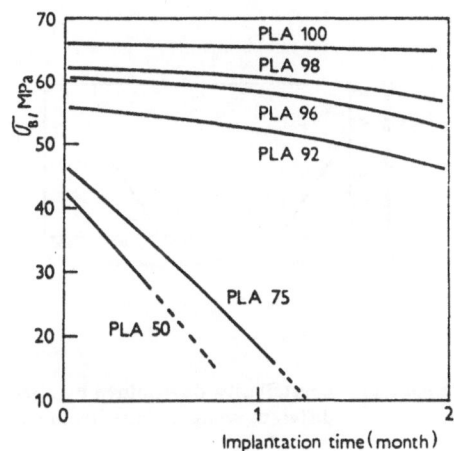

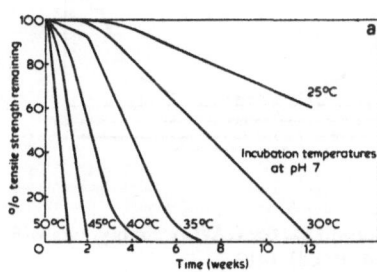

Figure 7. Tensile loss of Dexon[R] ('O'), PGA sutures in time after exposure to buffer (pH 7) at different temperatures from A.M. Reed and D.K. Gilding) (29).

Figure 8. Variation of tensile strength of PLA-PDLA copolymer implants, containing various amounts of PDLA, with the implantation time in tibias and femurs of sheep (from M. Vert et al) (38).

Vert et al. (38) have studied the biodegradation of PLA in rats and sheep and concluded that PLA prepared in the right way is very stable when used for bone surgery.

Factors influencing the biological stability are (a) the molecular weight, which must be as high as possible, (b) the presence of residual monomer and low MW compounds initially present or formed during the processing,(c) heating leads to degradation, (d) sterilization by β and γ-rays causes degradation, whereas ethylene oxide has no detrimental effects and,(e) annealing increases the crystallinity and therefore decreases the rate of biodegradation.

The incorporation of D,L lactic acid in PLA leads to a more rapid decrease in tensile strength after implantation of samples in tibias and femurs of sheep as shown in Figure 8 (38).

Christel et al. (39) used PGA reinforced PLA as resorbable materials for osteosynthetic purposes. Although promising results were obtained with bone plates, cracks were initiated at some screw holes were stress concentrations occurred.

Copolymers of GA and LA have also been prepared, but it was observed by Gilding and Reed (40) that the reactivity ratios r_g and r_l were quite different (r_g = 2.8 and r_l = 0.2 at 200°C), which implies that copolymers of glycolic and lactic acids will have broad composition ranges with glycolide always being preferentially polymerized at low conversions and lactide being incorporated to ever-increasing extents as the glycolide is depleted. In this respect it is also very important to notice that the crystallinity of the copolymers will be influenced by the incorporation of different amount of monomers (Fig. 9) (40).

The half-life in months of various copolymers of lactic- and glycolic acids implanted in rats was studied by Miller et al. (41). The results are given in Figure 10 (41). It can be seen that these data correlate with the data in Figure 9.

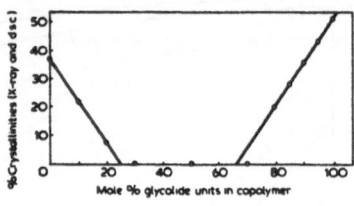
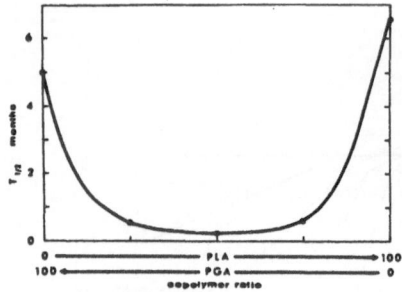

Figure 9. Crystallinity determined by X-ray and d.s.c. measurements for GA/LA copolymers with different compositions (from D.K. Gilding and A.M. Reed) (40).

Figure 10. Half-life of PGA/PLA copolymers after implantation in rat tissue (from R.A. Miller et al) (41).

A suture material composed of 90 % GA and 10 % LA monomer, Vicryl[R] was introduced by Wasserman and Levy (42). It was claimed that Vicryl[R] retains its tensile strength longer and is more rapidly degraded than Dexon[R]. The applications of the copolymers of GA and LA in medicine and biological technology were surveyed by Wise et al. (ref. 59).

Several other biodegradable polyesters with potential use for biomedical applications have been developed or are currently under investigation. These include poly-(hydroxy butyrate) (43); a ring opening copolymer of oxalic acid and propylene glycol, currently studied by Ethicon; biodegradable elastomers of poly(ethylene oxide) and poly(ethyleneterephtalate) (44,46); poly(orthoesters) (47,48) which are also used as bioerodible systems for the release of drugs; poly(dihydropyrans); poly(ε-caprolactone) (50), which could be enzymatically degraded at the surface when the segmented mobility of the polymer chains is sufficiently high to permit the required chain conformation for enzymatic attack and poly(dioxanon) (51) which has been evaluated as a suture material.

CHEMICALLY CONTROLLED RELEASE SYSTEMS FOR BIOACTIVE AGENTS

During the last decade several drug-release systems have been developed (reviews, ref. 3,4,52 and 53). These systems are either diffusion-controlled, chemically controlled, solvent activated or magnetically-controlled. In this section we will concentrate on one example of a chemically controlled drug delivery system, which may be representative for some of the problems encountered (57).

One of the area's which are very interesting for the development of water soluble high molecular weight prodrugs is the treatment of cancers. The drugs used for chemotherapy are usually very toxic and exert side effects. A typical example is the cytostatic agent adriamycin which has a specific toxicity on the heart (54). This side-effect may eventually lead to a lifethreatening congestive heart failure when a cumulative dose of 550 mg m^{-2} has been exceeded. A chronically low dose administration of the drug has been shown to increase the maximally tolerated dose and continuous infusion of adriamycin over 24 hours, repeated every 3 weeks in human results in equal therapeutic activity and decreased cardiotoxicity (55). An alternative method to prevent cardiotoxicity is the use of adriamycin-polymer conjugates, which are not taken up by heart muscle cells but are readily incorporated in tumor cells.

Macromolecular Conjugates of Adriamycin

Drugs can be combined with a polymeric system by different methods. We will further distinguish between systems which release the drug extracellularly or endocellularly.

Extracellular Release Systems

Drugs can either be mixed with a biodegradable matrix or covalently coupled to a polymeric system. In the former case the release rate of the drug might be determined by the diffusion of the drug through the matrix and/or by the rate of degradation of the matrix.

In the latter case the rate of release of the drug is frequently determined by the rate of cleavage of the bond between the drug and the polymeric system. In our application it has to be realized that plasma soluble delivery systems are required when necrosis caused by local release of adriamycin has to be avoided. Typical examples of extracellular release systems are the DNA-anthracycline complexes prepared by Trouet et al. (56) (Fig. 11).

Due to the reversibility of the DNA-anthracycline complex formation, the release of the drug from its carrier is, at least partly, governed by the rate of clearance of plasma from free anthracyclines. The release of covalently bound drugs from soluble carriers would be governed by solvolysis and enzymatic action (mainly esterases). Spacer groups between the carrier and the drug might increase the release from such systems.

Endocellular Release Systems

In this case the systems which we will call macromolecular prodrugs are not affected by solvolytic and enzymic processes in plasma and remain intact. Therefore the in-vivo distribution and transport of these conjugates are well defined and retained until they reach, by virtue of these properties, the target cell or tissue.

Tumor cells display a high uptake of macromolecules by endocytosis (Fig. 2), whereas normal tissue cells are poorly endocytotic. Carriers which have been utilized in this approach include; (a) proteins or synthetic macromolecules which have been shown to localize in tumor cells in-vivo, (b) lysosomotropic materials, which are substances showing a tendency to concentrate selectively in lysosomes, from which they can subsequently diffuse into other parts of the cells and (c) antibodies which specifically recognize antigenic determinants located preferentially on tumor cells.

The use of tumor specific antibodies is still problematic with respect to the specificity, the proper coupling techniques and low degree of substitution. Figure 12 shows the endocytosis and lysosomal digestion of adriamycin protein type conjugates. After internalization of the macromolecular substance by endocytosis, a phagosome is formed which fuses with a lysosome. The substance is exposed to about 40 digestive enzymes (58) which attack α-L-amino acid peptide bonds at a pH of 4-5. This

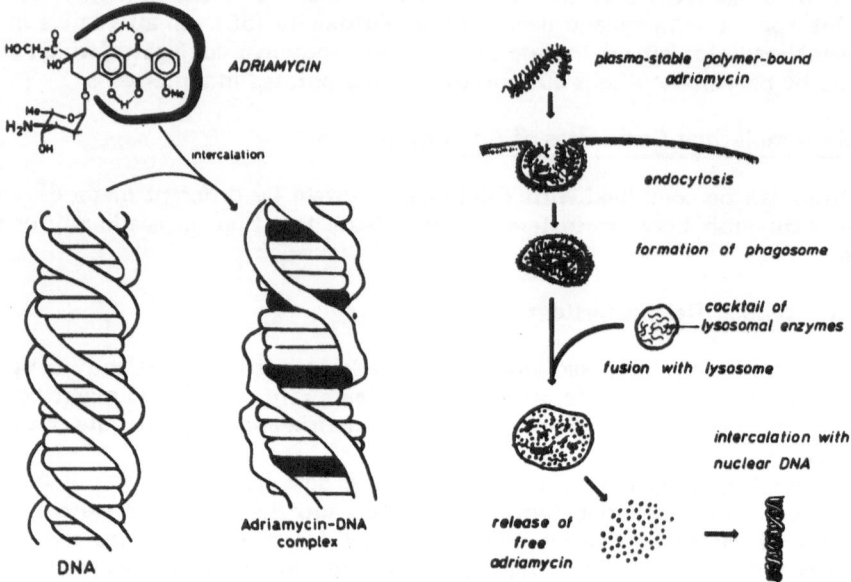

Figure 11. Intercalation of adriamycin with DNA. When the drug intercalates it results in a separation of the stacked bases and there is a local uncoiling of the helix. The complex has been used as a delivery system in cancer chemotherapy (56).

Figure 12. Endocytosis and lysosomal digestion of adriamycin-protein conjugates which may, depending on the type of carrier and covalent bonds used, ultimately result in the formation of free adriamycin.

results in a rapid degradation of the protein or poly(α-amino acid). It has to be realized that these processes in principle will also take place by cells of the reticuloendothelial system (RES). A direct comparison of uptake of macromolecular compounds by tumor cells or RES cells has not been made.

Two mechanisms in endocytosis can be distinguished; (a) fluid endocytosis, which is the slow uptake of fluid containing the macromolecule and (b) adsorptive endocytosis, which only occurs when a specific interaction takes place of the macromolecules with the cell membrane.

The real aim in prodrug design is to improve selectivity by delivering a greater amount of the drug to the tumor either by a more selective transport mechanism and or improved bioavailability of the drug in target tissue by virtue of a high enzyme level (i.e. γ-glutamyl transferase, γ-GT and plasmin). In this case the carrier systems have to be designed in such a way, that the higher levels of these enzymes occurring in some tumor cells would increase the rate of formation of the free drug.

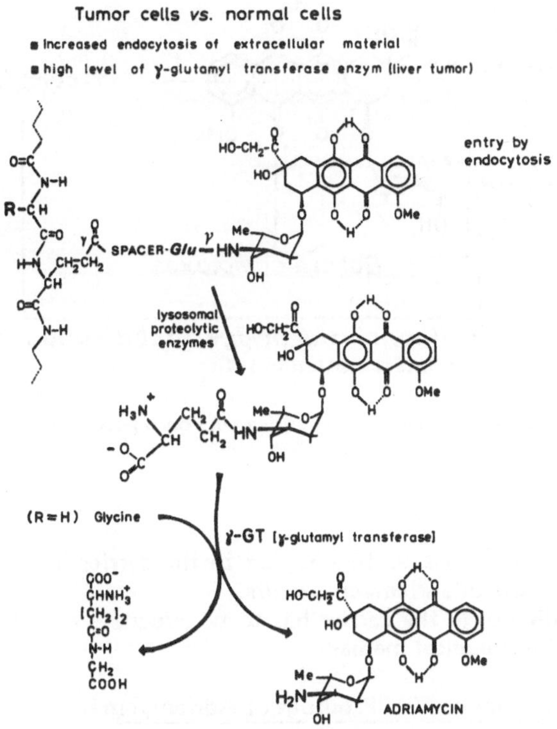

Figure 13. Tumor cells versus normal cells. In the design of the macromolecular prodrug we aim at two gradual differences found between normal cells and some tumor cells in the hope that these differences greatly add in selectivity.
Glutamic acid probably may also serve as a substrate for the γ-GT reaction.

A possible approach is depicted in Figure 13. After initial attack of the macromolecular prodrug by lysosomal enzymes, the γ-glutamyl derivative of adriamycin might be released followed by a rapid cleavage by γGT to free adriamycin. Summarizing the following conclusions can be drawn.

1. Biodegradable macromolecular carriers can in principle be used for a retarded non specific extracellular release of cytostatic agents.
2. A more promising approach would be the application of macromolecular carriers for a more selective endocellular delivery of non specific cytotoxic anticancer agents to tumors.
3. To improve the bioavailability of the drug in the target tissue conjugates have to be developed which are readily incorporated by tumor cells and which are poorly endocytosed by cells of the reticulo-endothelial system. Furthermore nontoxic low molecular weight prodrugs formed after lysosomal degradation of the conjugates should be rapidly cleaved by specific enzymes which are present in a higher concentration in the tumor cells as compared to other cells (for instance γGT and plasmin).

74

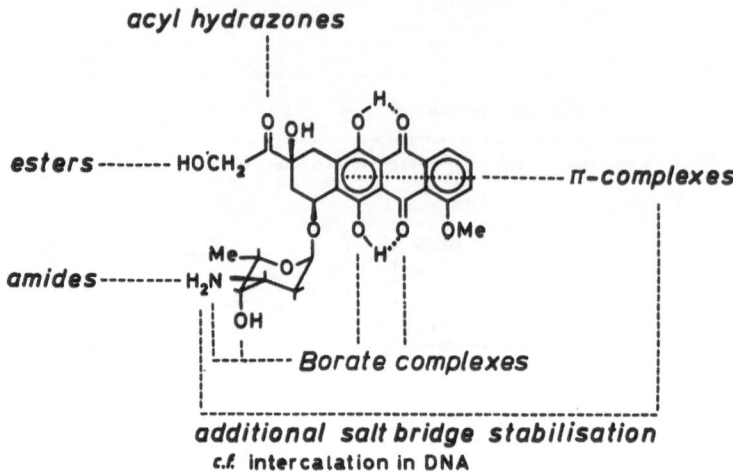

acyl hydrazones

esters -------- HOCH₂

amides -------- H₂N

π-complexes

Borate complexes

additional salt bridge stabilisation
c.f. intercalation in DNA

Figure 14.   Possible sites for the attachment of adriamycin onto polymeric carriers.

4. The cytostatic agent has to be coupled to the carrier in such a way that only endocellular release of adriamycin occurs.
5. The drug loading onto the carrier has to be adequate and the conjugate has to be soluble in physiological media.

Synthesis of Macromolecular Prodrugs of Adriamycin

We have concentrated on the use of poly(α-L-glutamic acid), PG, as a carrier because this polymer can be readily degraded by lysosomal enzymes, is rather plasma stable, and contains sufficient reactive groups for further derivatization. After partial derivatization the conjugate will still be soluble in water due to residual carboxylic acid groups. PG is not expected to be toxic in the quantities used in the carrier system and can be readily obtained with different molecular weight distributions, Figure 14 shows the possible sites for the attachment of adriamycin onto polymeric carriers.

Different conjugates of adriamycin and PG were synthesized by routes given in ref. 57. These include; (a) direct coupling of adriamycin onto PG via N-γglutamine bonds by using N-ethoxycarbonyl-2-ethoxy-1, 2-dihydroquinoline, EEDQ (Fig. 15), (b) coupling of adriamycin onto PG using peptide spacer groups (Fig. 16) or direct conjugation of adriamycin onto PG via an acylhydrazone linkage (Fig. 17). The degrees of substitution were varied between 1-20 weight % of adriamycin.

Anti-tumor Activity of Conjugates

The conjugates were tested for anti-tumor activity with a L1210 clonogenic assay. Some typical results are given in Table I.

The results from Table I show that direct coupling of adriamycin onto PG, yields conjugates (PA) with a very low activity. Fluorescence measured with a cell-sorter (FACS) after exposure of the L1210 cells to these conjugates shows that the

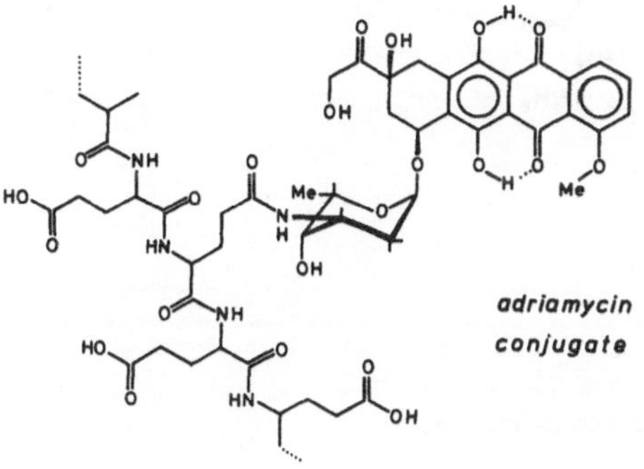

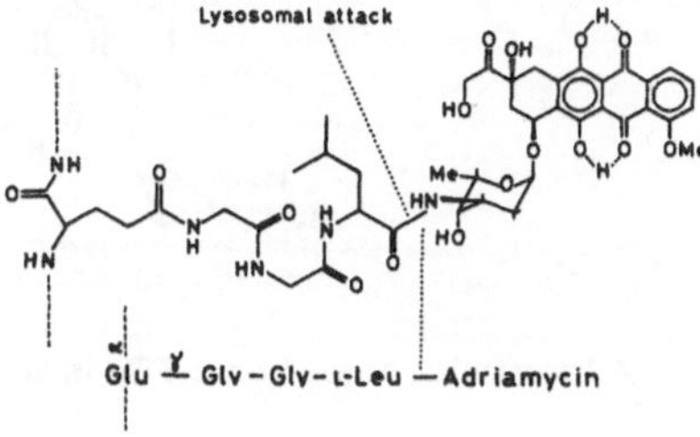

Figure 15. Adriamycin directly coupled onto PG via an amide bond.

Figure 16. Adriamycin coupled onto PG via a peptide spacer.

Table I. ID_{50} Values of Adriamycin and Adriamycin Conjugates Obtained with the L 1210 Clonogenic Assay.

Compound	Drug Code*	ID_{50} (ng.ml^{-1}) of conjugate	(ng adria.ml^{-1})
Free drug	Adriamycin	21-24*	21-24*
Conjugate (aminde)	P_2A_1	19030/25821*	3045/4131*
	P_2A_2	5100/5400*	1122/1188*
Conjugate (spacer-amide)	P_3-GGL$_2$-A$_1$	6725	201
Conjugate (hydrazone)	$P_3H_2A_1$	4455	71
	$P_3H_2A_2$	2062	53

* Results of two independent experiments : P denotes PG : A is adriamycin : G is glycyl : L is leucyl : H refers to acylhydrazone linkage : indices refer to different batches. ID_{50} means concentration of drug where 50 % inhibition of growth is reached.

conjugates are vividly internalized. This indicates that the low cytocidal action is attributable to a very slow degradation of the conjugate by endocellular enzymes. This was confirmed by the fact that treatment of these conjugates with papain did not yield any free adramycin.

Incorporation of a Gly-Gly-L-Leu spacer increased the activity by a factor of 5-10, which might be explained by a more rapid degradation of the conjugate, which was proven by the formation of adriamycin after papain treatment of P-GGL-A

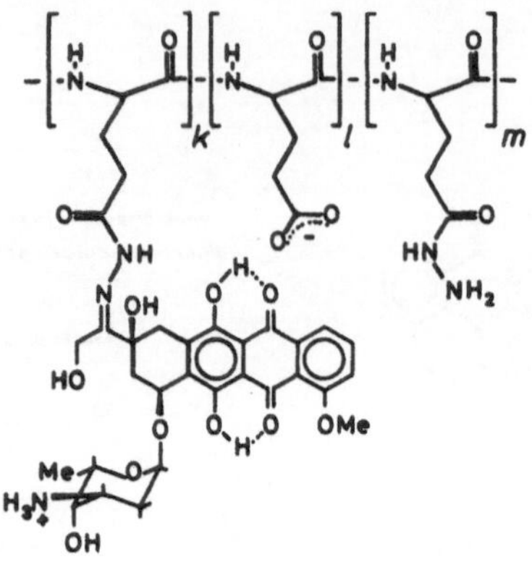

Figure 17.   Adriamycin coupled onto PG via an acylhydrazone linkage.

conjugates. The hydrazone conjugates show the highest activity which might be due to a rapid degradation of the conjugates after entering the cells.

These results are promising but further experiments have to be carried out to optimize the type and length of the spacer arm especially with respect to the intro-duction of structure elements which are prone to be cleaved by enzymes known to be elevated in various tumors like γ-GT and plasmin.

REFERENCES

1. Williams, D.F., in Fundamental Aspects of Biocompatibility, D.F. Williams, ed., CRC Press, Boca Raton, Florida, 1981.
2. Gilding, D.K., in Biocompatibility of Clinical Implant Materials, Vol. II, D.F. Williams, ed., CRC Press, Boca Raton, Florida, 1981.
3. Kim, S.W., Petersen, R.V. and Feijen, J., in Drug Design, Vol. 10, E.J. Ariens, ed., pp. 193, Academic Press, New York, 1980.
4. Langer, R. and Peppas, N., Rev. Macromol. Chem. Phys., C 23 (1):61, 1983.
5. Stenzel, K.H., Miyata, T. and Rubin, A.L., Ann. Rev. Biophysics and Bioengi-neering, 3:231, 1974.
6. Chvapil, M., Kronenthal, R.L. and Van Winkle Jr., W., Int. Rev. Conn. Tiss. Res., 6:1, 1973.
7. Ramachandran, G.N., Gould, B.S. and Milch, R.A., Treatise on Collagen, Academic Press, London, New York, 1967.
8. Yannas, I.V., J. Macromol. Sci., Rev. Macromol. Chem. C 7 (1):49, 1972.
9. Uitto, J.J. and Eisen, A.Z., Collagen in Dermatology in General Medicine, Fitzpatrick Ed. II, 1979.
10. Nishihara, T. and Miyata, T. Collagen Symp. (Japan), 3:66, 1962.
11. Drake, M.P., Davison, P.F., Bump, S. and Schmitt, F.O., Biochemistry, 5:301, 1966.
12. Gross, J. and Nagai, Y., Proc. Natl. Acad. Sci., 54:1197, 1965.

13. Seifter, S. and Harper, E., in The Enzymes, vol. III, P.D. Boyer, ed., pp. 649, Acad. Press, New York, 1971.
14. Milson, D.W., Steven, F.S. and Hunter, J.A.A. Connect. Tiss. Res., 1:251, 1972.
15. Steven, F.S., Torre-Blanco, A. and Hunter, J.A.A. Biochem. Biophys. Acta., 405:188, 1975.
16. Etherington, D.J., Connect. Tiss. Res., 5:135, 1977.
17. Harris, E.D. and Krane, S.M., N. Engl. J. Med. 291:557,605,652, 1974.
18. Burleigh, M.C., Quinby, W.C. and Bondoc, C.C., Surg. Clin. N. Am., 58:1141, 1978.
19. Salthouse, T.N., Williams, J.A.W. and Willigan, D.A. Surg. Gynecol. Obstet., 129:691, 1969.
20. Salthouse, T.N., Invest. Ophtal., 9:844, 1970.
21. Sawyer, N., et al., in Vascular Grafting, Clinical Applications and Techniques, C.B. Wright, R.W. Hobson II, L.F. Hiratzka and T.G. Lynch, eds., pp. 331, J. Wright, PSG Inc., Boston, 1983.
22. Horowitz, M.S., Goodman, D.J., Fogarty, T.J. and Harrison, D.C., J. Thorac. Cardiovasc. Surg., 67:885, 1974.
23. Salthouse, T.N., in Biocompatibility in Clinical Practice, D.F. Williams, ed., pp. 11, CRC Press, Boca Raton, Florida, 1982.
24. Alza., Br. Patent 1,372,944.
25. Gerendas, M., U.S. Patent 3,523,807, 1970.
26. Muzzarelli, R.A.a., Chitin, Pergamon Press, Oxford, 1978.
27. Schmitt, E.E. and Polistina, R.A., U.S. Patent, 3,297,033, 1967.
28. Casey, D.J., U.S. Patent, 3,902,497, 1975.
29. Reed, A.M. and Gilding, D.K., Polymer, 22:494, 1981.
30. Williams, D.F. and Mort, E., J. Bioengineering 1:231, 1977.
31. Schneider, A.K., U.S. Patent, 3,636,956, 1975.
32. Wooland, J.H.R., Yolles, S. Blake, D.A., Helrich, M. and Meyer, F.J., J. Med. Chem., 16:897, 1973.
33. Mhala, M.M. and Mishra, J.P., Indian J. Chem., 8:243, 1970.
34. van Dijk, J.A.P.P., Smit, J.A.M., Kohn, F.E. and Feijen, J., J. Polym. Sci., Polym. Chem. Ed., 21:197, 1983.
35. Schindler, A. and Harper, D., J. Polym. Sci. Polym. Chem. Ed., 17:2593, 1979.
36. Kulkarni, R.K., Pani, K.C., Newman, C.and Leonard, F., Arch. Surg., 93:839, 1966.
37. Kulkarni, R.K., Moore, E.G., Hegyeli, A.F. and Leonard, F., J. Biomed. Mater. Res., 5:169, 1971.
38. Vert, M.,et al., 26th Int. IUPAC Symp. on Macromolecules, Florence, Italy, 1980.
39. Christel, P., Chabot, F. Leray, J.L., Morin, C. and Vert, M., in Biomaterials 1980, Advances in Biomaterials, Vol. 3, G.D. Winter, D.F. Gibbons and H. Plenk Jr., eds., pp. 271, J. Wiley &Sons, Chichester, New York, 1982.
40. Gilding, D.K. and Reed, A.M., Polymer 20:1459, 1979.
41. Miller, R.A., Brady, J.M. and Cutright, D.E., J. Biomed. Mater. Res., 11:711, 1977.
42. Wasserman, D. and Levy, A., Can. Patent, 950,308, 1974.
43. Baptist, J.N., U.S. Patents 3,036,959, 3,044,942 and 3,225,766.
44. Reed, A.M. and Gilding, D.K., Polymer 22:499, 1981.
45. Gilding, D.K. and Reed, A.M. Polymer 20:1454, 1979.
46. Reed, A.M., Gilding, D.K. and Wilson, J., TASAIO, 23:109, 1977.
47. Choi, N.S., U.S. Patent 4,093,709, 1978.

48. Heller, J.H., Penhale, D.W.H., Helwing, R.F., Fritzinger, B.K. and Baker, R.W., AIChE Symp. Ser., 206:28, 1981.
49. Graham, N.B., Br. Polym. J., 10:19, 1978.
50. Schindler, A. and Pitt, C.G., Polymer Preprints 23(2):111, 1982.
51. Hein, P., Ethicon OP Forum 108: 4e quarter, 1981.
52. Kopecek, J. and Ulbrich, K., Prog. Polym. Sci., 9:1, 1983.
53. Duncan, R. and Kopecek, J., Advances in Polymer Science, 57:51, 1984.
54. Lefrak, E.A., Pitha, J., et al., Cancer Chemother. Rep., part III, 6:203, 1975.
55. Breed, J.G.S. Zimmerman, A.N.E. and Pinedo, H.M., Proc. Am. Cancer Res., 20:59, 1979.
56. Trouet, A., Baurain, R., Deprez-De Campeneere, D., Layton, D. and Masquelier, M., Recent Results in Cancer Research, 75:241, 1980.
57. van Heeswijk, W.A.R., Eenink, M.E., Stoffer, T., Potman, W., van der Vijgh, W.J.F., Pinedo, H.M., van der Poort, J. Lelieveld, P. and Feijen, J., Recent Advances in Drug Delivery Systems, S.W. Kim and J.M. Anderson, eds., Plenum, New York, (in press).
58. Trouet, A., Bull. Acad. Med. Bel., 135:261, 1980.
59. Wise, D.L., Fellmann, T.D., Sanderson, J.E. and Wentworth, R.L. in Drug carriers in Biology and Medicine, G. Gregoriadis, ed., pp. 235, Academic Press, 1979.

TAILOR MADE COMPOSITE MATERIALS FOR BIOMEDICAL USE

C. Migliaresi and L. Nicolais

University of Naples, Department of Materials and Production Engineering, Naples, Italy.

INTRODUCTION

The possibility of using polymeric materials for constructing artificial organs has been the object of many scientific publications and patents in the past years (1). However, polymers which are suitable for particular applications often display undesired side effects once implanted in the human body. In fact, the specifications which apply to polymeric materials used as substitutes for internal organs are very severe. Together with the specific physical properties which are required by the particular function, the material must show the following properties (2):

— high chemical and physical stability to biological environments;
— ability of being sterilized;
— absence of any kind of contaminant;

Moreover the polymer must not induce:

— tumor formation;
— antileukotactic response;
— thrombus formation;
— inflammatory encapsulation or cell modification in the surrounding tissue.

All these requirements strongly reduce the number of polymers which are potential candidates for biomedical applications. The most widely used polymers are: silicon rubbers, polytetrafluoroethylene (PTFE), polypropylene (PP), polyvinyl alcohol (PVA), polyvinylchloride (PVC), polyester resins (PET) and acrylic resins (AR). The silicon rubbers display high chemical and biological inertia coupled with mechanical properties similar to those of some natural tissues. They are used for plastic surgery and for making prostheses which are in direct contact with the blood.

One of the oldest uses of such material is in the Holter hydrocephalus check valves. Also pacemakers are generally coated with silicons in order to improve the resistance to biological environments. The main problem connected with this polymer is that the growing living tissue cannot adhere on it and consequently the formed fibrin cannot be transformed in fibrous tissue. As a concequence, occlusion of tubes will sometimes occur especially in the Holter valves. The PTFE based polymers are mainly used for surgery applications. They show high biomechanical stability and a high degree of porosity which permits good adhesion to the organic tissues. However the difficulties of processing strongly reduce their applications. The PVA has been widely used in the past, but since it has shown a tendency to promote calcification, its use is now limited. The PP and PET are widely used mainly in fiber form showing good biomechanical stability. The PVC is very common in artificial prostheses but only for short time applications due to its poor physico-chemical stability in living tissues. The AR are mainly used in small quantities for very specific applications and most of them are still under investigation for their in-situ long-term properties.

In the last years, a growing interest in a new class of biomaterials, the hydrogels, has been shown. These polymers are swollen extensively in water (30-70%) and display excellent biocompatibility also for long term applications (3). They are similar to the body's highly hydrated tissues and show strong biological interaction with them (4). In fact, hydrogels appear to absorb proteins and to adhere with cells more gently than lower water content foreign interfaces (4). Moreover, the water molecules included in the polymer seem to be associated within the three-dimensional network to form a quasi-organized structure similar to the one formed in the proteins (5). This enables rapid ingrowth of cells and capillaries and permits modeling of all tissue characteristics. In contrast with this high biocompatibility, the hydrogels generally display very poor mechanical properties reducing very much the possibility of their application as a material for artificial organs.

In the present paper the possibility of using the concepts of composite materials for designing artificial organs is investigated. Structural fiber composite materials with very high specific properties have been successfully utilized in many engineering applications. Because the fibers are so much stronger than ordinary polymeric materials, they normally impart strength to whatever matrix they are in. When the fibers are all aligned in one direction, maximum strength is achieved in the composite material along the direction of the fiber length. By purposely placing or weaving the fibers into specific directions, it thus becomes possible to tailor-make specific properties in specific directions and thereby satisfy the design requirements of structures subjected to a variety of multiaxial stresses.

It is precisely this ability to design materials to fit complex requirements combined with the improved specific properties that make fiber-reinforced composites so interesting.

Analogously the possibility of using polymeric substances specifically designed in the controlled release technology to solve a diversity of problems that have in common the application of some active agent to a system with the objective of accomplishing a specific purpose while avoiding certain other possible responses this agent might cause is becoming more and more attractive.

One of the common features of many of these techniques or formulations is the judicious selection of a polymeric material to act as a rate controlling device, container or carrier for the agent to be released.

PRINCIPLES OF FIBER REINFORCEMENT

All traditional structural materials have one thing in common: their actual strength is only a small fraction of their maximum theoretical strength based on the binding forces between atoms. It has been shown that the maximum theoretical tensile strength of a crystalline solid failing by en-masse cleavage across a crystallographic plane is approximatively one-tenth of its elastic modulus (i.e. $\sigma_{max} = 0.1$ E). The elastic modulus of glass, for example, is $\sim 10^7$ psi, which means its theoretical strength is roughly 10^6 psi. The elastic modulus of steel is 30×10^6 psi, which means its theoretical strength is roughly 3×10^6 psi. The actual tensile strength of a plate of glass is roughly 10,000 psi, while the strength of a plate of stainless steel can get up to 250,000 psi. In both cases the actual strength is at least an order of magnitude less than theoretical one. Modern theories on the ultimate strength of solids postulate that the reason for this is the presence of submicroscopic microcracks, fessures or other defects both at the surface and in the interior of all commonly produced materials. It is shown in the literature as an internal microcrack normal to an external load can cause large stress concentration at the crack tip.

In fact, if an elliptical defect is oriented so that the major axis (a) is perpendicular to the external load, the maximum stress at the crack tip is $\sigma_m = \sigma_o (1 + 2a/b)$, where b is the length of the minor axis. If there is a submicroscopic fissure where a = 1,000 Å and b = 10 Å (too small to see except with an electron microscope), the concentrated stress would be a factor of 201 times greater than the external load. Thus, the solid could fail locally and the crack could spread causing a further increase in stress concentration and ultimately a catastrophic failure.

When these submicroscopic defects are either removed or are oriented parallel to the stress directions, the material can approach its theoretical strength. A strong solid can in principle be made by forming very thin fibrous filaments. Very fine diameters limit internal defect sizes and orient other defects parallel to the fiber axis. Some of the fibers we have been discussing do indeed have strength approaching theoretical. The S-glass, for example, is very nearly at 70 percent of theoretical.

One of the major problems in utilization of these fibers is to imbed them in a matrix in such a way that they are in no way damaged either during fabrication or in service. Thus, the matrix must protect the surfaces of the individual fibers against abrasion or contact with the environment and it must separate the brittle fibers so as to prevent stress concentrations. Furthermore, since it is the fiber strength and stiffness that is being utilized, it is necessary to design the structure so that the fibers carry the external loads (Fig. 1).

Let us assume that all of the fibers are identical and all are aligned in the same direction parallel to an external load P_c. Further, assume that there is no slippage between the fibers and the matrix so that all components deform exactly the same amount. Then the load will distribute between the two components, P_f being carried by the fibers and P_m by the matrix (i.e. $P_c = P_m + P_f$). In terms of stresses σ_c, σ_m, and σ_f on cross-sectional areas A_c, A_m and A_f :

$$\sigma_c A_c = \sigma_m A_m + \sigma_f A_f$$

or

$$\sigma_c = \sigma_m \phi_m + \sigma_f \phi_f$$

where ϕ_m and ϕ_f are the volume fractions of matrix and fiber, respectively. Since the strains on both components are identical, the elastic modulus or stiffness of the

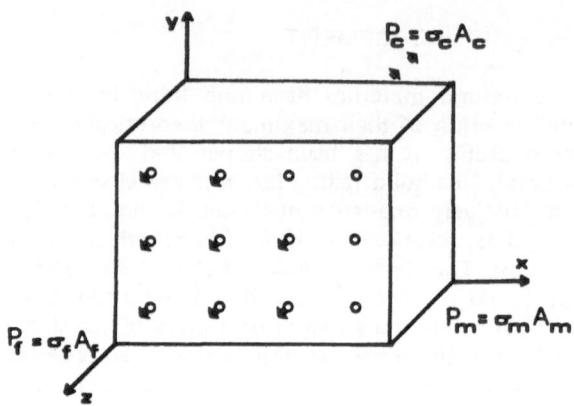

Figure 1. Schematic Representation of the Loading Conditions of a Composite Material.

composite parallel to the fibers (i.e. the longitudinal stiffness) is then :

$$E_c = E_m \ \phi_m + E_f \ \phi_f$$

For example, the elastic modulus of a typical plastic is about 0.5×10^6 psi while the stiffness of a boron fiber is 55×10^6 psi. If a unidirectional composite contains 50 percent by volume of boron, the longitudinal elastic modulus will be 27.75×10^6 psi or an increase of 55.5 times greater than the matrix alone. Also, the fibers will carry the major portion of the load ($P_f/P_c = (E_f/E_c) \ \phi_f$), or for the above case $P_f/P_c = 0.99$. Thus the fact that the plastic is weak is relatively unimportant since the fibers are carrying 99 percent of the load.

The longitudinal tensile strength is calculated in approximately the same way, and to a good order of approximation is :

$$\sigma_c = \sigma_m \ \phi_m + \sigma_f \ \phi_m$$

Thus, for the same case as above, the tensile strength of a typical plastic is about 10,000 psi, while the strength of boron fiber is 400,000 psi, and the longitudinal strength of a 50 percent by volume unidirectional composite is about 205,000 psi or a 20-fold increase over the matrix by itself.

If there is good adhesion between the fibers and the matrix, it is not necessary to have continuous fibers throughout a material to get substantial reinforcement. Thus, short fibers or even broken fibers can support a significant amount of the load. This is shown schematically in Figure 2 where two fiber ends exist in the matrix at the midsection.

When the material is stressed, the fiber ends attempt to separate, but are prevented from doing so by shear forces that are transmitted to the fiber by the adhering matrix. The nature of these forces is shown in more detail in Figure 2.

The tensile load on the fiber end is very low and builds up from the fiber end by interfacial shear in the matrix and at the interface. In order to utilize the fiber strength, the stress level must be able to reach the ultimate strength of the fibers. In order to accomplish this, both the matrix and the interface must be able to withstand the

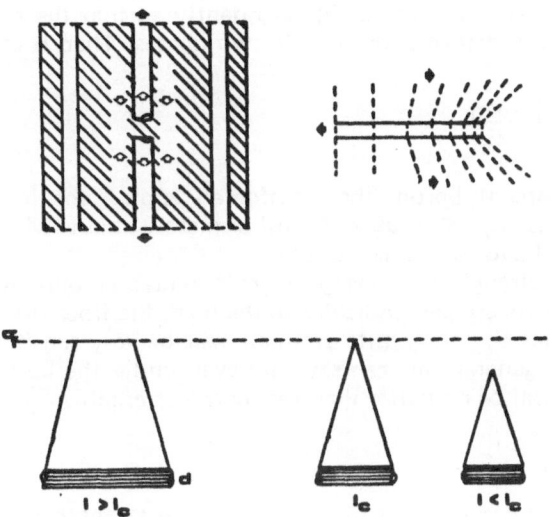

Figure 2. Schematic Representation of the Load Transfer Between Matrix and Fibers and of the Fiber Critical Length.

necessary shear forces to develop the fiber tensile load. It can be shown that for an ideal plastic matrix of yield strength τ_y or an interfacial bond strength of τ_y, a fiber of length l_c is needed to build the tensile stress level to σ_f in the fiber, where :

$$l_c = \sigma_f d_f / 2 \tau_y$$

where d_f is the fiber diameter. If the fiber is shorter than l_c, the stress level is less than the ultimate strength of the fiber and the composite fails by pulling the fiber out of the matrix rather than by breaking the fiber. Obviously, in this latter case, fiber strength is not being utilized to the maximum. One can see from the above equation that if the yield strength of the matrix or the interfacial bond strength is low, the critical fiber length required for good performance becomes very large.

This points to a most important area of research in the composites field. Two of the primary limiting factors in the performance of composite materials are the shear properties of the matrix and the adhesive bond strength between phases. Improvement of both of these characteristics is a continuing field of research.

Thus far, we have considered the strength and stiffness properties only in the direction of the fiber axis. In most structural applications the stresses are multi-axial so that the properties in other directions are also important. Consider, for example, the properties perpendicular to the fiber axis, called the transverse properties of the composite. Referring back to the schematic of the "unidirectional" composite, imagine a load being applied perpendicular to the fiber axes. In this case the matrix is free to deform without being constrained by the stiff fibers, so that the presence of the fibers does not do much good in this direction. The actual calculation of a transverse modulus is a complex problem, but one may get a lower bound estimate by using the series connected model.

The phases are assumed to act independently so that the total deformation is merely the sum of the deformations of the two phases. Than it can be shown that :

$$\frac{1}{E_c} = \frac{\phi_f}{E_f} + \frac{\phi_m}{E_m}$$

For the 50 percent boron fiber reinforced epoxy, the lower bound on the transverse modulus is $E_c \leqslant 0.99 \times 10^6$ psi or merely about twice the matrix modulus or only 1/28 of the longitudinal modulus.

The transverse strength is also very difficult to predict, but intuitively one should see that since the fibers are perpendicular to the load, the fiber strength is not utilized and furthermore that the composite strength will be very sensitive to the adhesion between phases. In general, one can say that even under the best circumstances the transverse strength will be no better than the matrix strength.

$$(\sigma_c)_{transverse} < \sigma_m$$

For the boron-epoxy composite the transverse strength will generally be less than 10,000 psi and experimentally it is often no better than 4,000 psi, which is only 2 percent of the longitudinal strength.

Here another of the truly serious difficulties with oriented composite structures; they are highly anisotropic, with the transverse properties being no better than the matrix or interfacial properties. One may calculate the stiffness and estimate the strength off the fiber axis in an unidirectional composite by using so-called transformation properties for anisotropic elastic bodies.

The strength properties are very sensitive to the angle of orientation. When the composite is loaded in tension at an angle θ to the fiber direction, three potential modes of failure must be considered. The first is failure by fracture of the fiber. If the fiber axis is at an angle θ to the external tension, the fibers will break at an external load $\sigma_c \sec^2 \theta$ where σ_c is the longitudinal ultimate strength of the composite. The second possible failure mode is by shear in the direction of the fibers on a plane parallel to the fiber axis, caused by a load $2 \tau \mathrm{cosec}\, 2 \theta$ where τ is either the shear strength of the matrix, the fiber or the interface. The third possible failure mode is by tensile failure transverse to the fiber axis, caused by a load $\sigma_u \mathrm{cosec}^2 \theta$ where σ_u is the transverse tensile strength of either the matrix, interface or fiber. Whichever mode requires the smallest breaking strength will cause the catastrophic failure.

The problems of off-axis failure leads one to an understanding of why fiber orientation, matrix shear and tensile strength, fiber-matrix interfacial bond strength, and the presence of voids or other imperfections are so important in determining composite strength.

One way to partially overcome the off-axis weaknesses of fiber-reinforced composites is to cross-ply a number of unidirectional layers, as shown in Figure 3, so that fibers are pointing in many different directions.

It can be shown that certain arrangements of multiple layers produce a so called "quasi-isotropic" laminate, which means that the stiffness and strength are approximately uniform throughout all angles. Naturally, whenever this is done one has to sacrifice the maximum level of the property in any one direction to obtain a lower, albeit uniform, level in all directions. Furthermore, by using multiple layers, one introduces new interfaces between layers that are sources for possible failure. Interlaminar shear failure is, indeed, one of the more severe difficulties with multilayered laminates.

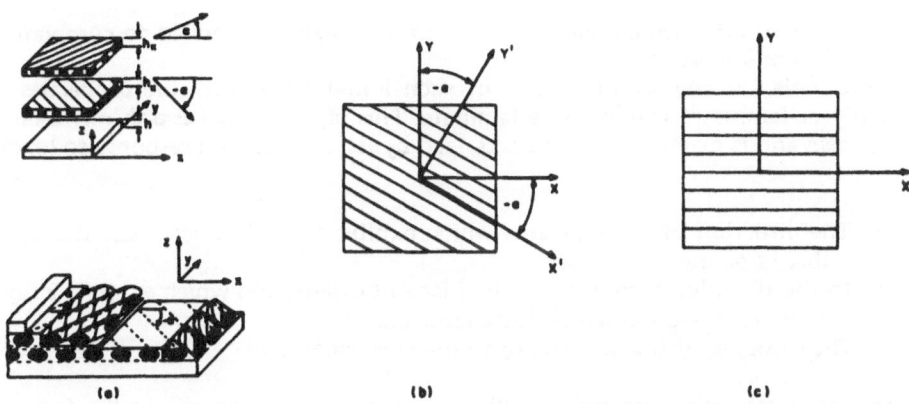

Figure 3. Illustration of a Continuous Fiber Composite Laminate.

Continuous fiber-reinforced structures can be fabricated in a number of different ways, but the contours and the complexity of the finished structure are usually severely limited by the available fabrication techniques. In general, one is limited to flat sheets, mildly curved surfaces, and simple shapes with an axis of rotation. As has been pointed out already, however, one can also use discontinuous (or short) fibers for effective reinforcement. It is clear, however, that there could also be engineering applications in which one is concerned with the electromagnetic or thermal conduction properties of the material. Instead of modulus and strength, one would then be interested in conductivity, dielectric constants, magnetic permeability and the like. Since many analogies exist between the various transport processes, an understanding of mechanical responses helps give a clearer understanding of the anisotropy of these others.

In the following sections we will very carefully examine the fundamental principles that are important in the mechanical behavior of composite materials consisting of an organic matrix and a stiff reinforcement.

CONSTITUTIVE RELATIONS FOR COMPOSITES

Current attitudes regarding composite materials emphasize the relationship of structural performance to the properties of a ply. A "ply" is a thin sheet of material consisting of an oriented array of fibers embedded in a continuous matrix material (Fig. 3). These plies are stacked one upon another, in a defined sequence and orientation, and bonded together yielding a laminate with tailored properties. The properties of the laminate are related to the properties of the ply by the specification of the ply thickness, stacking sequence, and the orientation of each ply. The properties of the ply are, in turn, specified by the properties of the fibers and matrix, their volumetric concentration, and geometric packing in the ply. Generally, the ply material is preformed and can be purchased in a continuous compliant tape or sheet form which is in a chemically semicured condition. Fabrication of structural items involves using this "prepreg" material and either winding it on to a mandrel or cutting and stacking it on to a mold after which heat and pressure or tension is applied to complete the chemical hardening process.

The basis for engineering design of such a material is then the properties of a cured ply or lamina as it exists in a laminate. This ply is treated as a thin two-dimensional item and is mechanically characterized by its strees-strain response to loadings in:

— The direction of the filaments which exhibit a nearly linear response up to a rather large fracture stress;
— In the direction transverse to the filament orientation which exhibits a significantly decreased moduli and strength; and
— The response of the material to an in-plane shear load.

By contrast with isotropic metallic materials, an oriented ply, in the form of a thin sheet, is anisotropic and requires four elastic (plane stress) constants (6-8) to specify its stiffness properties in its natural orientation :

$$\sigma_1 = Q_{11} \, \varepsilon_1 + Q_{12} \, \varepsilon_2$$
$$\sigma_2 = Q_{12} \, \varepsilon_1 + Q_{22} \, \varepsilon_2$$
$$\sigma_6 = Q_{66} \, \varepsilon_6$$

where $\sigma_6 = \tau_{12}$ and $\varepsilon_6 = \gamma_{12}$ or in matrix form

$$\begin{vmatrix} \sigma_1 \\ \sigma_2 \\ \sigma_6 \end{vmatrix} = \begin{vmatrix} Q_{11} & Q_{12} & 0 \\ Q_{12} & Q_{22} & 0 \\ 0 & 0 & Q_{66} \end{vmatrix}$$

where the plane-stress stiffness moduli are :

$$Q_{11} = E_{11} / (1 - \nu_{12} \, \nu_{21})$$
$$Q_{22} = E_{22} / (1 - \nu_{12} \, \nu_{21})$$
$$Q_{12} = E_{11} \, \nu_{21} / (1 - \nu_{12} \, \nu_{21})$$
$$Q_{66} = G_{12}$$

If, however, the ply is rotated with respect to the applied stress or strain direction two additional moduli appear which results in the indicated shear coupling rotation in simple expansion.

$$\begin{vmatrix} \sigma_1 \\ \sigma_2 \\ \sigma_6 \end{vmatrix} = \begin{vmatrix} \bar{Q}_{11} & \bar{Q}_{12} & \bar{Q}_{16} \\ \bar{Q}_{12} & \bar{Q}_{22} & \bar{Q}_{26} \\ \bar{Q}_{16} & \bar{Q}_{26} & \bar{Q}_{66} \end{vmatrix} \begin{vmatrix} \varepsilon_1 \\ \varepsilon_2 \\ \varepsilon_6 \end{vmatrix}$$

where

$$\bar{Q}_{11} = U_1 + U_2 \cos (2\theta) + U_3 \cos (4\theta)$$

$$\bar{Q}_{22} = U_1 - U_2 \cos(2\theta) + U_3 \cos(4\theta)$$
$$\bar{Q}_{12} = U_4 - U_3 \cos(4\theta)$$
$$\bar{Q}_{66} = U_5 - U_3 \cos(4\theta)$$
$$\bar{Q}_{16} = -(1/2) U_2 \sin(2\theta) - U_3 \sin(4\theta)$$
$$\bar{Q}_{26} = -(1/2) U_2 \sin(2\theta) + U_3 \sin(4\theta)$$

the variants, U_i to the rotation are :

$$U_1 = (1/8)(3 Q_{11} + 3 Q_{22} + 2 Q_{12} + 4 Q_{66})$$
$$U_2 = (1/2)(Q_{11} - Q_{22})$$
$$U_3 = (1/8)(Q_{11} + Q_{22} + 6 Q_{12} - 4 Q_{66})$$
$$U_4 = (1/8)(Q_{11} + Q_{22} + 6 Q_{12} - 4 Q_{66})$$
$$U_5 = (1/8)(Q_{11} + Q_{22} - 2 Q_{12} + 4 Q_{66})$$

In addition, lamination can result in up to 18 elastic coefficients and increased deformational complexities. But the additional coefficients can all be derived from the four primary coefficients using the concept of rotation and ply-stacking sequence (6,7). These complications are the result of geometric variables. If the laminate is properly constructed, the in-plane stretching of stiffness properties can still be specified by four elastic coefficients. We shall consider laminates of this nature.

The flow diagram of a typical calculation is shown in Figure 4. Note that both short and continuous fibers are handled in the same manner. These calculations, while tedious, are analytically simple. The "plane stress" stiffness, the Q_{ij} terms, are employed because lamination neglects the mechanical properties through the ply thickness. These stiffnesses are sometimes regrouped into new constants called "invariants", the U_i terms, for analytical ease. To compute the properties of the laminate one then sums the ply properties through the thickness of the laminate. For a balanced (same number of $\pm \theta$) and symmetrical ($+\theta$ or $-\theta$ at the same distance above and below the mid plane) the solution is :

$$A_{11} = U_1 + U_2 \cos(2\theta) + U_3 \cos(4\theta)$$
$$A_{22} = U_1 - U_2 \cos(2\theta) + U_3 \cos(4\theta)$$
$$A_{21} = U_4 - U_3 \cos(4\theta)$$
$$A_{66} = U_5 - U_3 \cos(4\theta)$$

Note the inverted A_{ij} terms yield the required elastic properties of the laminate in terms of the individual ply properties E_{11}, E_{12}, ν_{12}, and G_{12}.

$$E_{11} = \frac{A_{11} A_{22} - A_{12}^2}{A_{22}}$$

$$E_{22} = \frac{A_{11} A_{22} - A_{12}^2}{A_{11}}$$

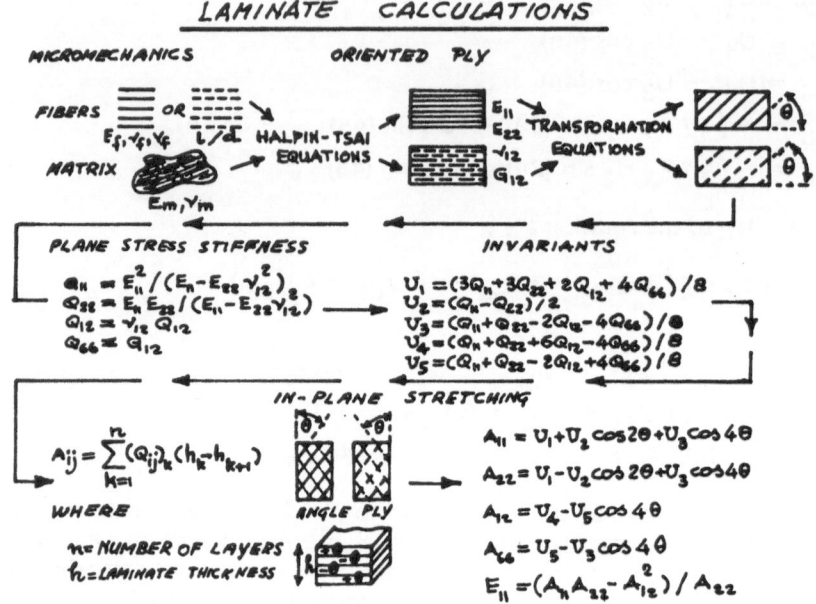

Figure 4. Laminate Calculations.

$$\frac{\nu_{12}}{E_{11}} = \frac{A_{12}}{A_{11} A_{22} - A_{12}^2}$$

$$G_{12} = A_{66}$$

These calculations have been throughly tested and agree closely with experiment.
The angle-ply laminate is predicted from the ply properties. The ply properties are in turn correlated with the transformation equations and the micromechanics. The micromechanics employed in this demonstration are based upon the "self-consistent method" developed by Hill (9). Hill rigorously modeled the composite as a single fiber, encased in a cylinder matrix, with both embebbed in a unbounded homogeneous medium which is macroscopically indistinguishable from the composite. Hermann (10) employed this model to obtain a solution in terms of Hill's "reduced module". Halpin and Tsai (11) reduced Hermann's solution to a simpler analytical form and extended its use for a variety of filament geometries :

$$E_{11} = E_f V_f + E_m V_m$$

$$\nu_{12} = \nu_f V_f + \nu_m V_m$$

$$\frac{\bar{p}}{p_m} = \frac{1 + \xi \eta V_f}{1 - \eta V_f}$$

where

$$\eta = (p_f / p_m - 1) / (p_f / p_m + \zeta)$$
$$\xi_E = 2 (1 / d) ; \qquad \zeta_{12} = 1 ; \qquad \zeta_{23} = 1 / (3 - 4 \nu_m)$$
$$\bar{p} = E_{22}, G_{12}, G_{23} ; \qquad p_f = E_f, G_f ; \qquad p_m = E_m, G_m$$

The short fiber properties are also given by the Halpin-Tsai equations where the module in the fiber orientation direction is a sensitive function of aspect ratio : 1/d at small aspect ratios and passes to the same properties as a continuous fiber composite at large but finite aspect ratios.

If the ply illustrated in Figure 5 is used in the construction of a balanced and symmetrical 0/90 laminate and is mechanically tested, a bilinear stress-strain curve is obtained and the stiffness is the sum, through the thickness, of the plane-stress stiffness of each layer. As the laminate is deformed, each ply possesses the same in-plane strain, and when the strain on the 90-deg layers reachs the strain level at which ply failure was experienced, the 90 layers crack. The failure in the laminate prevents the 90-deg layer from carrying their share of the load, Q_{ij} (90-deg) = 0. This load is transferred to the unbroken layers and results in a loss of laminate stiffness or modulus. Continual loading will ultimately produce a catastrophic failure of the laminate when the strain capability of the unbroken, 0-deg, layers is exceeded. For a 0/90 construction, employing the glass/epoxy material, the ratio of the ultimate failure stress to the crazing stress, the knee in Figure 5, is 6.1. Experimental data and a theoretical stress-strain curve are shown in Figure 8 for a $\pi/4$ (0 deg/±45 deg/90 deg) glass/epoxy laminate. Note the change in stiffness as the 90-deg and then the 45-deg layers craze and the correspondence of the theoretical ultimate strength of 52,000 psi with the experimental results of 50,500 psi. The ratio of ultimate stress to 90-deg ply failure is 4.5. While the strain for transverse ply failure is constant from laminate to laminate, the stress required to craze the system as well as final failure load is a function of laminate geometry because the construction of the laminate specifies the stiffness properties (crazing stress = stiffness x allowable transverse ply strain). It must be noticed that the area under the stress-strain curve is proportional to the impact energy. Therefore, lamination permits the engineer to tailor a fixed prepreg system to meet the conflicting stress/strain demands at different points in a structure.

A further point, the crazing strees of threshold is generally at or below the creep fracture or fatigue limit for all classes of composites (for glass/epoxy the fatigue limit lies between 0.25-0.30 of static ultimate strength). Boron and graphite are fatigue insensitive filaments, thus no fatigue damage is realized below first ply failure.

Thus, the material properties of a laminate are specified in terms of the ply engineering module, E_{11}, E_{22}, ν_{12} and G_{12}; the engineering strains to failure ε_1, ε_2 and ε_6; and the thermal expansion coefficients, ε_1 and ε_2.

APPLICATIONS

In the following, a few applications of composite materials in medicine are reported.

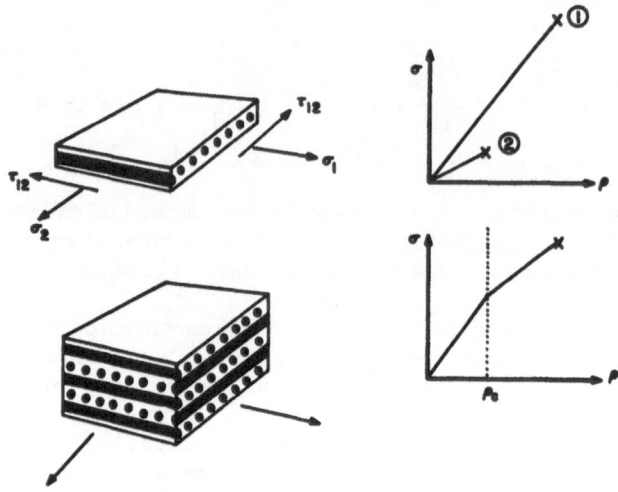

Figure 5.   Determination of Laminate Properties.

A Glass Bead Composite Acrylic Bone Cement

Acrylic bone cements introduced by Charnley in 1960 are today widely used in orthopaedics for bone prosthesis fixation. Nevertheless, high temperatures reached during the "in-vivo" polymerization, shrinkage and low dimensional stability of commercial cements are unacceptable faults which often cause necrosis of tissues surrounding the cements and loosening of the prostheses.

Although in the past many solutions have been proposed in order to reduce these inconveniens, such as addition of heat sinks or different formulations, no practical results have been obtained due to the decreased mechanical properties of the cements.

However, it is well assessed in polymer and composite technology that the use of crosslinking agents and reinforcing fillers can successfully improve both short and long term mechanical properties and dimensional stability, provided that opportune amounts of crosslinking agent are used and adhesion between fillers and matrix is achieved.

The physical characterization of a new glass bead composite crosslinked cement of composition reported in Table I, reveals an appreciable decrease of the reaction temperature with respect to that of a commercial cement, and a corresponding improvement of mechanical properties and dimensional stability (12).

Clinical evaluation of cements polymerized in-vivo in the iliac bone of rabbits and histological response at different implantation times, demonstrate that the composite cement is well tolerated and better adheres to bone than commercial cements.

Table I. Composition of the Composite Cement.

Phase 1 (40% by wt.)
- — 30% wt. solution of polymethylmethacrylate in methylmethacrylate
- — Ethylenedimethacrylate(2% by wt. referred to methylmethacrylate content)
- — Dimethylparatoluidine(2% by wt. referred to methylmethacrylate content)

Phase 2 (60% by wt.)
- — Glass beads
- — Benzoyl peroxide(1% by wt. referred to methylmethacrylate content in Ph.1)

A Composite Sheet for the Surgical Correction of Strabismus

In the last years a new class of polymeric materials for biomedical use, the hydrogels, has shown excellent biocompatibility also for long term applications (4), especially in ophtalmology. In fact, hydrogels are highly swollen in water and appear to absorb proteins and to adhere cells more gently than other polymeric substances; moreover the water molecules included in the polymer seem to be associated within the three dimensional network, to form a quasi organized structure, similar to the one formed in the proteins (5). This enables rapid ingrowth of cells and permits modeling of all tissue characteristics.

In contrast with this high biocompatibility, the hydrogels generally display very poor mechanical properties, reducing very much the possibility of their application as a material for artificial implants.

It has been shown that, by using the composite mechanics concepts, it is possible to reinforce opportunely the material in order to achieve the desired properties. In this application composite sheets obtained reinforcing Poly-2-hydroxyethylmeth-acrylate (PHEMA) with a Polyethyleneterephthalate (PET) net have been implanted in rabbits to test their potential application for the surgical correction of strabismus.

The load-deformation curve of a suture/composite sheet system and their appearence after the test, are reported in Figure 6. While a high mechanical resistence of the sheet is not required, the main rule of the net is to resist the suture, taking into account the dynamic condition of the applied load in-vivo. In the experiment, the applied load was concentrated on the stitches and the low resistence points were the knots of the suture which in all cases got either untied or broken under stress.

The histological examinations of the implant, inserted in the rectus superior muscle of the eye of rabbits for up to one year, reveals the excellent biocompatibility of the prosthesis. Never a reaction comparable to a rejection appeared, and normal connective elements, spreading into the PHEMA matrix and migrating freely around the single PET fibers, could be observed. Moreover, the presence of capillaries which grow inside the tissue entering the prosthesis furthermore indicate that the prosthesis is fully integrated in the natural tissue.

A Polyester Fiber Reinforced PHEMA Artificial Tendon

Tendons and ligaments, as with the most part of biological tissues, are composite structures where the overall properties are a well balanced compromise of the single component properties. In fact, they consist of collagen fibers and a matrix which contains gel-like acid mucopolysaccharides and fibroblast cells. The structure and

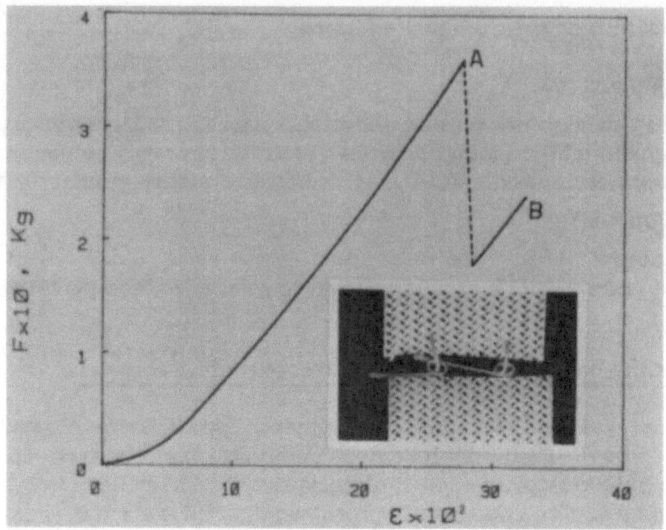

Figure 6.   Load-Deformation Curve of a Sutured PHEMA/PET Net Composite.

morphology of collagen fibers are rather complicated and not completely elucidated. However their waved shape and the elastic properties of the matrix are responsible for the characteristic tensile properties of ligaments which show low initial elastic modulus up to deformations of 4-6%, followed by a sudden increase in stiffness caused by the alignment of collagen fibers which further resist deformation.

While often tendon or ligament prostheses have been proposed without taking into account the relationships between morphology, properties and functionality, in the design of such a biocompatible prosthesis these conditions cannot be neglected.

By using the composite mechanics concepts it has been possible to realize a polyethyleneterephthalate fiber/poly-2-hydroxyethylmethacrylate composite (13) (see Fig. 7) for use as tendon or ligament prosthesis, where the amount and the orientation of fibers inside the hydrophylic PHEMA control both mechanical and viscoelastic properties.

In Figure 8 the tensile properties of such composite structures well compare with those of a natural tendon (13).

An Isoelastic Fiber Composite Plate for Fracture Fixation

The metal plates actually used in orthopedics for fracture fixation present an elastic modulus much higher than the bones to which they are connected. This difference of rigidity between plates and bones prevents the healing by proliferation of primary callus and results in lower strength of the repaired bone due to excessive stress protection.

Recently, a few papers have been published on the preparation and characterization of carbon fiber composite materials to be used as plates for fracture fixation. However, while this composite structure could be designed to fit the mechanical requirements, due to the electrical conductivity of the carbon fibers, corrosion problems cannot be avoided.

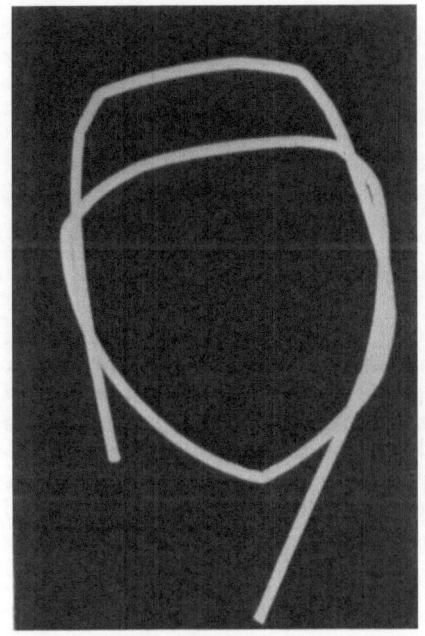

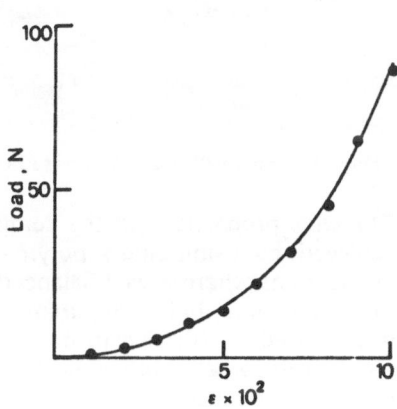

Figure 7.   Tendon Prosthesis.

Figure 8.   Load-Deformation Curve of a Natural Tendon (line) Compared to the Experimental Data (Full Circles) Obtained for a PHEMA/PET Prosthesis.

The micromechanics and the lamination theory can be used to design a composite laminate of desired mechanical properties. In particular, assuming that the tensile and flexural rigidity of the bone and the plate are equal, one can write :

$$E_b A_b = E_p A_p = E_p \, lt$$
$$E_b I_b = E_p I_p = E_p \, lt^3/12$$

where E is the Young modulus, A the area, I the inertia moment relative to a mass center longitudinal plane, the subscripts b and p refer to the bone and plate respectively, and l and t are the width and the thickness of the plate. From the solution of the previous equations, a value of the requested elastic modulus of the plate is calculated once the geometric parameter is opportunely fixed.

In particular, for a Kevlar/epoxy system, one can calculate the number of laminae at 0, 90 and ± 45 deg. to achieve the required characteristics.

The experimental result is shown in Figure 9 where a photograph of such plate is reported.

CONCLUSION

In the present paper the possibility of using the composite mechanics concepts to design biomedical prostheses with desired specific properties has been illustrated.

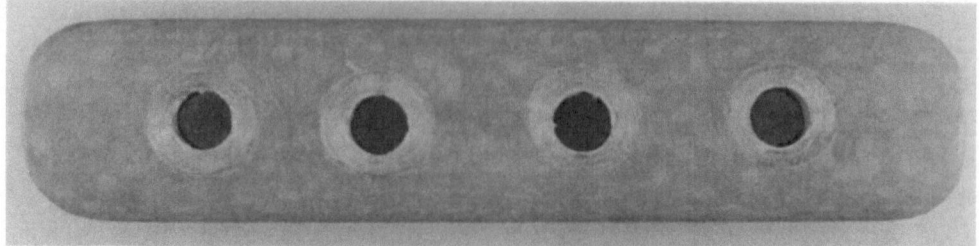

Figure 9.   Epoxy/Kevlar Composite Bone Fracture Fixation Plate.

The wide properties and the composite structure of natural tissues, which cannot be achieved by using single polymers, make composite materials very attractive for applications where a well balanced design of properties of the prosthesis should result in a biocompatibility requirement. The composite mechanics concepts, which are widely used for high performance applications, have brought a significative improvement in the area of biomedical applications of polymeric materials. The basics of the composite mechanics analysis have been reviewed and a few indicative examples of applications of polymeric composites have been reported.

REFERENCES

1.   Kronental, R.L., Oser, Z., Martin, E., Polymers in Medicine and Surgery, Plenum Press, New York, 1975.
2.   Lyman, D.J., Polymers in Medicine and Surgery, R.L. Kronental, Z. Oser, E. Martin, eds., Plenum Press, New York, 1975.
3.   Sprincl, L., Vacik, J., J. Biomed. Mater. Res., 7:123, 1973.
4.   Hoffman, A.S., Polymers in Medicine and Surgery, R.L. Kronental, Z. Oser, E. Martin, eds., Plenum Press, New York, 1975.
5.   Bruck, S.D., J. Biimed. Mater. Res., 7:387, 1973.
6.   Asthon, J.E., Halpin, J.C., Petit, P.H., Primer on Composite Materials: Analysis, Technomic Publ. Co., Stamford, CT, 1969.
7.   Tsai, S.W., Halpin, J.C., Pagano, N.J., Composite Materials Workshop, Technomic Publ. Co., Stamford, CT, 1968.
8.   Halpin, J.C., Nicolais, L., Ing. Chim. Ital., 7:173, 1971.
9.   Hill, R., J. Mech. Phys. Solids, 12:199, 1964.
10. Hermans, J.J., Proc. Konigl. Neder. Akadem. Weteschappen Amsterdam, 870:1, 1967.
11. Halpin, J.C., Pagano, N.J., Comp. Mat., 3:720, 1969.
12. Guida, G., Riccio, V., Gatto, S., Migliaresi, C., Nicodemo, L., Nicolais, L., Palomba, C., Biomaterials and Biomechanics, P. Ducheyne, G. Van der Perre, A.E. Aubert, eds., Elsevier Sci. Publ. B.V., Amsterdam, The Netherlands, 1984.
13. Migliaresi, C., Nicolais, L., Int. J. Art. Org., 3:114, 1980.

SYNTHETIC POLYMERIC MEMBRANES: CLASSIFICATION, PREPARATION, STRUCTURE AND TRANSPORT MECHANISMS

E. Piskin

Hacettepe University, Chemical Engineering Department, Ankara, Turkey

INTRODUCTION

Polymer films are generally employed as barriers to the free transmission of gases, vapors, liquids, ions and other substances. The term "membrane" has been applied to the polymer film used in the application where an exchange of matter between two environments separated by the membrane is concerned. In the most general sense, a membrane may be defined as an imperfect barrier, or an interphase between two phases which restricts the transport of various substances from one phase to another in a rather specific manner.

There are two different classes, namely biological membranes (biomembranes) and synthetic membranes.

The first group, biomembranes, are simply the functional boundaries between different spaces within the organism. There are several types of biomembranes which exist in the human body and other living organisms, such as plasma, or cell membranes, epithelial membranes, membranes of intracellular organelles, etc. These membranes are different in composition, structure or function. Although a lot of work has already been done on this subject, the facts and interrelationships between these three important properties are not understood throughly. Biomembranes do not only provide a barrier between the living and the inanimate world, but take up nutrients, eliminate waste, control environmental chemistry, regulate metabolism, act as transducers of chemicals, electricity, temperature and light into other energy forms. It is beyond the scope of this paper to discuss the biological membranes, thus, without going further in detail, mention should be made of prime importance of these membranes in the survival of organisms.

The second group of membranes, synthetic membranes, may consist of a large variety of materials including mostly natural and synthetic polymers, metals, ceramics, glass, carbons, or combinations of these materials with natural products such as collagen, albumin, etc. Much published data are available on methods of preparation and fabrication of synthetic membranes for specific applications.

A word of apology might be offered for the type of coverage sought in this and the following two chapters. No attempt has been made to make this an in-depth treatise. Nor has an effort been made to include a complete bibliography on the subject. Several excellent reviews already exist for this purpose. Instead, basic properties of synthetic polymeric membranes, preparation, structures and transport mechanisms (First Part); membrane separation techniques (Second Part); and biological applications (Third Part) are briefly reviewed in order to give an introductory idea to the reader about those aspects of the subject.

CLASSIFICATION AND CHARACTERIZATION OF SYNTHETIC MEMBRANES

There are many different ways of classifying membranes. Membranes may be;

— Homogeneous or heterogeneous;
— Symmetric or asymmetric in structure;
— Electrically charged or neutral;
— Solid or liquid;
— Etc.

Synthetic membranes may be characterized both by structure and by function. The former describes what they are, and the latter how they perform. Structural properties are their chemical nature their microcrystalline structure and their pore structure. Functional properties are permeability and perm selectivity. There are, of course other (secondary) properties such as mechanical properties, thermal stabilities, environmental hazards, etc. Here, our attention will focus on the membranes themselves, thus, they will be classified according to structure (Table I).

Table I. Classification of Membranes According to Structure.

SYNTHETIC MEMBRANES

        — HETEROGENEOUS
                — Symmetric
                — Asymmetric
                        — Integral Asymmetric
                                — With homogeneous skin
                                — With microporous skin
                        — Composite
                                — With homogeneous skin
                                — With microporous skin

        — HOMOGENEOUS

Synthetic membranes can be considered in two groups, namely heterogeneous and homogeneous, according to their micro-level (but not molecular level) structure. Different structures are schematically drawn in Figure 1.

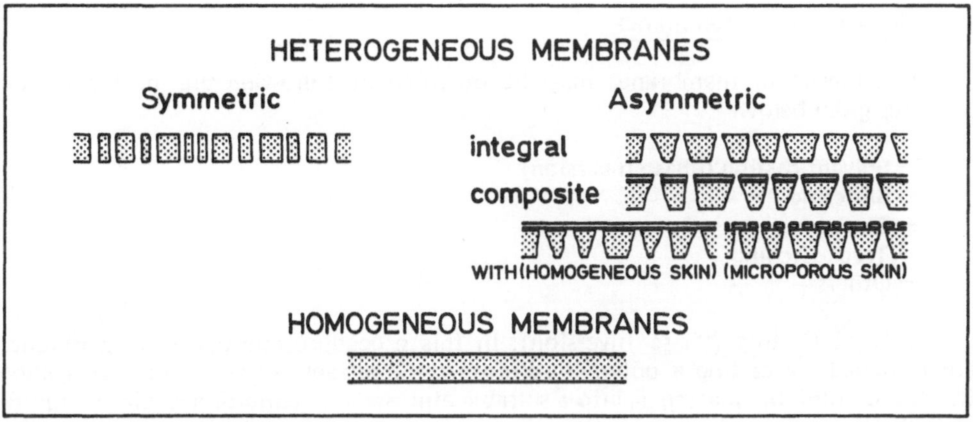

Figure 1.   Membrane Structures.

Heterogeneous membranes consist of a solid matrix with defined pores which have a diameter ranging from 5 nm to 50 nm. These membranes can be prepared as symmetric or asymmetric in structure. Asymmetric ones may be integral, or composite which refers to two different polymer layers composed in one membrane. Asymmetric membranes might have a "skin" layer on one side which might be again homogeneous or heterogeneous. It should be noted that the dense but thin polymer layer (skin layer) has a very important role in the permselectivity of these membranes.

The second group of the synthetic membranes, homogeneous membranes, are likely to be considered as a continuous media without any pores in it. However, it should be pointed out that these membranes must have also some kind of openings which permit the transfer of the permeating molecules. As it will be discussed in the latter part of this chapter, the free volume theory of diffusion through homogeneous polymeric structures declares the probability of finding enough local volume, while the activation energy approach emphasizes the need to create the free spaces. Here, we do not consider these free volumes (or free spaces) as micropores (or pores).

PREPARATION OF SYNTHETIC MEMBRANES

Synthetic membranes can be made from a wide variety of materials, including polymers, by following various specific ways and means which are described in patent literature (1-7). As mentioned above, homogeneous or heterogeneous with different structures, electrically charged or neutral, solid or liquid, etc. membranes may be prepared for specific applications. The main criteria for assessment of the membranes are selectivity and permeation rate of the preferentially permeating component. But, of course, further aspects such as mechanical strength, chemical and thermal stabilities, biocompatibility, environmental hazards, etc. should be considered in preparation of synthetic membranes for specific applications.

Here, putting the emphasis on heterogeneous membranes, some common general methods to prepare specific membranes are briefly reviewed.

Heterogeneous Membranes

Heterogeneous membranes may be obtained by following the most common methods given below.

- Solvent casting (Phase Inversion)
- Sintering
- Stretching
- Track-Etching
- Others

Solvent Casting (Phase Inversion). In this procedure microporous membranes are obtained by casting a polymer solution on a suitable surface and then gelling the liquid film by placing it into a suitable atmosphere (conditioned air or liquid) (4,6-9). During the gelling step, the polymer precipitates and the solvent evaporates. The procedural steps involved in membrane formation are as follows:

(1) Preparing a polymer solution, usually referred to as dope, (containing usually 10 to 30 % by weight polymer) by dissloving the polymer in a good solvent (or solvent mixture). Organic solvents such as acetone, DMF, and THF are usually used for this purpose.
(2) Casting the polymer solution into a film of typically 100-500 μm thickness on a proper surface (usually glass).
(3) Quenching (precipitation of polymer and evaporation of solvent) in a non-solvent, or mixture of some solvent which can also include some additives. Usually water is used as nonsolvent.
(4) Optionally, annealing in water for a certain period of time at 70°-80°C. This step is employed when a homogenous skin is expected.

Two limiting types of structures are achieved by following these steps depending on preparation procedure (Fig. 2). Finger type membranes give high transfer rates, but have low permselectivity, and they, are relatively weak. Low transfer rates with high selectivity are obtained in sponge (or foam) type membranes. These latter ones are rather mechanically strong.

Phase inversion membranes with different structures between these two limit structures and with different pore size and pore size distribution may be obtained by altering the system parameters. Factors which are effective on the membrane structure are given below.

- Polymer and its concentration in the casting solution
- Solvent systems
- Precipitant system
- Temperature of precipitation
- Pre and post procedures (annealing, etc.)
- Membrane thickness

The effects of several parameters on the resultant structure was examined by several investigators with all details (2,4,6-9). In conclusion, it can be said that high precipitation rates always lead to a finger type, slow rates lead to a sponge type, and very slow rates give a symmetric structure.

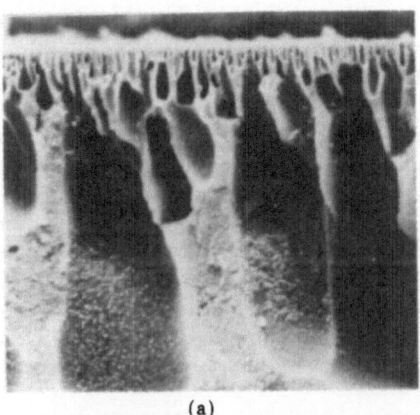 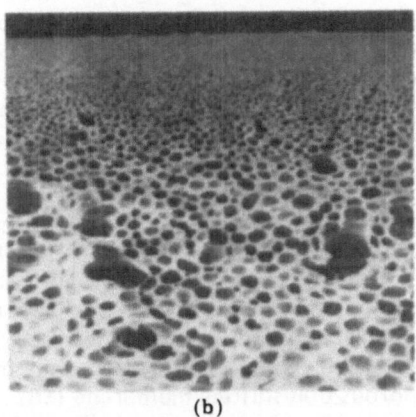

(a)   (b)

Figure 2.   Two Limiting Structures of Phase Inversion Membranes: (a) Finger Type, (b) Sponge
Type (Courtesy of Strathmann (7)).

The most important commercial microporous method. Both symmetric and
asymmetric membranes can be obtained. A wide variety of polymers, mostly cellulose
esters (e.g. CA, CN or CA + CN), and also PC, PVC, PAmids, PAcetal, PVF, PAcrylates,
cross-linked PVA, etc. can be used to prepare heterogeneous membranes by this
method. These membranes are used in microfiltration, ultrafiltration, reverse osmosis,
gas permeation, artificial kidney systems, drug delivery systems, etc.

Sintering. Sintered membranes are most simple symmetric membranes with
low porosity (10-40 %) which are made from metal, metal oxides or polymer powders
(2,10). In producing these microporous membranes by sintering process, finely divided
particles (spherical or fibrous in shape) are heated to a temperature at or below the
melting range of the material. As the exterior surface of the particles softens or melts
capillary pressure tends to rearrange the solid matrix. Sintered membranes have
irregular pore structure with an average pore diameter in the range of 0.05 to 100 μm.
The particle size of the initial powder is the main parameter determining the pore
sizes of the final membrane. PE, PP and PTFE are the polymers used most to prepare sintered membranes. They are used for filtration at elevated temperatures,
filtration of suspensions and aggressive solutions, air filtration, gas separation, etc.

Stretching. This procedure is also used to obtain microporous symmetric membranes (2,11,12). They are prepared by extrusion from polymer particles. The homogeneous films are then stretched perpendicular to the direction of extrusion. Thus,
permanent fractures (micropores) are induced in the film. The porosity of these membranes is very high (up to 90 %). The pores are relatively uniform and their average
diameter is in the order of 0.01 − 20 μm. These membranes exhibit good chemical,
thermal and mechanical stabilities. They are mostly hydrophobic, but with further
treatments wettable surfaces are also achieved. Partially crystalline polymers (e.g.
PE, PP, PTFE) are used to prepare this type of membranes. They are used for air
filtration, filtration of organic solutions, in membrane oxygenators, in drug delivery
systems, as vascular grafts, etc.

Track-Etching: Another relatively new procedure for preparing microporous
symmetric membranes is based on a process of irradiating a thin polymer film in the
field of α-particles and then etching the film chemically to produce essentially
straight through circular pores (tortuosity = 1) (13,14). These membranes are available

in pore sizes ranging from 0.03 to 8 μm. Polycarbonate and polyester films are usually used. With their very uniform thickness and pore size, they have found application in gravimetric aerosol filtration; microscopic analysis; blood rheology studies; artifical organs; steril filtration of biological solutions, etc.

Other methods. There are of course, many different procedures available to prepare heterogeneous membranes (2,4). Among these interesting approaches, most credit is given to the methods for preparation of composite membranes. They are now an important class of asymmetric, skin type, microporous membranes. They are prepared by depositing a very thin film (layer) onto the surface of a suitable, finely porous substrate. Skin layer gives permselectivity and substrate gives strength. There are exciting methods to make such kinds of membranes. One of them is based on interfacial polymerization of polyethylene imine with toluene diisocynate. This cross-linked structure creates a very thin membrane (250 - 500 Å) on the surface of finely porous polysulfone membrane (15).

Ionotropic gels are another group of heterogeneous membranes (4,16). They are prepared from polyelectrolyte sols containing polyanions (e.g. carboxymethyl-cellulose, alginic acid) or polycations (e.g. polyethyleneamine) by coagulation (or gelation) with electrolyte solutions. The factors which influence the resultant membrane structure are type, pH, and concentration of the electrolyte solution; type, concentration, and chain length of the sol, viscosity and temperature. These membranes have parallel pores, and are characterized by a very narrow pore-size distribution.

Homogeneous Membranes

Homogeneous membranes may be solid or liquid. Usually, a homogeneous membrane consists of a dense film where there are no pores in the structure. Therefore the mass transfer rates are rather low in these membranes. The most important advantage of these membranes is selectivity (which means here solubility). Thus, two species with different solubilities, but identical diffusivities can be separated by using these membranes.

Homogeneous membranes can be made from inorganic materials (e.g. glass, metals) or mostly from polymers (e.g. silicon rubber, PVC, PAN, PS, PVA, PE, PP, nylon 6, silicone-PC copolymer, polyphenyleneoxide). These membranes are generally made by casting from a solution or from a polymer melted by extrusion, blow and press molding (1-5,7). Different procedures may be applied depending on the membrane configuration desired (e.g. films, tubes, hollow fibers). In addition to the fabrication procedure, chemical nature of the polymer might be considered in order to obtain different microcrystalline structures. By changing polymer type (chemistry of backbone and side chains, substituents, etc.) polymer molecular weight, cross-link type, and density; by using mixtures of hydrophobic and hydrophilic polymers, and by including additives, microheterogeneity in the structure can be adjusted leading to membranes with different mass transfer and mechanical properties for specific applications such as gas separation, pervaporation, blood oxygenation, drug delivery, etc.

The most popular homogeneous membranes are ion-exchange membranes. They are charged membranes, which means they have fixed ions in the polymer matrix. Counter-ions, which are called mobile ions, can be bound by these fixed ions. Mobile ions can be exchanged with ions in the surrounding solution, mostly depending on charge and concentration of the specific ions in the solution. Fixed-ion groups are mostly sulfonic and rarely carboxylic, phosphoric, selenoic groups in cation-exchange membranes, and quaternary ammonium, phosphonium, etc. groups in anion-exchange membranes. The base carrier material (matrix) is usually polystyrene-divinylbenzene copolymer. These membranes are generally prepared by dispersing a conventional ion-exchange materials in a polymer matrix; or by polymerization of film-forming ionic monomers; or by introducing ionic groups into a film forming polymer (1,2, 17,18). The main applications of ion-exchange membranes is in electrodialysis and specific membrane electrodes.

STRUCTURE AND TRANSPORT MECHANISMS IN SYNTHETIC MEMBRANES

It has long been recognized that there is a close connection between the type of polymer membrane and the principle transport mechanism. The transport rate through membranes is determined by the driving force, and the concentration and mobility of permeate molecules in the polymer matrix. The concentration is primarily determined by chemical compatibility of the solute and the polymer. The mobility depends on factors such as the temperature the size and shape of solutes, and rather weakly on their chemical compositions as well as on the chemical nature, microstructure and morphology of the polymer.

There are essentially three different kinds of transport through membranes which are illustrated in Figure 3. First is called "passive transport" where membrane acts as a physical barrier. Solutes transfer through the membrane owing to the differences in the chemical potentials of the components on the opposite sides of the membrane, and diffusion takes place in the direction of the gradient. The chemical potential gradient is caused by differences in concentration, hydrostatic pressure, temperature, etc. In the second type of transport i.e. "facilitated" (or "carrier-mediated") transport, a carrier is confined to the membrane phase and interacts with solutes on both sides of the membrane. The carrier provides an additional mechanism of transport through the membrane and, in general, transport of a permeant through the membrane is selectively enhanced. This concept is also fundamental to understanding transmission through biological membranes. In biomembranes, transport is not only carrier-mediated but also "active" which is the third type of transport through membranes. Active transport is very selective and can occur against the gradient. Energy needs for this kind of transport are utilized by the several sources (usually ATP), which exist in the membrane.

Faced with so great a range of interlocking factors it is clear that a completely general treatment of transport through membranes is not easy at the present time. Excellent reviews of the various theoretical expressions of this physical fact have been offered by several investigators (1,19-23). This later section of the paper deals with some fundamental aspects of the structure and passive transport mechanisms in non-ionic membranes, and their formulation. Notice that due to very different behavior, transport through charged membranes is not included in this chapter.

Passive Transport Through Homogeneous Membranes

As mentioned before, structurally two different membranes are employed in membrane processes. Homogeneous membranes, i.e. non-porous membranes are so called because they have no identifiable voidage at colloidal level and species pass through them as if by diffusion through a solid phase. The following diffusion equa-

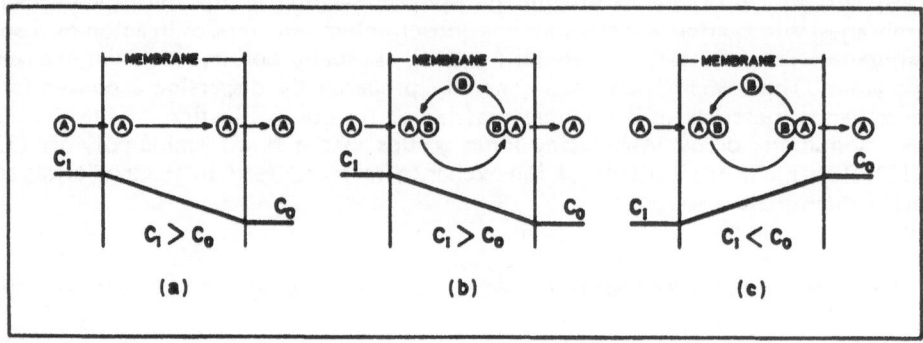

Figure 3. Transport Through Membranes: (a) Passive Transport; (b) Facilitated Transport; (c) Active Transport.

tion (Fick's Second Law) can be used to describe unsteady-state, one dimensional transport through these membranes (24).

$$\frac{\partial c}{\partial t} = \frac{\partial}{\partial x}\left(D \frac{\partial c}{\partial x} \right) \tag{1}$$

D and c are the diffusion coefficient and the concentration of dissolved penetrant, t is time, and x is a direction coordinate. The diffusion at steady-state conditions can be defined by Fick's First Law (by integration of Eq. (1)) (25).

$$J = -D \cdot \frac{dc}{dx} \tag{2}$$

where J is the flux of the penetrant within the polymer film. In this expression, it is assumed that diffusivity (D) is independent of concentration and direction. It is useful to mention here that this is not true, especially for liquid or vapor transport through homogeneous membranes, where solute - polymer interaction is appreciable (26). The solubility of most of the gases in polymer films is low, hence swelling and concentration (and also direction) dependence can be ignored. Thus, Eq. (2) is applicable to gas transport through homogeneous polymeric membranes. Further modifications are needed for vapor or liquid transport. Besides, the situation is further complicated by the fact that the transport of any substance in the membrane may be influenced not only by the presence of other species in the membrane but also gradients other than concentration gradients (e.g. temperature, etc.). These interactions are best discussed using the concepts of nonequilibrium thermodynamics and are not included here (19-23).

Transmission of a gas through a homogeneous membrane is shown diagrammatically in Figure 4. According to this model the so called "solution(or sorbtion)-diffusion" model, the concentration of penetrant in the inferface of the polymer film is related to the solubility and the partial pressure of the penetrant in the gas phase. It is assumed that each face of the membrane is in equilibrium with the gas phase.

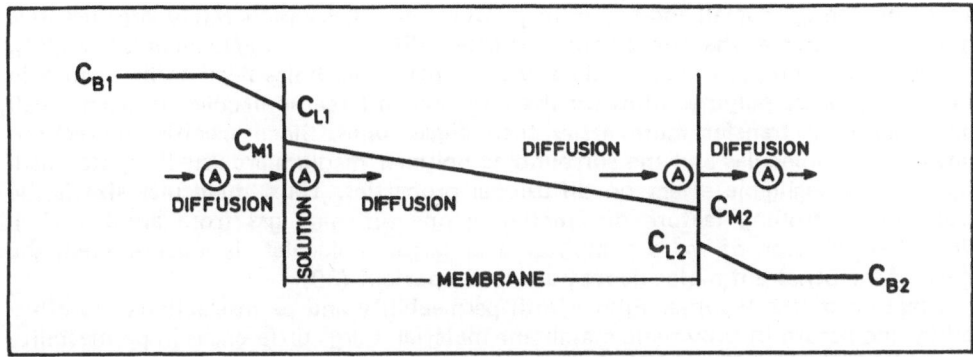

Figure 4.   Gas Transport Through Homogeneous Membranes: Solution - Diffusion Model.

The Henry's law constant (H), appearing in Eq. (3) characterizes the solubility (S) of a gas especially in rubbery state. Combination of Langmuir and Henry's law sorptions was proposed and formulated for the glassy state (27).

$$c = H.p \tag{3}$$

Here H is Henry constant, c and p are permeant concentrations in the polymer film and in the gas phase respectively. Using S instead of H, integration of Eq. (2) and substitution of Eq. (3) gives

$$J = \frac{D\,S}{\Delta x} \cdot \Delta p = \frac{P\Delta p}{\Delta x} \tag{4}$$

where Δx is the membrane thickness, P is "permeability" and Δp is the pressure gradient of the permeating component across the membrane. There is a considerable amount of permeability data in the literature. The parameters D,S, and P can be readily measured for simple gases by means of several methods, like the well-known time-lag method (28).

The solution-diffusion model is also employed for reverse osmosis where a symmetric membranes with homogeneous skins are used (29). In this process water or other liquids permeate through the membrane by the difference between the applied hydrostatic pressure and the osmotic pressure and the flux can be represented by

$$J_w = L_p (\Delta p - \sigma \Delta \pi) \tag{5}$$

Here J_w is water flux; L_p is the permeability coefficent; Δp and $\Delta \pi$ are the hydrostatic and the osmotic pressure gradients; and σ is the reflection coefficient.

There are several parameters which are effective on the transport through homogeneous membranes. Let us discuss them very briefly.

Temperature : Diffusion in polymeric membranes is an activated process, and in general both diffusivity and permeability increase with temperature, but when the activation energy is small and the enthalpy of solution has a moderately large negative value, P decreases as the temperature increases (diffusion through silicones) (20,23).

Nature of Gas : It is generally accepted that larger holes need to be formed in the homogeneous polymer films for the diffusion of larger molecules. It means small molecules may transfer more easily than bigger ones. Since specific interactions between gas molecules and the surrounding polymer medium are usually quite small, they have a negligible effect on diffusional properties. Thus, molecular size is the main rate-controlling feature differentiating one diffusing gas from another (27). When the diffusion of more complicated or larger molecules is encountered, the shape of the penetrant molecule may also be important (30).

Nature of the Polymer Film : Both permeability and permselectivity are affected by the nature of polymeric membrane material. Large differences in permeability are attributable to differences in interchain displacement and flexibility which in turn are causally related to intramolecular energy (chain flexibility, or chain stiffness) and intermolecular energy (cohesive energy). Chain flexibility and cohesive energy are two important parameters which affect diffusion inversely. Higher diffusivities are obtained by both increasing chain flexibility and decreasing cohesive energy.Both changes in polarity and steric effects result in changes in the chain flexibility and/or cohesive energy, hence leading to differences in transport properties (27,31).

Cross-linking (length of cross-linker, and cross-link density), the degree of crystallinity, additives (such as plasticizers, fillers, etc.) are also effective on the diffusion process. In general, as the degree of cross-linking increases, the chain flexibility and hence diffusion decreases (27,32-36).

Highly crystalline polymeric membranes are usually less permeable than amorphous ones.Percent crystallinty, crystalline size and orientation influence the mass transfer properties of the membranes (35-37). It should also be kept in mind that the crystalline and amorphous ratio is of great importance to the mechanical properties.

Crystalline regions in polymeric membranes exhibit resistance to plastic flow (or deformation). Like crystalline regions, fillers and other particle type additives introduce a heterogeneity at the microcrystalline level into the homogeneous polymer matrices.The geometry (shape, size and size distribution), concentration and concentration distribution, orientation, topology, composition, and other properties of the disperse phase is significantly effective on the transport through these membranes.

Usually, addition of a plasticizer to a polymer decreases the cohesive forces between the chains resulting in an increase in segmental mobility, hence, an increase in both diffusivity and permeability(34). In many polymer systems, water is an effective plasticizer. Polymers which swell greatly in water always have increasing diffusivity with increasing relative humidity (27,39).

Sorption and diffusion of vapors and liquids through homogeneous membranes are very complex problems, due to significant interactions between the permeates and the polymeric material. It is generally accepted that diffusion of vapors and liquids changes not only with their concentrations in the polymer matrix, but also is related to the concentration history at a special point.Diffusivity increases with the concentration of permeate in the membrane. Diffusion increases with temperature exponentially, which is more marked for the diffusion of larger molecules.The shape of the diffusant molecule is also important. Flexible molecules diffuse more easily. The diffusion of vapors and liquids is affected in the same way as the diffusion of simple gas molecules by changes in the nature of the polymer.However,it should be pointed that water is a very special character in homogeneous polymer films due to its high hydrogen bonding ability (23,27). Water diffusion through hydrophilic polymer films is the same as other liquid-polymer systems. However, the diffusion coefficient of water in hydrophobic membranes decreases with increasing water concentration in the matrix (e.g. silicone), just the opposite to other liquids. This is usually explained by the clustering (or polymerization) of water in the polymer. Permeability is almost constant even though the diffusion constant decreases.

Passive Transport Through Heterogeneous Membranes

As mentioned above a heterogoneous membrane has interconnected voidage or pores through which species can pass through. There are several theoretical models to determine or explain the transport properties and mechanisms within the heterogeneous (microporous) membranes. These models assume sieve-like behaviour, which means species are retained depending on the particle size cutoff of the membrane. This is simply a sieving mechanism according to the size of particles (Fig. 5). Permeability and permselectivity within these membranes depend on the pore size and pore size distribution of the membrane as well as particle size, shape, charge, and maybe the chemistry of the particle.

The phenomenological equations to describe membrane processes can be written in terms of the differences in composition, pressure and temperature between the solutions on the other side of the membrane. These equations are integrated over the membrane to determine the average flows and forces.

There are three important expressions as partial differential equation of continuity (conservation of mass), the equation of motion (conservation of momentum), and the equation of energy (conservation of energy) (40). According to the membrane processes, by making the necessary assumptions, these partial differential equations can be simplified and integrated in order to find the relations between the fluxes and the driving forces.

In most of the membrane processes, the equation of continuity and the equation of motion are solved simultaneously. If the solution behaves as an incompressible Newtonian fluid of constant density, ρ, and constant viscosity, μ, and if the flow velocities are low and are in a laminar region, the Navier-Stokes equation can be employed. This equation is obtained by simplification of the equation of motion (by means of the equation of continuity), and is given below.

$$\rho \frac{Dv}{Dt} = -\nabla p + \mu \nabla^2 v + \rho g \tag{6}$$

| mass per unit volume times acceleration | pressure force on element per unit volume | viscose force on element per unit volume | gravitational force on element per unit volume |

This equation, again, is not solved by analytical methods, hence further assumptions are need for applications in modelling of membrane processes. The simplest model for transport through a porous medium (like microporous membranes) is an assembly of straight circular capillary tubes in which all capillaries are parallel and equal length. When the Navier-Stokes Equation is integrated for the laminar, unidirectional flow of isothermal fluid through a straight circular capillary of radius ,r, and length, l, Hagen-Poiseuille's equation is obtained. The assumptions that are implied in the derivation of this equation are : (a) The flow is laminar, Newtonian

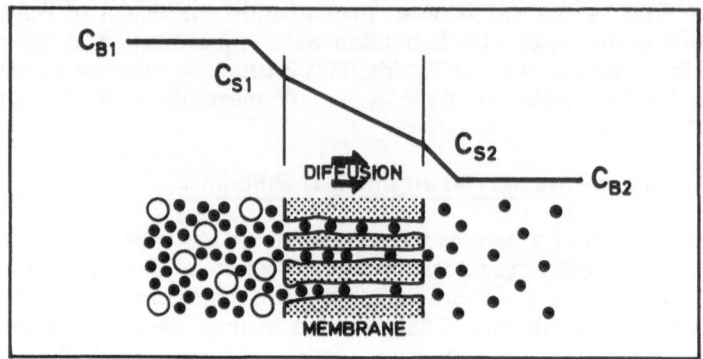

Figure 5.   Sieve - Like Transport Through Heterogeneous Membranes.

and steady state; (b) the density is constant; (c) end effects are neglected; and (d) fluid behaves as a continium.

$$J = \frac{\pi r^4}{8 \mu \ell} \cdot \Delta p \qquad (7)$$

If the number of pores per unit area is N, and the liquid content of porous structure is expressed as ε ($\varepsilon = N \pi r^2$) which is called the void fraction (or porosity), Eq. (7) can be written as follows

$$J = \frac{\varepsilon A r^2}{8 \mu \ell} \cdot \Delta p \qquad (8)$$

Here, A is the total cross-sectional area of the assembly normal to the flow direction, J is the convective transport rate (flux) of solution resulting from a pressure difference (Δp) across the membrane. If the first group at the right side of the equation is lumped together into a membrane constant (P_H), the following expression is obtained.

$$J = P_H \cdot \Delta p \qquad (9)$$

Here, P_H may be called the hydrodynamic permeability of the membrane. Notice that this form of the equation is exactly the same as Darcy's equation Darcy's Law is generally obeyed for the flow of a fluid through a porous medium and can be derived again from the equations of continuity and the equation of motion. Hydrodynamic permeability is replaced by Darcy's Law permeability of the membrane as given below.

$$J = P_D \cdot \Delta p \qquad (10)$$

To carry the capillary anology further, microporous membranes may be assumed as consisting of porous assemblies of solid particles which characterize the polymer matrix. The specific surface area A_o of the particles can be defined as,

$$A_o = \frac{\text{surface area of the solid particles}}{\text{volume of the solid particles}} \qquad (11)$$

We can combine this definition with the modified Hagen-Poiseuille formula to obtain

$$J = \frac{\varepsilon A}{K A_o^2 (1-\varepsilon) \ell} \cdot \Delta p \tag{12}$$

This equation is called the Kozeny-Carman equation, and K is known as the Kozeny constant. Again, the same treatment can be repeated for this equation and the terms in the right side (except Δp) can be lumped together in a membrane permeability constant which may be determined experimentally :

$$J = P_{KC} \cdot \Delta p \tag{13}$$

The pore models discussed above are suitable for ultrafiltration, microfiltration where the selectivity of a porous membrane is a consequence of its sieve-like behaviour, and the driving force is the pressure difference.

If solute rejection by the membrane is significant, osmotic pressure must also be considered, like in reverse osmosis where microporous asymmetric membranes can be employed. The water flux in these systems is proportional to the difference between the applied hydrostatic pressure and the osmotic pressure (Eq. (5)).

When there is no hydrostatic pressure difference across the membrane, if the chemical potential gradient is utilized only by the concentration difference for species (such as in dialysis) solute transport can be given as the following equation:

$$J = P_m \cdot \Delta c \tag{14}$$

Where J is the solute flux, Δc is the concentration difference across the membrane and Pm is the membrane permeability.

Another general expression to evaluate the mass transfer properties of microporous membranes is Knudsen equation. It can be noticed that as in the derivation of Hagen-Poiseuille's formula, it is assumed that the fluid behaves as a continuum. This assumption is not valid if the molecular mean free path of the permeate molecules is comparable to the pore diameter. Knudsen's formula, which is employed in calculating gas transfer rates through microporous membranes at certain conditions, is as follows :

$$J = \frac{4}{3} \cdot r \, \varepsilon \cdot \left(\frac{2 \, RT}{\pi M}\right)^{1/2} \cdot \frac{\Delta p}{\ell \ RT} \tag{15}$$

Where J is the molar flux. This equation again can be simplified and expressed as follows;

$$J = P_K \cdot \Delta p \tag{16}$$

here, P_K is the proportionality constant and is related to membrane permeability.

Conclusion

The phenomena arising across a membrane separating two fluids (gas or liquid) of different concentration are considered by focusing on the transport through membrane matrix. However, the design equations for calculation of mass transfer through membranes must include the transport mechanisms in the adjacent solutions and interfacial resistance to mass transfer at fluid-membrane interfaces. Whatever the nature of the diffusing species, a feature common to all these diffusion processes is the role the fluid films adhering to the membrane faces play in controlling the overall rates of permeation of the species across the membrane. The resistances at both sides of the membrane surface have an important contribution in order to lead to an overestimation of the specific permeation rates in membrane processes. Usually, in studies involving diffusion, the bulk solutions on either side of the membrane are kept very well stirred. Despite this, the existance of a fluid zone of finite thickness on either side is accepted. Under these conditions, the total mass transfer rates may be controlled either by the membrane or by the fluid layer. Generally it is agreed that the layer across which the slowest rate of flow occurs determines the overall rate of diffusion. Besides these extreme conditions, both resistances might be effective on controlling the rate of permeation across the membrane. Without going any further, it can be concluded that all parameters which do influence the diffusion in these adjacent fluid films must be taken into consideration for an effective module design where either homogeneous or heterogeneous membranes are employed.

REFERENCES

1. Lakshminarayanaiah, N., Transport Phenomena in Membranes, Academic Press, New York, 1969.
2. Keller, P.R., Membrane Technology and Industrial Separation Techniques, Noyes Data Corporation, New Jersey, 1976.
3. Rogers, C.E., Permselective Membranes, Marcel Dekker, New York, 1971.
4. Kesting, R.E., Synthetic Polymeric Membranes, McGraw-Hill, New York, 1971.
5. Hwang, S.T. and Kammermeyer, Membranes in Separations, John Wiley & Sons, New York, 1975.
6. Sourirajan, S., Reverse Osmosis and Synthetic Membranes, National Research Council, Ottawa, Canada, 1977.
7. Strathmann, H., J. Memb. Sci., 9:121, 1981.
8. Loeb, S. and Sourirajan, S., Ad. Chem. Ser., 38:117, 1962.
9. Strathman, H., Kock, K., Amar, P. and Baker, R.W., Desalination, 16:179, 1975.
10. Nordberg, M.E., J. Amer. Chem. Soc., 27:299, 1944.
11. Bierenbaum, H.S., Isaacson, R.B., Druin, M.L. and Plovan, S.G., Ind. Eng. Chem. Prod. Res. Develop., 13:2, 1974.
12. Gore, R.W., U.S. Patent, 3, 953, 566, April 27, 1976.
13. Fleischer, R.L., Brice, P.B. and Walker, R.M., Science, 149:383, 1965.
14. Price, P.B. and Walker, R.M., U.S. Patent, 3, 303, 085, February 7, 1967.
15. Cadotte, J.E., U.S. Patent, 4, 039, 440, August 2, 1977.
16. Thiele, H. and Hallich, K., Kolloid Z., 163:115, 1959.
17. Wyllie, M.R.J. and Patnode, H.W., J. Phys. Colloid. Chem, 54:204, 1950.
18. Juda, W. and McRae, W.A., J. Amer. Chem. Soc., 72:1044, 1950.
19. Kedem, O. and Katchalsky, J. Gen. Physiol., 45:143, 1961.
20. Crank, J. and Park, G.S., Diffusion in Polymers, Academic Press, New York, 1968.
21. McGregor, R., Diffusion and Sorption in Fibers and Films, Academic Press, London, 1974.

22. Meares, P., Membrane Separation Processes, Elsevier Scientific Publ. Co., Amsterdam, 1976.
23. Sweeting, O.J., The Science and Technology of Polymer Films, Vols. I.II, Wiley-Interscience, New York, 1976.
24. Crank, J., The Mathematics of Diffusion, Clarendon Press, Oxford, 1975.
25. Fick, A., Pogg. Ann., 94:59, 1855.
26. Harris, F.W. and Seymour, R.B., Structure-Solubility Relationships in Polymers, Academic Press, Inc., New York, 1977.
27. Park, G.S., in Characterization of Coatings: Physical Techniques, R.R. Myers and J.S. Long, eds., pp. 473, Marcel Dekker, New York, 1976.
28. Daynes, H.A., Proc. Roy. Soc., Ser. A., 94:286, 1920.
29. Lonsdale, H.K., Merten, U., Riley, R.L., J. Appl. Polym. Sci., 9:1341, 1965.
30. Stannett, V., in Diffusion in Polymers, J. Crank and G.S. Park, eds., Chap. 2, Academic Press, New York, 1968.
31. van Amerongen, G.J., J. Polym. Sci., 5:307, 1950.
32. Barrer, R.M. and Skirrow, G., J. Polym. Sci., 3:549, 1948.
33. Barrer, R.M., Barrie, J.A. and Wong, P.S.—L., Polymer, 9:609, 1968.
34. Barrer, R.M., Mallinder, R. and Wong, P.S.—L., Polymer, 8:321, 1967.
35. Barrer, R.M., in Diffusion in Polymers, J. Crank and G.S. Park, eds., Chap. 6, Academic Press, New York, 1968.
36. Barrer, R.M. and Chio, H.T., J. Polym. Sci., 10:111, 1965.
37. van Amerongen, G.J., Rubber Chem. Tech., 37:1065, 1964.
38. Barrie, J.A. and Machin, D., J. Macromol. Sci. Phys., 3:673, 1969.
39. Ito, Y., Kobunshi Kagaku, 18:158, 1961.
40. Bird, R.B., Stewart, W.E. and Lightfoot, E.N., Transport Phenomena, John Wiley &Sons, Inc., New York, 1960.

SYNTHETIC POLYMERIC MEMBRANES: SEPARATION VIA MEMBRANES

E. Piskin

Hacettepe University, Chemical Engineering Department, Ankara, Turkey

INTRODUCTION

Membrane separation has recently been added to the available separation processes. Improvements over the recent years have greatly enhanced its attractive economics and applicability. It has already captured the attention of several industries such as chemical technology, pharmaceutical, medical and food industries, biotechnology, water purification and demineralizations, etc. Many new applications for today's membranes are opening new horizons in the research, clinical and processing fields.

Membrane processes offer significant advantages over conventional separation techniques, i.e. distillation, sorption, crystallization, extraction, etc. They are modest in their energy requirements. They do not produce waste products. They have acceptable recoveries and product purities. In most cases they are more economical, more efficient and relatively faster. Separation can be performed at moderate feed temperatures.

The literature bearing upon the membrane separation processes is enormous and widely spread over different fields. There are excellent reviews and books dealing with these processes. This chapter covers conventional, or most common, membrane processes in general. It is aimed, here, to discuss the fundamental aspects of the membrane processes, namely microfiltration, ultrafiltration, reverse osmosis, dialysis, electrodialysis, gas permeation and pervaporation. To this extent it is hoped that this chapter will give a basic knowledge about the membrane separation techniques, as well as essential differences between them.

MICROFILTRATION

Fundamentals

The general concept of filtration is to remove unwanted or harmful contaminants from a flow of a gas or a liquid by mechanical means. A pressure gradient is usually

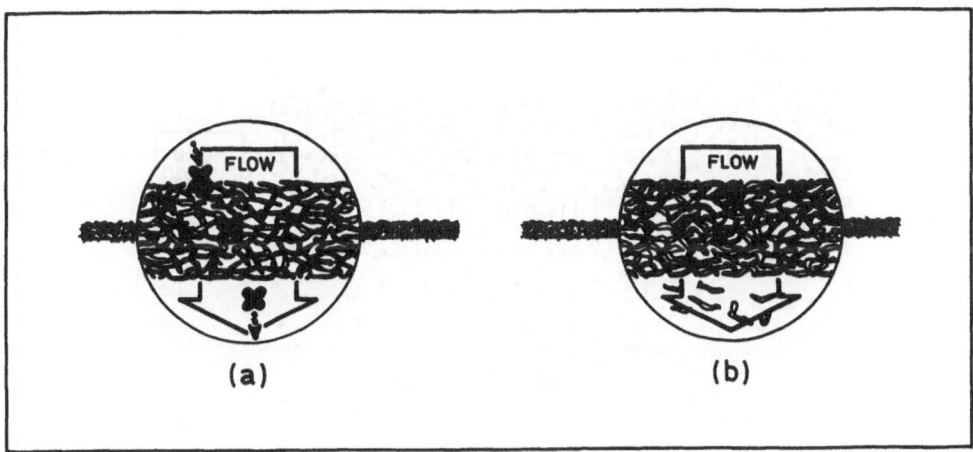

Figure 1.   Depth Filters: (a) Filtration; (b) Media Migration.

applied in order to maintain a fluid flow through the filtration media.

Conventional filters, so called depth filters are composed of a random mat of fibers, such as glass fibers, asbestos ceramics and metals, often bound together with resins (Fig. 1). Fiber filters rely upon the depth of the fiber mat to trap particles. Particles entering a depth filter stop at the point where resistance encountered is equal to the driving force. High fluid velocities or pressures can allow to drive them deeper in the filter. This mode of particle capture is called a depth retention. In other words, particles do not only accumulate at the feed side surface of the filtrate, but also are arrested within the medium. These conventional filters have an important limitation, as they always exhibit media migration. Fibers, particles or fragments can escape during filtration. Although, because they are less expensive than other filters, they are employed today usually as prefilters prior to a final filter in order to enhance the final filter service life.

Membrane filters are usually plastic films with pores or holes of controlled size. Particles that are larger than even the largest pores of the pore-size distribution of a microfiltration membrane are retained upon its surface with absolute efficiency. This mode is likely characterized as sieve-type retention (Fig. 2). The pore diameter determines the degree of separation. Neither the number of particles, nor the magnitude of the applied differential pressure have an important effect. The main advantage of membrane filters is that these filters do not contain fibers which can work loose during filtration and contaminate the filtrate. Membrane filters consist of about 20 % volume of solid, the rest of the volume is pore space or void. Due to their highly porous structure, membrane filters offer high flow rates.

Solvent flux (J) through a microfiltration membrane is usually expressed in terms of the hydrostatic pressure difference across the membrane (Δp) and the hydrodynamic resistance of the membrane (Rm).

$$J = \frac{\Delta p}{R_m} \tag{1}$$

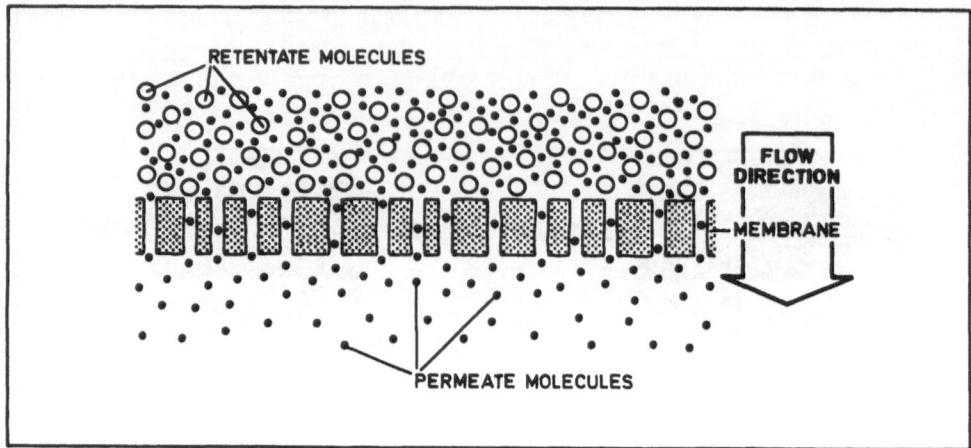

Figure 2.　Sieve-Like Retention.

According to the type of the membrane, several factors such as pressure, membrane area, viscosity, temperature, type and concentration of the suspended substances, and application and condition of a prefilter, influence the flow rate (1). In microfiltration, the suspended particles which are increasingly retained by the membrane gradually block its pores. This results in a progressive lessening of the rate of solvent flow. In order to maintain a constant solvent flow, the applied pressure should be increased.

Microfiltration usually employs symmetric microporous membranes having pores with nominal size rating in the range of 0.2 to 10 μm (200 to 100,000 Å). According to molecular weight designation MF membranes retain substances typically in the molecular weight (MW) range between 300 and 300,000. Therefore, microfiltration is carried out comparatively lower than applied differential pressures in the range of 0.1 to 2 bar (or 2 to 30 psi).

Membranes and Filtration Systems

The earliest microfiltration membranes were developed by Richard Zsigmondy (Nobel Prize winner) (2). They were made from cellulose acetate and cellulose nitrate by a solvent, casting procedure. Following this original technique, symmetric, heterogeneous microfiltration membranes with rated pore size and pore size distribution were prepared from cellulose derivatives and are now manufactured by several companies. Besides cellulosic membranes, today, membranes which are made of polypropylene, polycarbonate, acrylic copolymers, polyvinyl chloride, polyamide, polytetrafluoroethylene and polyvinylidene are utilized for microfiltration. These membranes are made by quite different procedures such as streching, track-etching and others (3-7).

Filtration through membrane filters is maintained by either positive pressure or vacuum systems. In general, pressure filtration is employed in process applications (production) in contrast to vacuum systems which are utilized for analytical applications (quality control).

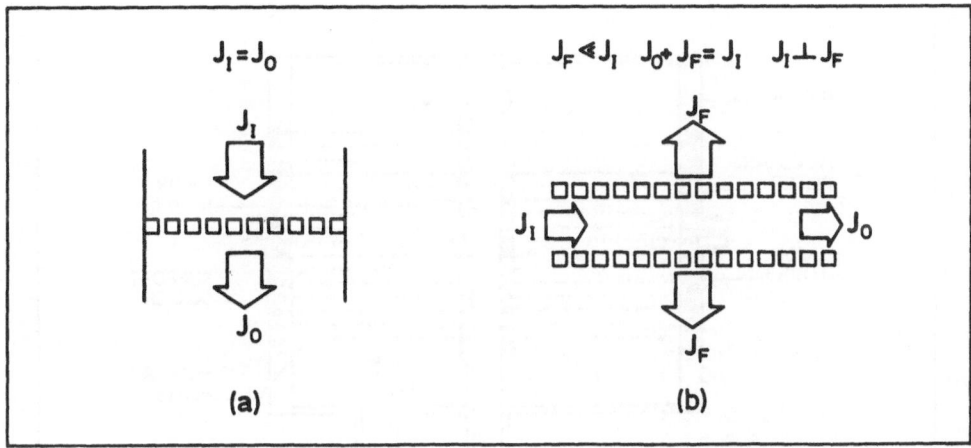

Figure 3.   Microfiltration: (a) Through Flow Filtration; (b) Cross Flow Filtration.

Microfiltration is applied either in batch fashion or in continuous fashion. Two types of physical microfiltration are in use (Fig. 3): (a) Through flow filtration (Dead-end); (b) cross flow filtration. In through flow filtration, permeate and feed flow directions are the same. It is an inherently unsteady-state operation and usually requires backwashing. Filtrate flows in a perpendicular direction to that of the feed flow in cross flow filtration. Particulate accumulation on the surface of the membrane may be controlled rather easily by shear induced by the feed flow.

The plate-and-frame modules utilizing discs of membrane material are one of the most widely used desings of systems on the microfiltration market (Fig.4a).Very high filtration rates (up to 10,000 gallons per hour) can be achieved with these units. However, the equipment and the maintaining costs are high. The pleated cartridge configuration is the other most commonly used system design (Fig. 4b). Membrane pleating enables the cartridge to contain a high surface area per unit size. Compounding of cartridges in a single housing offers flow rates to meet almost any industrial need, with relatively low cost.

Applications

The history of the application of the microfiltration was started with the bacteriological analysis of water (8). Today, there are numerous analytical applications as well as large scale industrial applications. The world wide market size (about 300 million/ year in 1982) is half of the total market for pressure-driven membrane processes, i.e. microfiltration, ultrafiltration and reverse osmosis. (1,9-11). The technologically important applications of microfiltration are given below.

- Production of ultrapure water for electronic industry in order to control contamination problems in all phases of fabrication.
- Clarification and sterile filtration of pharmaceutical, medical and biological, heat sensitive solutions and beverages.

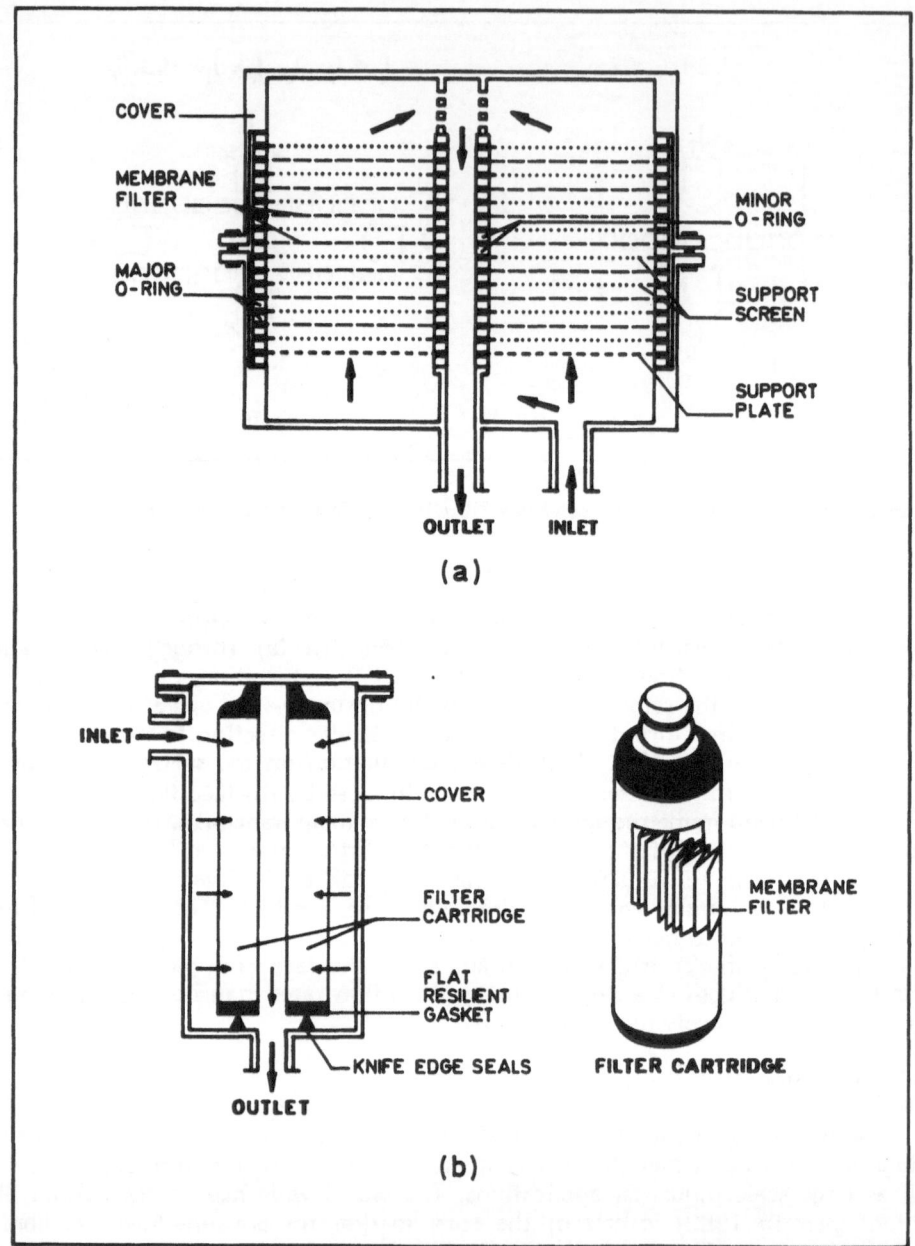

Figure 4.   Microfiltration Modules: (a) Plate - and - Frame Module; (b) Pleated Cartridge.

— Removal of particles from gas and liquid streams for chemical, food, pharmaceutical and biological industries, as well as for several analytical applications.
— Product purification, process solvent recovery, gas filtration, and environmental analysis in chemical industry and in biotechnology.
— Microbiological, analytical and biological control.

ULTRAFILTRATION

Fundamentals

Ultrafiltration (UF) is membrane separation process which is grouped together with two other pressure-driven filtration processes, namely reverse osmosis (RO) and microfiltration (MF) (9-15). In these three distinct levels of filtration processes, the liquid being treated is brought into contact with a membrane which allows preferential passage of the solvent or certain dissolved species under a driving force of hydrostatic pressure difference. Ultrafiltration covers the zone between the other two processes; the solvent and the solutes of low molecular weight can pass through the membrane whereas the solute particles of larger molecular dimensions are retained. Ultrafilters are used for removal of species ranging in size from 0.001 μm (10 Å) to 0.02 μm (200 Å). According to molecular weight designations, UF membranes retain substances typically in the molecular weight (MW) range between 300 and 300,000. In contrast to RO where molecules with MWs greater than about 300 as well as with MWs less than 300 are retained, UF membranes are freely permeable to molecules with MWs of 1000. In other words, UF membranes exhibit low rejection for osmotic pressure generating solutes (e.g. salts) which are roughly 5-20%. Therefore, it is agreed that UF membranes act as molecular screens that reject substances at the membrane solution interface, with retention or cutoff levels expressed in terms of molecular weight. Notice that microfiltration membranes are also MW cutoff (or sieve-type) membranes, but with different range of applications. It should also be noted that the lines of differentiations between these three regimes of filtration are not sharp, and the classification is rather arbitrary.

Ultrafiltration membranes can be characterized by their cutoff, i.e. their capability to retain larger molecules than those of stated size and to pass smaller species as well as solvent. It must be noted that, however, the rated cutoff is not an accurate value but an approximation. Like microfiltration membranes, UF membranes are microporous membranes with a pore size distribution (except track-etching membranes) as shown in Figure 5. Diffuse molecular weight cutoffs are usually observed, rather than sharp cutoffs (Fig. 6), which means precise separation is not achieved in most cases, especially in the case of macromolecules. Such factors as molecular size, charge and shape determine the extent of rejection, or passage, of substances by the ultrafiltration membrane. When total rejection is required a membrane with cutoff well below the desired solute should be selected.

From a practical point of view, UF is further differentiated from RO and MF by the level of applied transmembrane pressure. As mentioned above, osmotic effects are small in UF. Besides, UF membranes are highly porous and have extremely high water permeability, hence ultrafilters operate at modest pressures, generally between 1 to 7 bar (or 15 to 100 psi). Solvent fluxes typically achieved in these filters are in the range of 10 to 200 liters / m^2. hr.

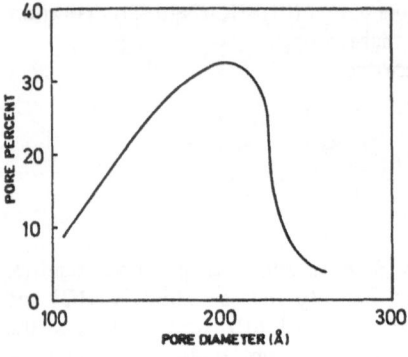

Figure 5.   Pore Size Distribution.

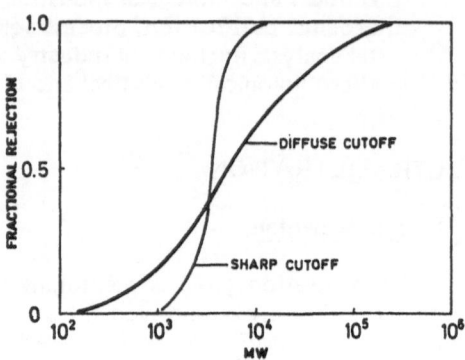

Figure 6.   Molecular Weight Cutoff.

Transport Properties

The separation mechanism in UF membranes, like in MF membranes, is based on a sieving effect under an applied pressure gradient. Various models of the sieving process have been proposed to explain the variations observed and to determine the design characteristics of these membranes (9-15). Early models are based on Hagen-Poiseuille's law, where filtration flux increases almost linearly with increasing the hydrostatic pressure difference as shown in Figure 7 in arbitrary units, and the filtration rate through the membrane can be expressed as given in Eq. (1). However, especially when macromolecules are being treated, due to concentration polarization phenomenon these models are not valid (16-19). At low applied pressures, the filtrate flux rises linearly with the hydrostatic pressure difference. But as the transmembrane pressure increases, the filtrate flux increases rather slowly and finally reaches a with a plateau value.With further increase in applied pressure no change in flux is observed.

The conventional model encountered the concentration polarization in ultra-filtration can be described by using Figure 8. During ultrafiltration of any solution containing a retained solute, a region of high solute concentration, a so called concentration polarization appears at the upstream (or feed) surface of the membrane. In this pre-gel polarized region, there is a solute back transport from the membrane through the bulk of the feed. The total resistance to mass transfer is equal to the sum of the boundary-layer fluid film resistance and the membrane resistance. The permeate flux rises linearly in this pre-gel region. Further increase in the local concentration of rejected solutes on the surface eventually lead, to the formation of a gel layer which resists the passage of solvent and acts as a secondary membrane. This situation is called the gel polarized region. At this point the limiting filtrate flux has been reached, and it does not change with transmembrane pressure. The following expression derived from the boundary-layer models are used to formularize the solvent flux for total reflection cases:

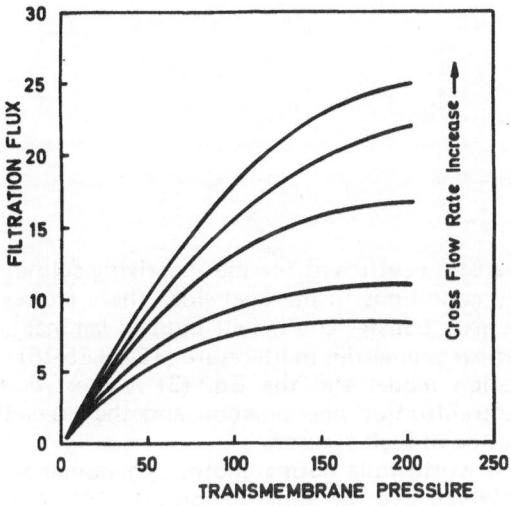

Figure 7. Filtration Flux Versus Transmembrane Pressure in UF Membranes.

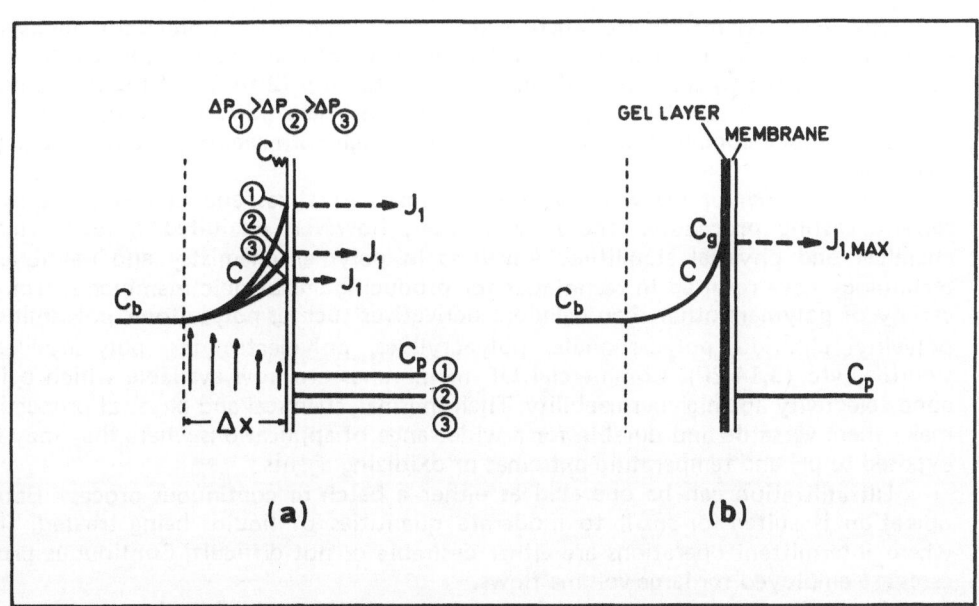

Figure 8. Concentration Polarization in UF.

for pre-gel region:

$$J_w = K.\ln \frac{C_w}{C_b} \qquad (2)$$

for gel region:

$$J_w = K.\ln \frac{C_g}{C_b} \qquad (3)$$

Here K is the mass transfer coefficient for the polarizing solute, and is evaluated for various hydrodynamic conditions in the feed side. There are several empirical equations to correlate the mass transfer coefficient both in laminar and in turbulent flow regimes, for different flow geometries in literature (12,13,15-19).

The gel polarization model and the Eq. (3) is most commonly used in the explanation of the ultrafiltration phenomenon and the prediction of filtrate flux, but it is unlikely to not be of high accuracy.

At this point it is worthwhile noting another phenomenon, membrane fouling, which is usually considered with gel polarization (18, 19). The limiting permeation flux is time-dependent, or in other words, declines steadily with time. This observable trend is called membrane fouling, which is not simply explained in terms of gelation, but rather may be due to changes in the chemical nature of the gel layer with time.

These adverse effects can not be eliminated completely, but may be controlled by maintaining high flow rates and by creating secondary flows at the feed side surface of the membrane.

Membranes and Modules

Ultrafiltration membranes are heterogeneous, symmetric, or preferentially asymmetric in structure. These asymmetric (or anisotropic) membranes consist of a very thin (0.1 to 1.5 μm) skin layer of finely porous texture (2 to 100 Å) upon a much thicker (50 to 250 μm) layer of highly porous body. The skin and porous structures provide a unique combination of permselectivity, high permeability, and non-clogging characteristics.

Early UF membranes were made of cellulose derivatives, and were prepared by a solvent casting procedure. These membranes, however, exhibited limited thermal, chemical and physical stabilities. Advances in polymer chemistry and membrane technology have resulted in techniques for producing anisotropic membranes from a variety of polymers other than cellulose derivatives such as polysulfone, polyamides, polyvinyl chloride, polycarbonate, polyacrylates, polyelectrolytes, polyvinylidene flouride, etc (3,14,20). Commercial UF membranes are now available which offer good selectivity and high permeability. Their thermal, chemical and physical properties make them versatile and durable for a wide range of applications where they may be exposed to pH and temperature extremes or oxidizing agents.

Ultrafiltration can be operated as either a batch or continuous process. Batch operation is suited for small to moderate quantities of liquids being treated, and where intermittent operations are either desirable or not difficult. Continuous processes are employed for large volume flows.

As mentioned before, two basic system are employed in filtration processes. In the dead-end approach, a stirring assembly is also installed for minimizing concentra-

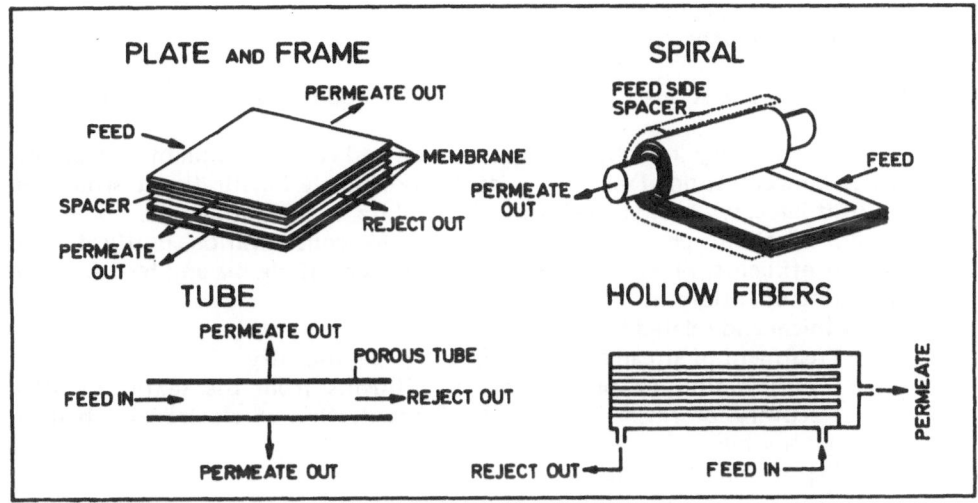

Figure 9. UF Module Design.

tion build-up near membrane surface. This batch-type UF cell is found particularly useful for the treatment of relatively small volumes(up to 10 liters) of dilute solutions (0.01 to 5 % solids by weight). For higher capacites, cross-flow approach which utilizes usually modular structures is used. In this approach, the fluid is channeled over the membrane and progressively depleted of solvent as well as microsolutes. It is important, here, to ensure a sufficient flow rate past the membrane surface in order to control the formation of concentration polarization layer. Recirculation of the feed flow is usually needed in order to satisfy minimum flow requirements.

Today, there are four different basic module designs used in large scale ultrafiltration units (Fig. 9). In tubular modules, the fluid flow can be adjusted and, thus, concentration polarization and membrane fouling can rather easily be controlled, and they can be also easily be cleaned. However, these units have relatively high investment and operating costs. The plate-and-frame modules provide a larger membrane area per unit module volume than the tubular modules, but it is difficult to control the concentration polarization. Costs are generally lower than tubular units. The other two module designs, namely spiral-wound and hollow fiber units,seem generally not to be suitable for ultrafiltration. They provide very high membrane surface area per module volume (up to 1200 m^2 / m^3), and investment and operating costs are low. However, clogging, concentration polarization and membrane fouling are severe problems associated with these modules.

Applications

Ultrafiltration membranes have found many analytical applications in laboratory scales such as:

— Concentration of proteins, enzymes, viruses, hormones, etc.
— Separation of proteins, hormones, nucleic acids, etc.

— Purification of proteins, enzymes, etc.
— Clinical and biochemical analyses

Ultrafiltration is also used for a large variety of applications in many industries.

— In food and diary industries for purification and concentration of macromolecules, concentration of milk and related products; sterile filtration, clarification
 of fruit juice, wine, etc.; treatment of egg white, fermentation, etc.
— In biological and pharmaceutical industries for concentration, purification of
 several effluents, removal of pyrogens, treatment of plasma and blood, manu-
 facturing of antibiotics.
— In chemical and related industries :
  — Treatment of streams in the pulp and paper industry
  — Concentration or purification of effluents from the textile industry
  — Recovery of rinse, water and reconcentration of electropaint bath in
   automobile industry
  — Separation of oil and water
  — Treatment of other industrial waste water

REVERSE OSMOSIS

Fundamentals

To define reverse osmosis, we must first give the basic demonstration of osmosis.
When equal volumes of water and an aqueous solution are separated by a semipermeable membrane, osmosis occurs as water (solvent) permeates the membrane to dilute
the solution (Fig. 10). The semipermeable membrane is one which allows the water
to pass through it, but not other components (solutes). This action is called osmosis
and the amount of hydrostatic pressure required to equalize the volumes again, or, in
other words, to stop water flux after equilibrium has been reached, is called the
osmotic pressure. This phenomenon has been recognized for a long time, and was first
described mathematically by van't Hoff for dilute solutions as follows:

$$\pi = \phi RTc \qquad\qquad (4)$$

here π is the osmotic pressure of a solution; c is the molar solute concentration, T is
the absolute temperature: R is the gas constant; and ϕ is the osmotic coefficient
which goes to unity for ideal solutions.

It is possible to reverse this natural phenomenon (osmosis) by applying pressure
on the concentrated solution side of the membrane. If a pressure is applied in excess
of the osmotic pressure, reverse osmosis (RO) occurs as water molecules are forced to
pass through the membrane, while the solute molecules are rejected and concentrated
in upstream (Fig. 10).

A reverse osmosis membrane does essentially reject all classes of species including
dissolved inorganics and organics, particles, bacteria and pyrogens. Membrane mechanisms for preventing the molecules passing through the RO membranes are based on
the processes related to their size, shape, ionic charges and also interactions between
the solutes and the membrane itself.

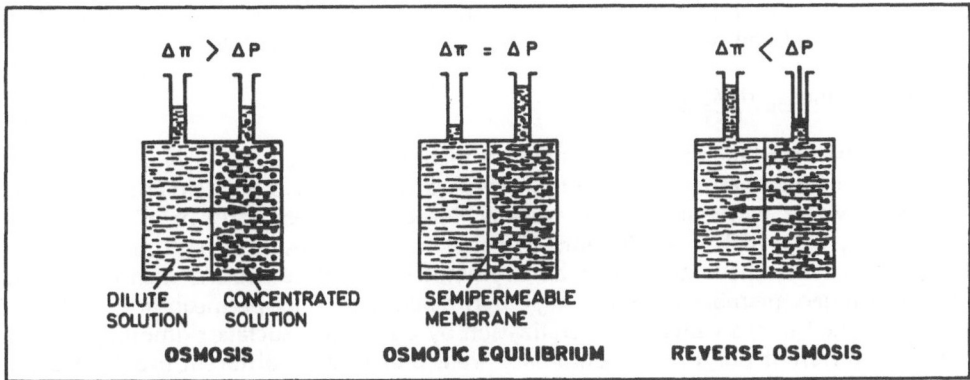

Figure 10. Osmosis and Reverse Osmosis.

There are many different models to try to explain the semipermeability of RO membranes, and mathematical studies of water and solute transfer through membranes. Recent approaches are developed on the thermodynamics of irreversible processes (21-24). However, among the others most credit has been given to the solution-diffusion model (25). This simplest model that gives adequate results is widely used in reverse osmosis plant design. The mathematical expression as of the model for solvent and solutes are given in the previous chapter of this book.

In reverse osmosis, the membrane separation properties are generally represented by solute rejection (or retention), R (%), defined as:

$$R = (1 - \frac{Cs_2}{Cs_1}) \times 100 \tag{5}$$

where Cs_1, and Cs_2 are the solute concentrations in the feed (or retentate) and in the permeate (or filtrate) solutions.

Percent solute passage (% S.P.) is also used to define separation performance and is related to rejection as follows:

$$\% \text{ S.P.} = 100 - R \tag{6}$$

In comparing the RO membranes or modules, care is needed because the values for rejection or percent solute passage given in the technical literature are for standard conditions of solute type and concentration pressure temperature, flow rate, and recovery rate.

As mentioned before, concentration polarization is a general phenomenon observed in mass transfer through membranes. Causes of concentration polarization in reverse osmosis are the same as in ultrafiltration. Increase in the local concentration of solutes results in an increase in osmotic pressure, thus reducing the water flux, and also promoting solute flux which means a decrease in the product quality. Severe deposition on the surface, known as membrane fouling, might cause plugging of the feed flow channels. This is usually observed in solutious containing large quantities of suspended or colloidal particles. These kind of solutions should be treated with tubular or more likely with plate-and-frame reverse osmosis modules.

Membranes and Modules

Studies regarding the reverse osmosis technique go back as early as the 1930s. However, this membrane separation process was first defined by Reid and coworkers (26). Low water permeation rates were achieved with these early membranes, even though they have high salt rejections. The first successful result came from the UCLA group (27). They have produced an asymmetric cellulose acetate membrane (the Loeb-Sourirajan membrane) with high permselectivity and permeability, and thus have succeeded in sea water demineralization by a so called surface skimming process. Later on, different polymeric membranes were prepared by different procedures and were examined in reverse osmosis modules. The, literature on these studies is extensive. Here, only some important membrane types with specific module design are included.

One of the most widely used membranes is asymmetric cellulose acetate membrane based on Loeb-Sourirajan phase inversion technique. These membranes are available in flat sheets which are employed in spiral wound membrane modules tubes, and hollow fibers.

These kind of membranes have high salt rejection (average 97 % for NaCl) and high water flux (3,11,24) The water flux declines with time and the membranes are also somewhat sensitive to chemical attacks. In practice, pH control and pre-treatments are recommended to minimize the membrane fouling and to increase the use-life (or long term stability).

The second popular group of membranes are made of aromatic polyamides (28,29). These membranes have relatively less water permeability, but are more salt retentive than CA membranes. Polyamide membranes are employed in commercially available hollow fiber modules. Membrane fouling is also observed in these modules, but generally hydraulic stabilities of these membranes are high.

The alternative composite membranes are also in commercial use. These membranes are usually prepared by following an interfacial polymerization procedure and are currently sold in the form of spiral wound modules (30,31). They have a very high rejection (α 98-98.5 % for NaCl), and water flux through these membranes is close to the values of those obtained with CA membranes. Their chemical stability is a matter of polymer material used. Some of them are very sensitive, especially to free Cl_2 and need a careful pre-treatment procedure.

Other membrane materials are being developed or under investigation for specific reverse osmosis applications where high chemical stability or high rejections, etc. are required (3,11,20,24,32). However, generally speaking, these are not still competative with the established ones given above.

Research in reverse osmosis is not only centered on finding membrane materials with high permeability for water with high rejection for salts and with long time stability, but also on suitable design of modules. It should be pointed out that in reverse osmosis aqueous solutions with very high osmotic pressures (e.g. for sea water = 25-40 atm, for orange juice = 25-100 atm) are handled and thus a driving force as pressure difference, typically 100-800 psi is applied. Therefore packing membranes in such a way that they have a high surface area per unit volume of module is aimed. This is nicely achieved, especially in hollow fiber units, and to a lesser extend with spiral winding. Spiral wound modules have wider application possibilites due to the fouling consideration. This configuration provides higher water flux and longer membrane life than hollow fibers. It is diffucult to clean the hollow fiber units once they are fouled. The other two module designs in use, namely tubular and plate-and-frame modules, are preferentially employed only when solutions with high concentrations of suspended and colloidal species are treated.

Applications

Reverse osmosis is a membrane separation technique where salts and microsolutes are separated from macromolecules. Its range of application in terms of particle size is 0.0001-0.001 μm (or 1-10 Å). Solutes with molecular weights more than 300 Daltons are wholly retained by reverse osmosis membranes. This technique has a very wide range of possible applications to aqueous solutions. Some of these applications are briefly given below.

- Production of potable water from;
  - sea water;
  - brakish water.
- Water for industries:
  - Rinse water for electronic industry.
  - Deionized or softened water for chemical industry.
  - Sterile deionized and pyrogen free water for medical and pharmaceutical industries.
- Waste water treatment:
  - Recovery of valuables from food industry effluents.
  - Treatment of effluents in sugar industry, and in paper and pulp industry.
  - Treatment of municipal and other industry wastes in order to decrease the pollutant load.
- Concentration of
  - food products, such as fruit juices, milk and other syrups;
  - solution in pharmaceutical industry (e.g. amino acid solution);
  - streams in chemical industry.

DIALYSIS

Fundamentals

The concept of dialysis was first proposed by Thomas Graham, in 1861 (33), who is conceded to be the discoverer of dialysis. Dialysis is a membrane separation process in which very large molecules (colloids) are separated from small ones (crystalloids) in response to differences in chemical potential between the liquids (Fig. 11) (34-38). The kinetic movements of the solute molecules tend to drive them through the dialysis membrane in the direction of high concentration to low concentration. It is an unaugmented process. In contrast to other membrane processes, the energy necessary for separation comes only from intrinsic free energy of the solute molecules. In should be noted at this point that in practice, dialysis is accompanied by other membrane processes such as osmosis, ultrafiltration electrodialysis. In such processes, transport is also further complicated owing to membrane-solution interactions

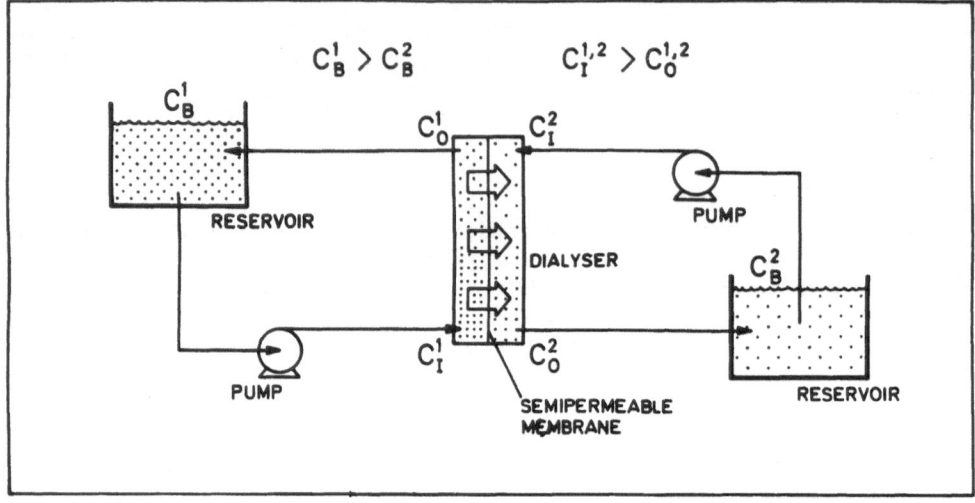

Figure 11. Dialysis.

involving ionic, covalent and hydrogen bonding, chemisorption, physical sorption and other effects. The purpose of this section is to deal particularly with the aspects of simple dialysis where the membrane is considered as a rigid, non-polar sieve and clearly operates by the pore mechanism. As mentioned before if a membrane operates by this mechanism it has more of the characteristics of a simple sieve and will allow solutes of various sizes to diffuse through differentially according to their size. In this very simple, but practical approach, solutes are assumed to transfer from one fluid to another through the pores of the dialysis membrane as a result of concentration gradient, simply by diffusion.

The diffusion of any single solute in a dialyzer may be considered in two rate controlling steps (a) Diffusion of solute through the adjacent fluid films on both faces of the membrane; (b) diffusion of solute into the pores of the membrane. Thus, the diffusion rate in a dialyzer may be expressed with the following equation which includes these rate controlling steps.

$$N = K.A.\Delta c \tag{7}$$

Where N is the solute diffusion rate in molar units; K is the overall mass transfer coefficient, A is the total surface area for mass transfer, and Δc is the driving force for mass transfer in mole fractions.

The reciprocal of the overall coefficient can be considered to be the overall resistance and composed of three resistances in the series.

$$\frac{1}{K} = \frac{1}{k_1} + \frac{1}{k_n} + \frac{1}{k_2} \tag{8}$$

The individual terms on the right-hand side of this equation represent the individual resistances of two adjacent fluids ($1/k_1$ and $1/k_2$) and of the membrane ($1/k_n$).

It is generally agreed that the mass transfer rates attainable in dialysis are often limited to a major extent, by the resistances of the fluid phases. Liquid film mass transfer coefficients in contemporary dialyzers are not nearly large enough to be negligible. Therefore, the individual resistance of boundary layers should be considered together with the membrane resistance for the evaluation of mass transfer in dialyzers.

The film diffusion rate limitation is a function of hydrodynamic conditions in the dialyzer. The liquid boundary layers on the membrane surfaces can be reduced in thickness by increasing the local velocity of fluid flow and this should have important implications for the design of dialyzers. The mass transfer rates are further augmented by introducing secondary fluid motion caused, for instance, by pulsation of the fluid phases. In practical design of dialyzers, transverse (or radial) mixing are promoted by changing fluid channel geometry, and by using flow deviators. Several designs of flow deviators have been proposed in order to create an intercirculation patern. It should be noted that turbulent flow is not achieved in dialyazers, and thus turbulent mixing is not considered in these units.

In design computation of dialyzers, the membrane itself is, of course the basic component of the system which controls the mass transfer rates. The nature of the dialysis membranes is of very great importance in determining both the rate and the results of dialysis. Such factors as the existence of pores, pore size, pore size distribution, type of pores, membrane-solute-solvent interactions, and membrane thickness are effective on dialysis operation.

Membranes and Modules

Dialysis membranes are a heterogeneous, usually symmetric, type of membranes (36). They are usually prepared by casting or extruding of a polymer solution into a thin film, and then solvent evaporation or precipitation of polymer in a suitable atmosphere (either in air or in solution). Further physical or chemical modifications, such as streching, annealing at elevated temperatures or treating with chemicals, are also applied in order to achieve the desired microporous structure.

The principal source of membrane materials for use in dialyzers is regenerated cellulose. Cellophane (or Visking) membrane is one example of a regenerated cellulose which was used in the mid 1930s. Another regenerated cellulose membrane, namely Cuprophane is prepared by cellulose via a cuprammonium intermediate, and finds a very wide market in hemodialysis units (39).

In addition to Cellophane and Cuprophane, membranes based on cellulose, such as cellulose acetate and cellulose nitrate, are also in the dialysis market.

A number of other new, non-cellulosic membranes for dialysis have been prepared and partially characterized. These membranes are made of crosslinked water soluble polymers (e.g. poly-N-vinylpyrrolidone and polyvinyl alcohol), polypeptides (e.g. collogen), block copolymers (e.g. copolyether-ester, copolyether-polycarbonate, and copolyether-urethane), polyacrylonitrile, nylon / epoxy, etc. Several types of these membranes have been commercialized (20,36,40-44). But it should be noted that during the past experience, cellulosic membranes have kept the first place in dialysis market.

Early dialyzers were bulky, expensive and not very efficient. The most nearly classical design is the filter-press arrangement the so called the plate-and-frame design.

Tubular membrane modules have also been used, especially in hemodialyzers. The capillary membrane module design may be considered as a breakthrough in dialyzer module design. Recently, due to their good flow control and a large membrane surface area per unit volume, much credit has been given to these modules, again, in artificial kidney technology.

Applications

As mentioned above, dialysis is very slow process and it is not highly selective. These two disadvantages of dialysis limit its applicability in industrial separations. However, the passivity of the process has some advantages, when the absence of external energy sources offers protection to a solution of sensitive substances like in food, biological, medical and related industries.

The classical application of dialysis is in the recovery of caustic soda from hemicellulose solutions generated during the manufacture of rayon. Recent years have seen new application of dialysis to treatment of several effluents in the metal refining and finishing industries. Waste treatment and processing of foods and biological material are other potential application of dialysis. The most important and dominant use of dialysis today is, of course, the supplementing or replacing human kidney function. In this treatment, blood of patients with kidney failure is extracorporeally circulated through dialyzer units periodically, in order to remove exogeneous and endogeneous toxins from blood. The potential market for hemodialyzers is extremly wide, perhaps it is in the first place in worldwide market of the membrane-based industries with a market size of about $ 200 million per year.

ELECTRODIALYSIS

Fundamentals

Electrodialysis is a membrane separation process where ion selective membranes are utilized in order to separate ions from electrolyte solutions under an applied electric gradient (45-49). Electrodialysis units consist of compartments (or cells) which are separated by alternating cation-permeable and anion-permeable permselective membranes. These compartments are assembled in a multicompartment electrodialysis unit (also called as stack). Each stack consist of an anode and a cathode and typically 50-200 membrane pairs (one cation-exchange, one anion-exchange). Figure 12 illustrates a general design of an electrodialysis apparatus. As seen here, the feed solution is pumped between the membranes. The terminal compartments are bounded by electrodes, for passing direct current through the whole stack. When the electrodes are connected to a direct current source, ions in the solutions begin to migrate toward the electrodes with opposite charge. Due to ion selective membranes, as an overall result, the electrolyte concentration decreases in alternate cells, while ion depletion occurs, simultaneously, in the other compartments.

In general, when an electrical field acts on an electrolyte solution, cations move to the cathode and anions move to the anode. If the electrolyte solution is separated by membranes, transport of ions and solvent is further limited. The existence of charged groups allows the membrane to act as a permselective barrier. This is a highly complex transport phenomenon in which transfer of ions is completely governed by the nature of the membrane. Most of the current teories of membrane transport behav-

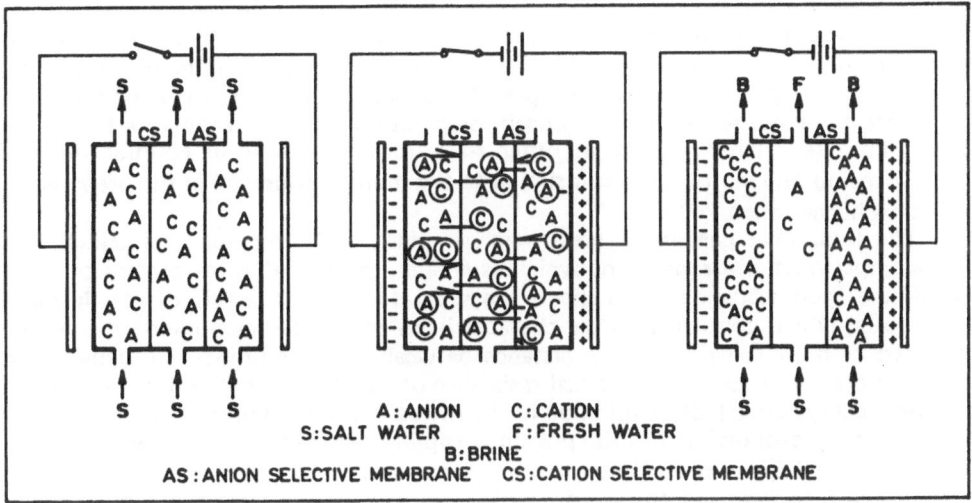

Figure 12. Electrodialysis.

ior are based on Nerst-Planck flux equation or modified forms. There are also other theories using the principles of irreversible thermodynamics or utilizing the concepts of the theory of rate processes. All of these theories are treated for several systems and a number of relations have been derived for a better description and understanding of transport phenomena in these membranes. Detail definitions of these approaches are found in several books and reviews (21,22,36,50-53).

Membranes and Equipment

Ion selective membranes are, in fact, ion exchange materials, and chemically similar to conventional ion exchange resins. They have fixed charged groups in the matrix to which mobile ions with opposite charge are attached in order to maintain the electrical equilibrium. When these membranes are placed into an electrolyte solution and electrical current passes through them by the motion of the mobile ions which exist in the matrix, the ions with same charge as of the mobile ions are picked up on one face and released at the other.

The most important properties of ion exchange membrane are, of course, their selectivity for oppositely charged ions and their ion permeability. They should have a high ion permeability, or in other words, a low electrical resistance in order to minimize the d.c. power dissipation and thus the energy requirements. The ion selective membranes are usually the most sensitive parts of electrodialysis systems. Like many other membrane separation processes, membranes can loose their mechanical strength, as well as their permselectivity and permeability due to fouling and chemical or mechanical attrition. This, again, means higher power cost. Therefore it is further required in the selection of suitable membranes for electrodialysis, that they should have high form stability.

A large amount of work is concerned with the preparation and the manufacturing of electrodialysis membranes with good chemical and mechanical stabilities and favorable electrical performance (47,54-59). There are basically two approaches of making ion selective membranes. In the first one, ion exchange resins are incorporated into a polymer membrane matrix by different techniques (e.g. molding, calendering or solvent casting). In the second approach membranes are first made of polymers which are the materials originally used in preparation an ion exchange resins. Then, these films are further treated in order to introduce anionic or cationic moietes into the membrane matrix, which is similar to the method followed in the preparation of ion exchange resins.

The functional part in an electrodialysis plant is the membrane stack. In this multicompartmental arrangement which is similar to that of filter presses or plate -and-frame modules, membrane sheets are separated by the sheets of plastic mesh (or spacers) which control the flow characteristics across the membrane surface. The thickness of these spacers, i.e. the distance between the membranes is usually 1 mm or less in order to lessen the electrical resistance of the fluid layer and thus reduce the electrical energy cost. Notice that due to the increase in the pumping energy cost, this cost is directly proportional to the pressure drop in the membrane stack which increases when the thickness of the flow path is decreased.

In order to decrease the mass transfer and also to minimize the concentration polarization in electrodialysis stacks, liquid flow velocities, generally, as high as 10 to 100 cm/sec are maintained. Further improvements on this subject are achieved by using well designed spacers with uniform flow distribution.

Most of the electrodialysis stacks are designed as one of two basic types: tortuous-path or sheet flow (Fig 13). The tortuous-path type of spacers consists of a flow channel that makes several 180° bends, and thus provides a long liquid flow path. This gives an opportunity to work at relatively high flow velocities. The turbulence in the flow pattern is promoted with the cross-straps introduced in the channels. In the sheet flow, liquid is allowed to flow from one side to another side in an uninterrupted manner. Plastic screens are used to ensure the turbulence in the fluid phase. Low linear velocities are found in this type of design, but pressure drops in sheet flow systems are considerably less than obtained in tortuous path sacks. In conclusion, it can be said that all these criteria must be taken into consideration for a suitable selection of electrodialysis sack design for specific application.

Applications

The dominant use of electrodialysis to date has been for the purification of brakish water. In recent years it has also been adapted for demineralization of sea water. In principal, it is applicable wherever recovery or removal of ions is required. Thus, it is also used in metal plating, food and pharmaceutical industries for the treatment of effluents (or solutions).

GAS PERMEATION

Fundamentals

Gas permeation is a membrane separation process used for the separation of gaseous species via membranes, and is based on the principle that some gases permeate much more rapidly than others due to differences in their mobilities or solubilities in the membrane matrix (Fig. 14). The principles of this separation technique were

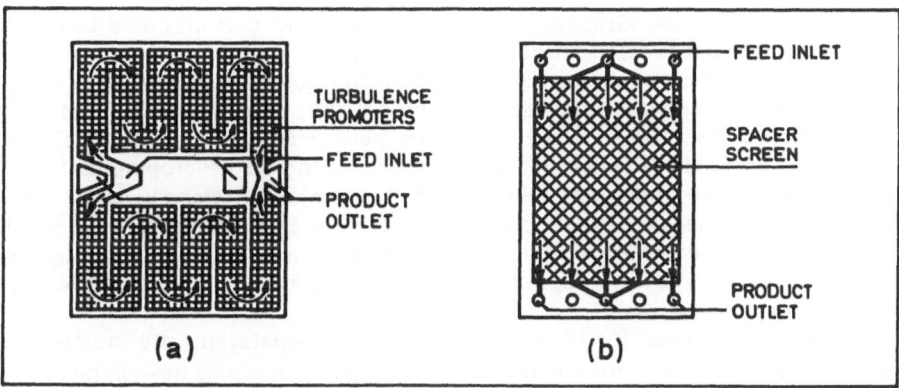

Figure 13. Electrodialysis Stack Design.

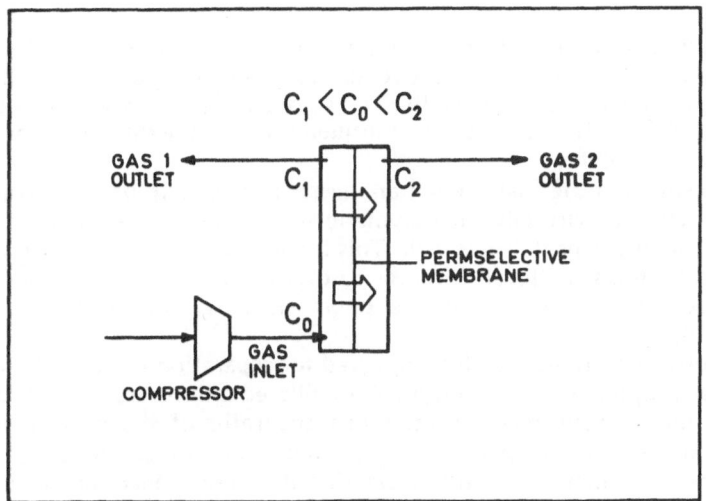

Figure 14. Gas Permeation.

first suggested by Thomas Graham in 1866, who reported that air could be enriched in O_2 by selective permeation through a natural rubber membrane (60). In spite of this very early discovery of gas permeation, this technique has not competed with the conventional gas separation processes (e.g. cryogenics, adsorption, absorption) for many years. This is because of the unsufficient permselectivity and permeability of the earlier membranes. However, very recent technological developments have advanced membranes to the point where their large-scale commercial use is feasible (61-63). Membrane systems are simple, straightforward and, therefore, easy to operate and maintain. Membrane gas separation has shown economic advantages over conventional methods both in capital and operating costs. It also requires less space than competing processes.

The membranes used for technically relevant gas separations are mostly homogeneous, or, heterogeneous with a non-porous skin layer. Equations describing gas transport through these membranes, which are given in the previous chapter in this book, are based on the sorption-diffusion model, i.e. a combination of Fick's law of diffusion and Henry's law relating solubility of gases in polymeric membranes. According to this model, flow rate across the membrane is proportional to area and pressure difference, and inversely proportional to thickness. The product recovery varies also with membrane permeability which is a direct polymer characteristic. The permselectivity of these type of membranes, can be represented by the ratio of permeabilities of species i and j in the membrane, respectively.

$$\alpha_{ij} = \frac{P_i}{P_j} \tag{9}$$

Where α_{ij}, so called separation factor or relative permeation rate, indicates the polymeric membrane's ability to separate two species i and j; P_i and P_j are the permeabilities of these two species. Permeability and separation factor are unique to a membrane polymer. Notice that factors which influence either the diffusivity or solubility also influence permeability.

It is interesting to note that there is an inverse relationship between permeability and permselectivity for virtually all polymeric membranes. Selectivity of the membranes is low, if their permeability is high. This is a limiting point in the application of gas permeation at industrial level. In order to overcome low fluxes, large membrane areas are utilized, and to overcome the poor selectivity multistage processes are necessary (64-68).

Microporous membranes are also employed for separation of gases. As mentioned in the previous chapter, Knudsen and/or Poiseuille equations are used to define the flow through microporous membranes. When the ratio of the pore radius of the membrane to the mean free path of the gas molecule is close to unity, Knudsen flow is applicable. When this ratio is significantly larger than unity, Poiseuille's equation is used to determine the flux. In some cases both equations are concerned in a simultaneous mode.

Separation factors with Knudsen flow are represented as follows;

$$\alpha_{ij} = \left(\frac{M_j}{M_i}\right)^{1/2} \tag{10}$$

where M_i and M_j are the molecular weights of two species i and j. It should be pointed out that although the separation factors obtained in microporous membranes are lower than those observed in homogeneous membranes, they are accompanied with significantly higher permeabilities.

Membranes and Separators

The most important element in the gas permeation process is, of course, the membrane itself. In contrast to other membrane separation processes, here, the resistance of the fluid films adjacent to the membrane surfaces may be omitted in most cases. In order to maintain the competition between gas separation and conventional methods, we need such membranes in which high fluxes can be achieved with high permselectivity. These two polymer properties determine the separating capabilities. System capability with operating environment must also be considered. Notice that, in gas permeation, the membrane must withstand substantial pressure differentials (200 to 2000 psig). Thus, membrane durability to mechanical, temperature or chemical changes must be taken into consideration, as well as membrane permeability and permselectivity, in order to achieve a favorable gas separation application.

Earlier membranes for gas separation were not successful simply owing to their poor selectivity and low permeability. Progress in synthesis of asymmetric, skin type membranes made gas separation attractive again in very recent years (64, 69-72). This asymmetric structure allows for high rates while retaining permselectivity of the membrane. The highly porous, thick polymer substrate layer give the membrane mechanical strength while the very thin homogeneous skin layer provides permselectivity.

Today, asymmetric cellulose acetate, and asymmetric composite polysulfone membranes are most widely used in gas permeators. These membrane are usually prepared by solvent casting, plasma discharged polymerization and many other attractive methods. CA membranes are now being manufactured as flat sheets and are available as spiral-wound modular design. Hollow fiber modules which consist of composite fibers having a polysulfone substructure and a silicon rubber skin layer have also found a large scale of industrial application.

Applications

Separation and/or purification of mixed gas streams found in refineries, chemical plants and natural gas resorvoirs are the potentially feasible applications of gas permeation. Examples include purification of natural gas containing CO_2 and H_2S, recovery of CH_4 from biogas, recovery of He from natural gas, H_2 purification and recovery in the petrochemical industry and in ammonia plants, etc. One of the most specific applications of gas permeation is membrane oxygenators. Blood oxygenators are used to supply O_2 to the blood and to remove excess CO_2 from it during open-heart surgery.

PERVAPORATION

Another type of membrane separation of growing interest is pervaporation, where a liquid mixture is separated by removing permeated product (permeate) in the vapour state (61,64,73-75). In pervaporation, the feed is in liquid form and the permeate is vapour. The partial pressure of permeate in the downstream side of the membrane is lower than its saturation pressure. This is usually maintained by applying

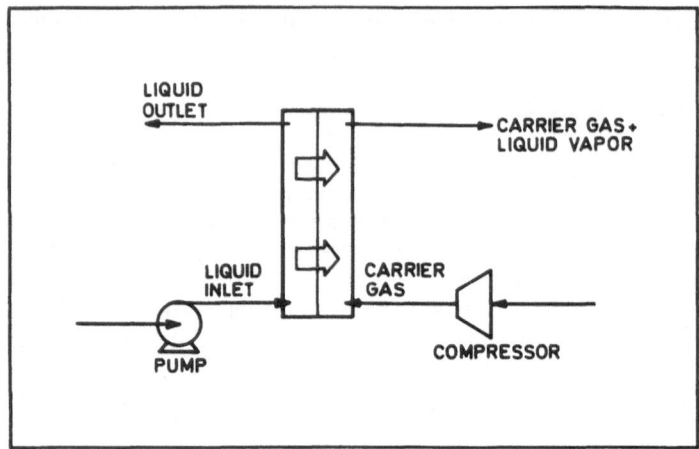

Figure 15. Pervaporation.

a vacuum or by employing a carrier gas. Schematic representation of pervaporation is given in Figure 15.

Transport phenomena in pervaporation are not understood throughly. Transfer of species within the pervaporation membranes is much more complicated than occurs in the membranes which are employed in other membrane separation techniques. This is due to the anisotropic swelling of the pervaporation membrane, i.e. sorption of liquid on the feed side of the membrane produces a significant swelling, while vapour side is kept dry by vacuum or carrier gas. The anisotropic swelling is the characteristic feature of pervaporation membranes and leads to change in both diffusivity and solubility with permeate concentration in the membrane matrix. Therefore, the models used to describe the performance of pervaporation membranes are based on the calculations accounting concentration-dependent diffusion and sorption coefficients.

Both permeability and permselectivity of pervaporation membranes are strongly dependent on the composition of the feed. A very complex, coupled transport occurs in these membranes. In general, the pervaporation flux increases when the temperature is raised. It has been reported that the product side pressure is also effective on the selectivity and the permeation flux. The chemical nature of polymer matrix, and the microcrystalline structure of the membrane are also important properties.

Unfortunately, in contrast to other membrane processes, there is not an established criteria for membrane preparation and equipment design in pervaporation. Furthermore, a serious practical problem with this technique lies in the need to transport large amount of heat required for evaporation of the permeating species. This enthalpy of vaporization poses an additional cost and difficulties in separator design.

It is generally agreed that the membrane processes encountered in the previous sections of this chapter are economical and reliable in most cases when applied to the separation of aqueous solutions and gaseous mixtures. In contrast to these membrane separation techniques, pervaporation is still in the early stages of development and it is not employed on the industrial scale yet, due to problems discussed above. It should be noted that better understanding the transport phenomena, novel models of operations (e.g. continuous column approach), better equipment design and developments in more selective and permeable membranes could open up a variety of new applications in the chemical and related industries in the future.

Pervaporation is potentially applicable to mixtures that are difficult to separate by conventional techniques, such as azeotropic mixtures or mixtures of close-boiling components, heat sensitive products, etc.

REFERENCES

1. Dutka, B.J., Membrane Filtration, Marcel Dekker, New York, 1981.
2. Zsigmond, R., U.S. Pat., 1, 421, 341, 1922.
3. Kesting, R.E., Synthetic Polymeric Membranes, McGraw-Hill, New York, 1971.
4. Nordberg, M.E., J. Amer. Chem. Soc., 27:299, 1944.
5. Thiele, H. and Hallich, K., Kolloid Z., 163:115, 1959.
6. Fleischer, R.L., Brice, P.B., and Walker, R.M., Science, 149:383, 1965.
7. Bierenbaum, H.S., Isaacson, R.B., Druin, M.L. and Plovan, S.G., Ind. Eng. Chem. Prod. Res. Develop., 13:2, 1974.
8. Goetz, A. and Tsuneishi, N., J. Amer. Water Works Assoc., 43:943, 1951.
9. Schweitzer, P.A., Handbook of Separation Techniques for Chemical Engineers, McGraw-Hill, New York, 1979.
10. Stannett, V.T., Koros, W.J., Paul, D.R., Lonsdale, H.K. and Baker, R.W., Adv. Polymer Sci., 32:99, 1979.
11. Lonsdale, H.K., J. Memb. Sci., 10:81, 1982.
12. Michaels, A.S., in Progress in Separation and Purification, Vol. I, E.S. Perry, ed., Interscience Publ., New York, 1968.
13. Cooper, A.R., Ultrafiltration Membranes and Applications, Plenum Press, New York, 1980.
14. Strathmann, H., J. Memb. Sci., 9:121, 1981.
15. Turbak, A.F., Synthetic Membranes, Vol. I and II, ACS Symp. Ser., American Chemical Society, Washington, D.C., 1981.
16. Flinn, J.E., Membrane Science and Technology, Plenum Press, New York, 1970.
17. Porter, M.C., Ind. Eng. Chem. Prod. Res. Develop., 11:234, 1972.
18. Matthiasson, E. and Sivik, B., Desalination, 35:59, 1980.
19. Fane, A.G., Fell, C.J.D. and Waters, A.G., J. Memb. Sci., 9:245, 1981.
20. Keller, P.R., Membrane Technology and Industrial Separation Techniques, Noyes Data Corp., New Jersey, 1976.
21. Lakshminarayanaiah, N., Transport Phenomena in Membranes, Academic Press, London, 1969.
22. McGregor, R., Diffusion and Sorption in Fibers and Films, Academic Press, London, 1974.
23. Lonsdale, H.K. and Podall, H.E., Reverse Osmosis Membrane Research, Plenum Press, New York, 1972.
24. Sourirajan, S., Reverse Osmosis and Synthetic Membranes, National Research Council, Ottawa, Canada, 1977.
25. Lonsdale, H.K., Merten, U. and Riley, R.L., J. Appl. Polym. Sci., 9:1341, 1965.
26. Reid, C.E. and Kuppers, J.R., J. Appl. Polym. Sci., 2:264, 1959.
27. Loeb, S. and Sourirajan, S., Adv. Chem. Ser., 38:117, 1962.

28. Richter, J.W. and Hoehn, H.H., U.S. Patent, 3, 567, 632, March 2, 1971.
29. McKinney, R., Separation and Purification Methods, 1:31, 1972.
30. Riley, R.L., Fox, R.L., Lyons, C.R., Milstead, C.E., Seroy, M.W. and Tagami, M., Desalination, 19:113, 1976.
31. Cadotte, J.E., King, R.S., Majerle, R.J. and Petersen, R.J., J. Macromal. Sci. Chem., A 15:727, 1981.
32. Lonsdale, H.K. and Podall, H.E., Reverse Osmosis Membrane Research, Plenum Press, New York, 1972.
33. Graham, T., Phil. Trans. Roy. Soc., 151:1836, 1861.
34. Lane, J.A. and Riggle, J.W., AIChE Chem. Engr. Prog. Symp. Ser. No. 24, 55:127, 1959.
35. Leonard, E.F. and Bluemle, L.W., Trans. N.Y. Acad. Sci., 21:585, 1959.
36. Tuwiner, S.B., Diffusion and Membrane Technology, Reinhold, New York, 1962.
37. Michaels, A.S., Trans. Amer. Artif. Intern. Organs, 12:387, 1966.
38. Leonard, E.F., in Kirk-Othmer Encyclopedia of Chemical Technology, Vol. 15, pp. 1, John Wiley &Sons, New York, 1981.
39. Bandel, W., Osterreich, Chemiker-Zeitung Jahrgang 65, 1964.
40. Lyman, D.J., Loo, B.H. and Crawford, R.W., Biochemistry, 3:985, 1964.
41. Barbour, B.H., Bernstein, M., Cantor, P.A., Fisher, B.S. and Stone, Jr., W., Trans. Amer. Soc. Artif. Intern. Organs, 21:144, 1975.
42. Klein, E., Nephrology, 9:131, 1978.
43. Lyman, D.J., in Replacement of Renal Function of Dialysis, W. Drukker, F.M. Parsons, J.F. Maher, eds., pp. 69, Martinus Nijhoff Publishers, The Hague, 1979.
44. Klein, E., Holland, F.F. and Eberle, K., Kidney Int., 18:18, 1980.
45. Meyer, K.H. and Strauss, W., Helv. Chim. Acta, 23:795, 1940.
46. Nachrod, F.C. and Schubert, J., Ion Exchange Technology, Academic Press, New York, 1956.
47. Wilson, J.R., Demineralization by Electrodialysis, Butterworths, London, 1960.
48. Spiegler, K.S., Principles of Desalination, Academic Press, New York, 1966.
49. Lacey, R.E. and Loeb, S., Industrial Processing with Membranes, Wiley-Interscience, New York, 1972.
50. Katchalsky, A. and Curran, P.F., Nonequilibrium Thermodynamics, Harvard Univ. Press, Cambridge, Massachussetts, 1965.
51. Helfferich, F., Ion-Exchange, McGraw-Hill, New York, 1962.
52. Shaffer, K.S. and Minta, M.S., in Principles of Desalination, K.S. Spiegler, ed., Academic Press, New York, 1966
53. Meares, P., Membrane Separation Processes, Elsevier Scientific Publ. Co., Amsterdam, 1976.
54. Mason, E.A. and Juda, W., AIChE Chem. Engr. Prog. Symp. Ser. No. 24, 55:155, 1959.
55. Wyllie, M.R.J. and Patnode, H.W., J. Phys. Colloid Chem., 54:204, 1950.
56. Juda, W. and McRae, W.A., J. Amer. Chem. Soc., 72:1044, 1950.
57. Clarke, J.T., U.S. Patent, 2,780,604, February 5, 1957.
58. Connolly, D.J. and Gresham, W.F., U.S. Patent, 3,282,875, November 1, 1966.
59. Grot, W., Chem.-Ing.-Tech., 47:617, 1975.
60. Graham, T., Phil. Mag., 32:402, 1866.
61. Hwang, S-K. and Kammermeyer, K., Membranes in Separations, John Wiley, New York, 1975.
62. Schell, W.J. and Houston, C.D., Chem. Eng. Prog., 33, 1982.
63. Schell, W.J., Hydrocarbon Processing, 63:47, 1983.

64. Kammermeyer, K., Chem.-Ing.-Tech., 48:672, 1976.
65. Hwang, S-T. and Kammermeyer, K., Can. J. Chem. Eng., 43:38, 1965.
66. Burnett, L.J. and Riley, R.L., Gas Separation Membranes: Technology and Applications, UOP, Inc., San Diego, California, 1977.
67. Hwang, S-T. and Thorman, J.M., AIChE J., 26:558, 1980.
68. Berry, R.I., Chem. Engr., 88:63, 1981.
69. Gantzel, P.K. and Merten, U., Ind. Engr. Chem. Process Des. Devel., 9:331, 1970.
70. Ward III, W.J., Browall, W.R. and Salemme, R.M., J. Memb. Sci., 1:99, 1976.
71. Gardner, R.J., Crane, R.A. and Hannan, J.F., Chem. Engr. Prog., 73:76, 1977.
72. Hennis, J.M.S. and Tripodi, M.K., J. Memb. Sci., 8:233, 1981.
73. Hagerbaumer, D.H. and Kammermeyer, K., AIChE Chem. Eng. Prog. Symp. Ser. No. 10, 50:25, 1954.
74. Kammermeyer, K. and Hwang, S-T., Can. J. Chem. Engr., 82, 1966.
75. Rautenbach, R. and Albrecht, R., J. Memb. Sci., 7:203, 1980.

SYNTHETIC POLYMERIC MEMBRANES: BIOLOGICAL APPLICATIONS

E. Piskin

Hacettepe University, Chemical Engineering Department, Ankara, Turkey

INTRODUCTION

Exceptional advancement in polymer science and membrane technology during the past decades has made possible an enormous variety of biological applications for membrane-moderated devices. As mentioned in the previous chapter, conventional membrane separation techniques has opened new horizons in separation science. These young processes are nicely employed in concentration, purification, separation, fractionation or steril filtration of effluents which contain biologically active substances. Today, a suitable membrane separation device is available for almost all these separation problems. In this chapter, it is not attempted to give any further details of these processes and applications. Instead, our emphasis in this section is on the description of the other novel and very exciting applications of membrane moderated systems that have emerged in biological and related fields. Of course, only some of the most common applications, including blood oxygenators, artificial kidney systems (i.e., hemodialysis and hemofiltration), plasmapheresis, hemoperfusion, and other membrane-moderated systems as carrier of biologically active substance, are considered by giving some insight into the subject.

BLOOD OXYGENATION

Physiological Principles of Gas Exchange Process

All living cells require to get oxygen and to get rid of carbon dioxide. In man, the cardiovascular and the respiratory systems are responsible to supply the necessary amount of oxygen to all the tissues of the body, and to remove the metabolic waste, i.e. carbon dioxide. Blood transports these respiratory gases to and from all tissues. The venous blood returning from tissues enters the right heart cavities, and is brought to the lungs by the pulmonary artery (Fig. 1). Its branches distribute blood to capillaries which are in close contact with respiratory surfaces, i.e. the functional units

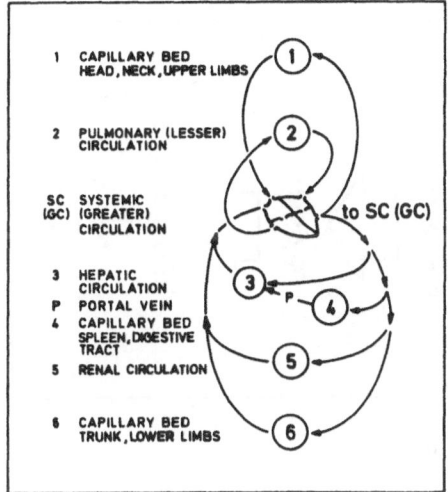

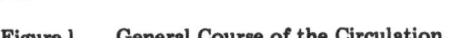

Figure 1.   General Course of the Circulation.

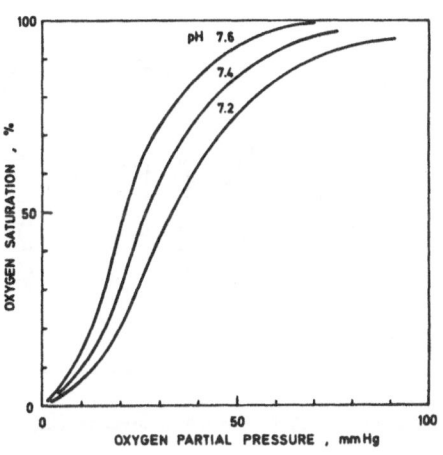

Figure 2.   Oxygen Dissociation Curve.

of the lung, namely the alveoli. Gas exchange takes place between the blood passing through the pulmonary capillaries and the inspired air in the alveoli. The pulmonary capillaries which link to form branches of the pulmonary veins convey freshly oxygenated blood to the left heart cavities. Arterial blood is then distributed to the body tissues. During its passage through the capillary beds of the body, the arterial blood gives up oxygen, and takes up carbon dioxide. Then, the blood becomes again unoxygenated, and returns to the heart as the venous blood.

Carriage of O_2 and CO_2. Under normal conditions, the solubility of oxygen in blood is low, and thus the amount of dissolved oxygen may be neglected as far as oxygen supply to the tissues is concerned. About 90 % of oxygen is carried as oxyhemoglobin. According to the famous intermediate compound hypothesis of Adair (1), combination of hemoglobin (Hb) with O_2 takes place in four stages:

$$Hb_4 + O_2 \longrightarrow Hb_4O_2$$
$$Hb_4O_2 + O_2 \longrightarrow Hb_4O_4$$
$$Hb_4O_4 + O_2 \longrightarrow Hb_4O_6$$
$$Hb_4O_6 + O_2 \longrightarrow Hb_4O_8$$

A blood of completely reduced Hb contains only Hb_4 molecules, whereas the blood of fully saturated oxyhemoglobin consists entirely of Hb_4O_8. Partially saturated blood, it is assumed, contains also the intermediate compounds. Oxygen saturation is usually used to express oxygen content of the blood. It is a function of the partial pressure of the O_2 in the immediate environment. This relation is given by an S-shaped curve, i.e. the oxygen dissociation curve (Fig. 2). It is also influenced by the partial pressure of CO_2 or pH, and by temperature.

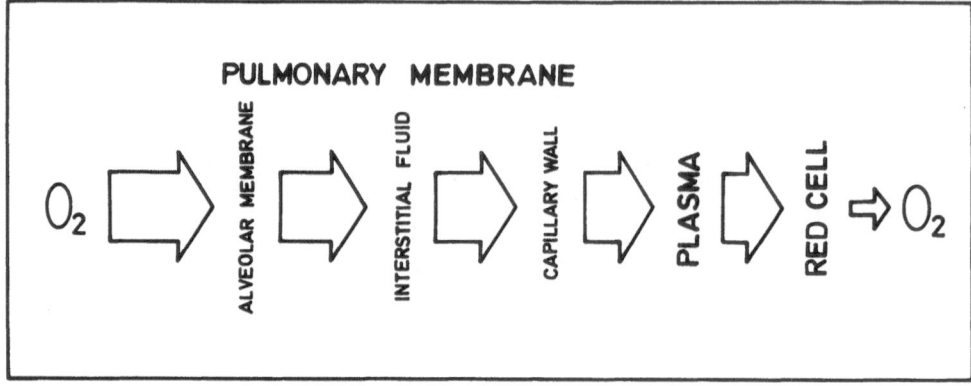

Figure 3.   Diffusion Resistances to Oxygen Transport in Lungs.

Carbon dioxide is carried in the blood in three ways. The bulk of CO_2 is carried as bicarbonates in the plasma and in the red cells. To a lesser extent, CO_2 forms carbamino compounds with hemoglobin.

The solubility of CO_2 in plasma is about 25 times of the oxygen solubility. However, again, only a small part of CO_2 is carried by this way.

Uptake and Release of O_2 and CO_2 in the Lungs. When the venous blood flows through the pulmonary capillaries it is exposed to a high oxygen partial pressure (about 100 mm Hg in alveolar air), and a low carbon dioxide partial pressure (about 40 mm Hg in alveolar air). Therefore, oxygen diffuses into plasma where O_2 tension is about 40 mm Hg (oxygen saturation of 70%), and carbon dioxide diffuses out of plasma where CO_2 tension is about 46 mm Hg. In the arterial blood leaving lungs for tissues, the O_2 and CO_2 tensions are about 100 mm Hg and 40 mm Hg, respectively.

During the natural process of blood oxygenation, there is no direct contact between gas and blood in lungs. The gas transfer occurs through the pulmonary membrane which consists of: the alveolar membrane, the interstitial fluid, and the capillary wall. Oxygen transport in the lungs from alveoli to the hemoglobin is affected by a series of resistances given in   Figure 3. The mass transfer resistance attributable to the pulmonary membrane is a significant fraction of the total resistance for O_2 (about half). Diffusion in plasma gives about 20 % of the total resistance for O_2 transport. The total mass transfer resistance of the red cell membrane and inter cellular fluid is one of the dominant components for oxygen transport. It is generally agreed that, the rates of the chemical reactions of O_2 with hemoglobin are extremely high, hence chemical reactions are not limiting steps for the rate of uptake of O_2 in the lungs.

In contrast to O_2 transport, studies have shown that the influence of diffusional steps on the over-all rate of the CO_2 transfer process in the lungs is not significant. The chemical reactions offer more than 80 % of the total resistance for CO_2 transport.

Conclusion. The lungs can oxygenate up to 30 liters of venous blood per minute. up to 2400 ml (STP) of oxygen can be taken up. Basal conditions for a resting healthy adult man at $37^{\circ}C$ are: Blood flow rate = 5 liters / min; O_2 required = 250 ml (STP)/

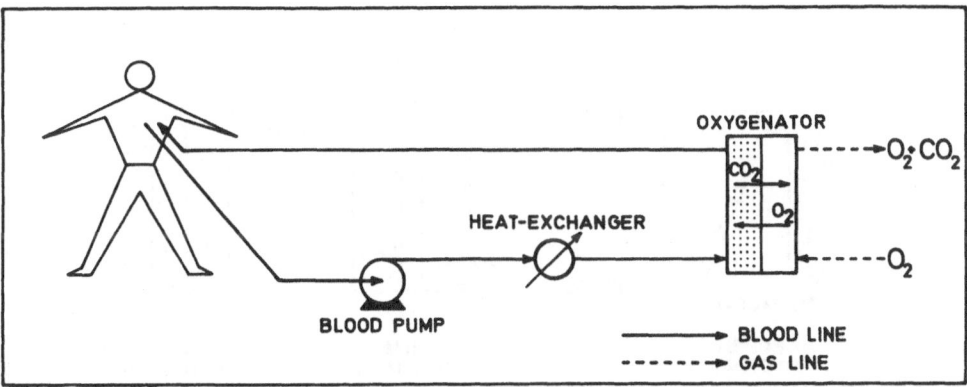

Figure 4.   Heart - Lung Machine.

min; and CO_2 produced = 200 ml (STP)/min. It should be noted that these are also nominal design requirements for total respiratory support with an artificial oxygenation system.

Artificial Oxygenation

The concept of artificial oxygenation originated as early as 1868, but it took more than a century to develop an artificial gas exchange device at commercial level for oxygenation of blood in an extracorporeal circuit. Even today, it is not possible to oxygenate blood in extracorporeal circulation for prolonged periods without creating harmful effects. At this moment, blood oxygenators are not generally used as replacements for diseased or failing lungs, but usually are used to simplify open-heart surgery by enabling a surgeon to make the operation of intracardiac abnormalities under direct vision in a bloodless area.

An artificial cardiorespiratory device (Fig. 4), i.e. the heart-lung machine, which consists of a mechanical pump for oxygenation of blood and removal of carbon dioxide (instead of natural lungs), and a heat exchanger in order to keep the blood temperature at constant value, is used during open-heart surgery.

Most important functional component of this extracorporeal circuit is, of course, the oxygenator. A succesful oxygenator must provide efficient gas - blood contact to permit adequate O_2 supply to the blood stream and CO_2 elimination. As mentioned above, it must be able to oxygenate up to 5 liters of blood per minute to nearly 100% saturation. Simultaneously, it must remove a proper amount of CO_2 to maintain pCO_2 levels in physiologic range without causing respiratory acidosis (CO_2 retention) or respiratory alkalosis (CO_2 depletion). An ideal oxygenator should have also low priming volume; should not create harmful effects (e.g. trauma to the blood cells, denaturation of plasma proteins and micro-bubbles or particulate micro-embolisation); should be of simple design, easy handling and reliable sterilization.

A large variety of devices have been developed for blood oxygenation. The earliest types of oxygenators were direct gas-liquid contactors such as bubble, sreeen and rotating disc devices (Fig. 5) (2). Perhaps the most popular are the so-called bubble oxygenators, which are widely used even today. In these devices nearly pure oxygen is in-

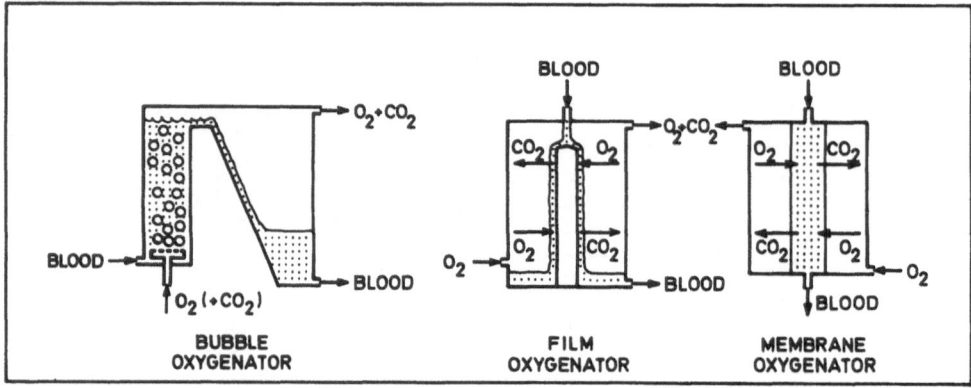

Figure 5.   Different Type of Oxygenators.

troduced into the blood directly in the form of bubbles. The direct contact methods produce efficient mass transfer rates of O_2 and CO_2, but the resultant trauma restricts their use to short-term procedures (about one hour). It should also be pointed out that significant irreversible lipoprotein denaturation occurs at the large blood-gas interfaces in direct contact devices. The formation of the microemboli produced by micro-bubbles must also be prevented which is achieved by using debubblers with very large hold up. It is also necessary to use convenient surfactants, which can be potential hazards, to ensure the removal of micro-bubbles in these devices.

Membrane Oxygenators

In membrane oxygenators, a permselective membrane is interposed between the blood and gas phases in order to prevent the deleterious changes noted in direct contact devices. These oxygenators reduce the trauma and presumably denaturation of blood proteins found in oxygenator designs that employ a blood-gas interphase. Membrane oxygenator design eliminates also oxygenator-produced micro-bubbles which cause micro emboli. Unfortunately, interposition of the membrane between the phases also drastically reduces the gas transfer efficiency both by adding an additional resistance in series, and by causing a relatively stagnant blood region near the wall. Because the additional resistance increases the surface area required for adequate gas transfer, this in turn results in increased size and priming volume.

The majority of efforts for developing a better oxygenator have been directed toward fashioning more efficient devices that would have membranes with high permeating rates for O_2 and CO_2, and would provide a thin layer of blood over the membrane and breaking up the boundary layer.

Gas transfer across the membrane depends upon the nature of the membrane materials and its thickness, and the partial pressure difference of the diffusing gases on opposite sides of the membranes.

In the case of natural lung, the partial pressure of O_2 in venous blood is about 40 mm Hg, which needs to be brought to about 100 mm Hg for arterial blood. If air at 760 mm Hg (atmospheric air) is used, then the average driving force for oxygen is about 80 mm Hg. The CO_2 content of venous blood is about 45 mm Hg and this is the maximum driving force for removal, considering that the inspired air has negligable amount of CO_2. In the case of oxygenators, since usually pure oxygen is used, the driving force for O_2 is about 690 mm Hg. Since the partial pressure of CO_2 in blood is not more than 50 mm Hg, the driving force of CO_2 in oxygenators is as same as in the case of natural lung. It can be concluded that in order to get an equal transmission of O_2 and CO_2, the membrane should be at least twelve times more permeable to CO_2.

Various membranes have been utilized for membrane oxygenator. The earliest membranes, Cellophane membranes with typically 10 ml/min. m^2 of oxygen transfer rates were used by Kolff and Balzer in oxygenation of venous blood through hemodialysis (3). Other early non-porous, relatively hydrophobic membranes such as polyethylene (4), ethyl cellulose (5) and even polytetrafluoroethylene (Teflon) (6,7) have been used, but not with much success. These early membranes were replaced by silicone rubber which has far favourable gas permeability. Silicone rubber is known as the most permselective homogeneous (non-porous) membrane. It has 4-5 times more permeability for carbon dioxide than for oxygen. However, as mentioned above, it was still very far from the requirements for an ideal oxygenator membrane. However, it has been utilized in most of the earlier industrial development of membrane oxygenators. Most silicone polymers have little strength, thus they have been incorporated with fillers (8), or have been reinforced with textiles, e.g. dacron, (9), or have been made as copolymers, e.g. silicone-polycarbonate (10), where in the later case polycarbonate increases the strength. They have been available both in the form of sheets and hollow fibers. Studies have indicated that silicone rubber membranes provide a moderate oxygen transfer rate but are inefficient in terms of carbon dioxide elimination. At that time it was agreed that CO_2 transfer is limited by the chemical nature and the thickness of the polymer membrane, but O_2 transfer is primarily limited by the adjacent blood film, thus by the geometry of the blood path.

The milestone of membrane development for blood oxygenation, which is worth remembering, is the concept of using heterogeneous (microporous) hydrophobic membranes. One of the most popular microporous membrane used for oxygenators is tetrafluoroethylene, which can be prepared by a technique for expanding of PTFE uniaxially and biaxially in forms such as sheets and tubes (11-14). More recently, stretched-polypropylene membranes have been offered, again in the forms of sheets and hollow fibers. Only these few porous, hydrophobic materials have so far yielded high enough gas transfer rates for O_2 and also for CO_2. The membranes have very high gas transfer rates, i.e. about fourth times those found with Cellophane membranes (typically 400 ml/min. m^2 of oxygen transfer rate). The membrane resistance, thus becomes not dominant, even for CO_2, in contrast to the case with non-porous membranes, e.g. silicone rubber.

However, in the case of an oxygenator based on microporous membrane technology, there are some disadvantages dictated. There is evidence that microporous membranes can cause far greater platelet and red cell damage than, for example, polydimethylsiloxane coated membranes. It was also noted that over prolonged periods the gas channels in the membrane may become flooded with fluid, and thus may cause progressive reduction in the gas transport across the membrane. It should be also noted that the transmembrane pressure must be kept in some limits to avoid the ultrafiltration, or reversely microbubble emboli.

In order to eliminate these drawbacks associated with microporous membranes, several interesting approaches have been proposed, such as coating of the blood side surface of the membrane with non-thrombogenic, very thin homogeneous membranes

(15,16), or treatment of membrane surfaces with bioactive agents, e.g. albumin (15).

As it was mentioned above, not only the membrane, but also the adjacent blood film is one of the most dominant factor which limits the gas exchange in the membrane oxygenators. Especially in the oxygenators utilizing microporous membranes, it is important to control the flow geometry and blood film thickness in order to achieve adequate O_2 and CO_2 transfer rates. Most of the solutions which have been proposed are based on implying high blood shear rates at the membranes, which are usually created by increasing high blood flow rates or by secondary flows (2,17-20). It is important to emphasize that the augmentation of the gas transfer can be achieved in this way, but high blood shear rates seem to be the main reason for trauma, which again must be avoided.

In conclusion, it can be said that, today, there are nicely designed disposable membrane oxygenator modules in the form of spiral-wound, plate-and-frame, and hollow fibers, which fulfill many of the basic requirements for blood oxygenation in short-term applications, such as open-heart surgery, but it seems that much more effort must be expended to investigate the concept of long-term respiratory assistance in man.

ARTIFICIAL KIDNEY

The Kidneys in Natural Excretory System

The kidneys are the chief excretory organs of the body with the respiratory system and the skin. The kidneys excrete waste products of metabolism (e.g. urea , uric acid, creatinine and others), and adjust the loss of water and electrolytes from the body in order to keep body fluids relatively constant in amount and composition. The kidneys are also responsible for maintaining the pH of the blood, and thus the body fluids at a relatively constant value.

About 20-25 % of the left ventricle's total output of blood in each cardiac cycle is distributed to the kidneys by the renal arteries. The renal arteries divide into several branches, and lastly give rise to afferent arterioles which bring blood to the functional unit of the kidney, the so-called nephron. Each kidney contains approximately one million of these functional units (Fig. 6). The afferent arteriole divides into glomerular capillaries which are surrounded by Bowman's capsule, i.e. an expansion of the nephron. Here about 15-25 % of the water and solutes (i.e. non protein solutes, crystalloids, such as Na^+, K^+, Cl^-, glucose, urea) are filtered from plasma through the renal tubule. The filtered blood leaving the Bowman capsule flows in the efferent arteriole. The efferent arteriole divides again to form peritubular capillaries which surround the renal tubule. Here, most of the water and other substances in the glomerular filtrate diffuse back into the blood flowing in peritubular capillaries. These substances are partially or totally reabsorbed, or not reabsorbed according to their thresholds. Some substances are secreted into the lumen of the nephron from peritubular capillaries during formation of the urine. In contrast to simple sieve-like filtration in the glomerulus, reabsorption and secretion occur via complex transport mechanisms, mostly active transport. The peritubular capillaries finally converge into veins in order to leave the kidneys. The renal tubule carrying the urine joins a collecting duct which opens into renal pelvis.

The urine amount and composition varies from specie to specie, time to time, but it usually contains sodium, calcium, potasium, chloride, phosphates, sulphates,

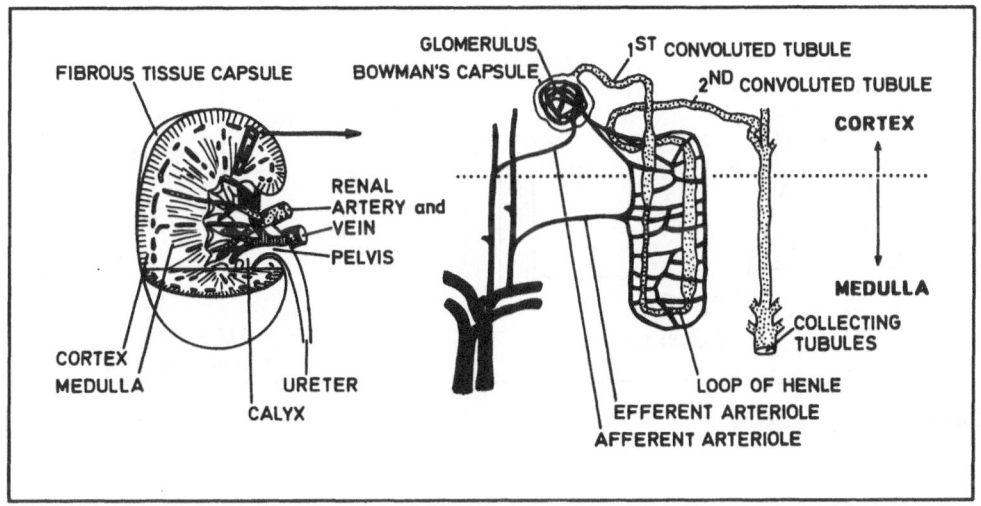

Figure 6.　Nefron.

ammonia, and the major metabolic waste materials, such as urea, uric acid, creatinine, etc. The kidneys are perfused by 500-600 ml of plasma mer minute, and 1-1.5 liters of urine are excreted per day, which varies with fluid intake and with fluid output from other routes (i.e. skin, lungs, gut), and with diet.

As kidney function decreases various substances which are normally excreted by the kidneys will accumulate, thus leading to morbidity and disability. At this point the loss in excretory capacity has to be matched by exogenous means, i.e. artificial kidney systems, in order to keep the overall mass balance in the body.

Artificial Support

Today, artificial kidney systems are not yet able to compensate for normal renal functions, for instance the kidney's endocrine or metabolic activities. Instead, a part of the kidney's excretory function can be replaced by these systems to some extent. Principally, in artificial kidney system waste or toxic metabolic products normally excreted by the natural kidney, are removed from the blood. In other words, artificial kidney therapy is applied to the patients with renal insufficiency in order to keep the concentrations of potentially harmful endogeneous or exogeneous substances below certain levels to avoid organ toxicity.

There is no longer any restriction as to the kind of renal failure which can be treated by the artificial kidney. There are many indications for artificial kidney therapy, which can likely be considered in two main categories, i.e. acute renal failure and chronic renal diseases. In the treatment of an acute patient, the artificial kidney therapy is applied mostly 2-5 times in order to keep the patient alive until their immediate problem is corrected and their own kidneys begin to function normally. In the case of chronic renal insufficiency, the kidneys of the patient are damaged irreversibly and would never return to normal function. In this case, the artificial support becomes a routine procedure and must be utilized several times a week for

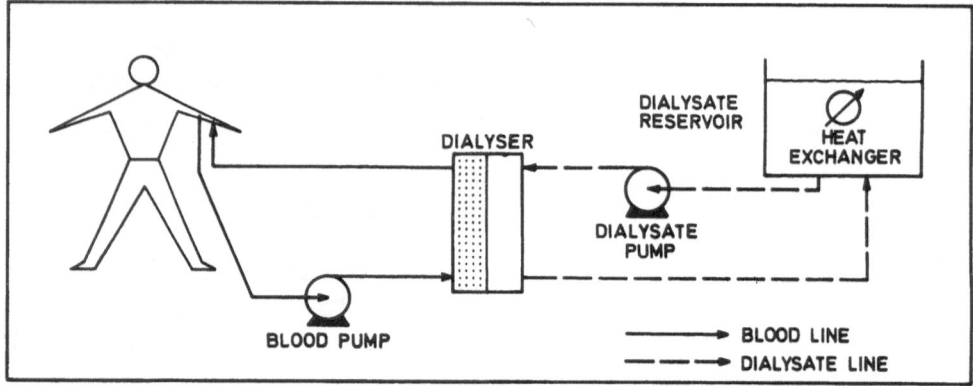

Figure 7.   Hemodialysis.

the rest of the patient's life or until such time as a kidney transplantation can be performed.

There are three artificial kidney systems that are in use today, namely peritoneal dialysis, hemodialysis and hemofiltration.

In peritoneal dialysis the semipermeable dialysis membrane is the peritoneum which is the membrane lining the wall of the abdomen. The dialysate solution is placed into the peritoneal cavity by a special catheter. Solutes diffuse from blood in peritoneal capillaries to dialysis solution in the peritoneal cavities. Since our main interest in this paper is synthetic membranes and their biological applications, we would not deal with attitudes of peritoneal dialysis. Without going further, let us point out that, recent breakthroughs in controlling infection with better catheter design, make this technique increasingly comparable with standard hemodialysis.

Hemodialysis

Hemodialysis is an extracorporeal system where arterial blood from the patient is pumped through a dialysis unit consisting of a semipermeable dialysis membrane (Fig.7). The blood is passed over one side of the dialysis membrane while a dialysate solution containing a suitable solution of ions (Na^+, Ca^{++}, Mg^{++}, acetate or bicarbonate, arbitrarily K^+, and dextrose) is circulated on the other side. Thus, waste or toxic products from blood are removed. The dialysate compositions is adjusted to maintain the correct electrolyte concentration in blood. Excess water can be ultrafiltered by applying a hydrostatic pressure difference between blood and dialysate side. A typical hemodialysis session usually lasts from 4 to 6 hours. Patients with chronic renal insufficiency must undergo two or three times each week.

The results of the first experimental attempt to use hemodialysis in animals, which was undertaken by Abel, Roundtree, and Turner, was reported in 1913 (21). In this first hemodialysis application, they used collodion membranes. The first clinically successful application of hemodialysis was reported by Kolff, who had designed a rotating hemodialysis unit consist of Cellophane tubing (22). A breakthrough in the wide range use of hemodialysis especially in chronic renal failure occurred in 1960, when Scribner introduced the famous arterial-venous shunt made of Teflon (23). Afterwards, hemodialysis technology has rapidly improved, and the relevant industry has completed the necessary technical preparations. Today, it can be said that about 20 million such procedures are succesfully applied each year all around the world, and hemodialysis still offers the best possible method for acute and chronic renal failure.

Membranes. Cellulose nitrate (collodion) was the first membrane used in hemodialysis (21). Cellophane (or visking tubing) was then utilized in early devices. Cellophane is a type of regenerated cellulose (24). In the preparation process, cellulose is dissolved in aqueous alkali (i.e. NaOH) by reaction with carbon disulfide to form the xanthate, and when this solution is extruded in film or fiber into aqueous acid, the acid destroys the soluble xanthate and reprecipitates the high molecular weight cellulose in the form of Cellophane film or rayon fiber.

Cuprophane membrane is also a type of regenerated cellulose which is made by the cuoxam process (25). In this process, cellulose, usually derived from cotton linters is dissolved in ammonia solution of cupric oxide, then this complex is extruded into an acidic solution to yield the regenerated cellulose. Different kinds of Cuprophan membranes in the form of sheets and tubes in earlier hemodialyzers and as hollow fibers in recent devices, have been used to a large extent. Even though a number of new synthetic membranes have been developed over the last years in competition with Cuprophane it is widely accepted that Cuprophane membranes (especially in the form of hollow fibers) still seem to be the material of choice today, although there are very recent reports about its undesirable effects on the complementary system (26,27).

Developments in reverse osmosis membrane technology for water desalting has opened up ways to prepare new hemodialysis membranes. With a variety of pore structure cellulose acetate membranes based on the phase inversion technique whereby the polymer is dissolved in a solvent system, then the resulting solution is either used to cast a film or to spin a hollow fiber, and finally the membrane is precipitated in a non-solvent system, are considered for hemodialysis and marketed mostly in the form of hollow fiber units (28).

After the "middle-molecules" hypothesis proposed by Babb and Scribner (29), investigations on production of hemodialysis membranes have been focused on improving the membrane permeabilities by having membranes with more open pore structure, and thus having higher clearance rates for bigger molecules and higher ultrafiltration rates. Several such membranes having finely or coarsely porous structure have been made of a variety of polymers. As alternatives to the existing regenerated cellulose and cellulose acetate membranes, membranes with high hydraulic and diffusive permeabilities which provide adequate clearance of middle molecules, with low hydrophilicity, and mostly symmetric structure such as polysulfone, polyamide, polycarbonate, polyacrylonitrile, and polymethylmethacrylate (30-33) have already been commercialized.

There are a variety of block-copolymer membranes which consist of several combinations of hydrophilic segments to impart biocompatibility, water swellability and selectivity, and hydrophobic segments to increase the mechanical strength of the resultant membrane. Such membranes have been made from polyethylene oxide-polyterephthalate, polyethylene oxide-polycarbonate, polyether-urethane, and have been investigated for possible hemodialysis applications (34-36).

The membranes have also been prepared from a variety of water-soluble polymers (e.g. polyvinylpyrrolidone, polyvinylalcohol, polyethyleneglycol and polyhydroxyethylmethacrylate) which have been cross-linked with different chemicals (37).

Besides several of the membranes described above, other recent approaches for preparing better hemodialysis membranes such as polyelectrolyte membranes (38), polyaminoacid membranes (39), and collagen membranes (40), with high biocompatibilities, good mechanical properties and improved dialysis rates would trigger the future of hemodialysis.

Modules. In the previous chapter in this book, the importance of the module design on the performance of membrane separation process has already been discussed. Notice also that the mass transfer rates attainable in hemodialyzers is, of course a function of the membrane active area and the permeability of the dialysis membrane. It is also showed that the liquid films adjacent to the membrane in the blood and the dialysis solution sides, especially the blood side resistance are also effective. It should also be noted that the membrane takes on an increasing fraction of the total resistance as the molecular weight of the permeant molecules increases. Therefore, in order to attain higher mass transfer rates, or in a broader term high "clearance rates", not only the selection of the membrane is important, but design of the dialyzer module must also be taken into consideration.

The first disposable dialyzer was designed in 1956 by Kolff and Watschinger (41). It was a tubular, or coil type dialyzer (so-called Twin Coil Dialyzer) and consisted of Cellophane tubing wound around a central plastic core. Kiil introduced the first flat-plate dialyzer in 1960 (42), which was a modification of Skeggs and Leonard's original design utilized sheets of cellulose membrane. Mahon and coworkers reported the capillary kidney in 1964. The first hollow fiber dialyzer utilizing regenerated cellulose acetate fibers was based on this original development, and was marketed later on (28). During the next years a variety of hemodialysis units were explored, but these three principal designs remained essentially the same. Reduction in size has been achieved. A number of different designs with similar external appearance but varying internal construction have been marketed throughout the world. Successful flow distribution, low flow resistance, a wide range of ultrafiltration, and low residual blood volume have overcome many of the objections to the use of early devices. In conclusion, among the others hollow fiber dialyzers utilizing Cuprophane seem to be the most attractive dialyzers in the hemodialysis market today.

Hemofiltration

Ultrafiltration of blood across synthetic membranes was proposed back in the 1930's (43). Skeggs, Leonards and Kahn introduced the use of ultrafiltration to remove excess fluid from the blood of normal and edematous dogs (44). Henderson reported removal of toxins from blood by so called peritonel ultrafiltration dialysis (45). The first substantial clinical application of hemofiltration was reported by Quellhorst and coworkers (46). Then, many reports have documented that hemofiltration can be considered as a further therapeutic alternative to hemodialysis for the treatment of patients suffering renal diseases. Unfortunately, despite the advantages over hemodialysis in respect to elimination of intermediate or middle molecular weight substances with higher rates due to convective transport, hemofiltration is not widespread.

Hemofiltration is a membrane process by which uremic toxins in the blood are removed by means of convective flow under a transmembrane pressure gradient (Fig. 8). With a filtration rate of up to 40 % of the blood flow, blood is filtered in hemofiltration separators. The ultrafiltrate formed contains microsolutes, e.g. all electrolytes in plasma, urea, creatinine, uric acid, glucose, etc., but no proteins

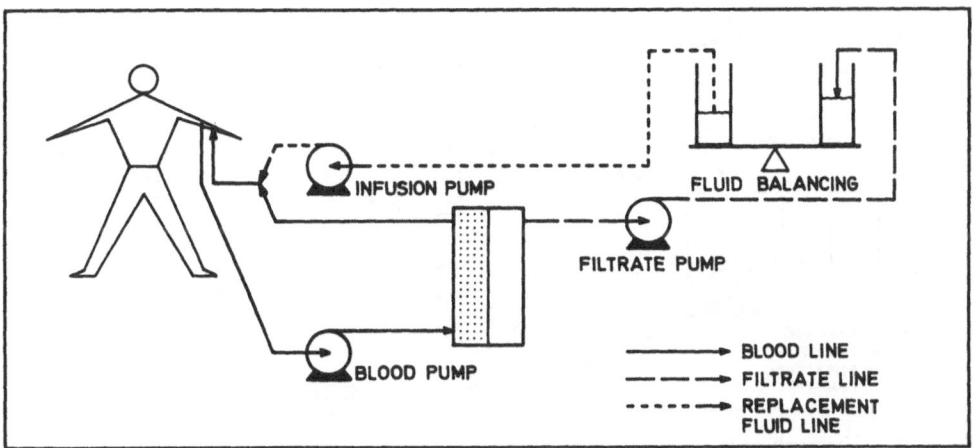

Figure 8.   Hemofiltration.

and cellular elements of the blood, is discarded. In order to maintain patient fluid balance a corresponding volume of sterile physiological solution is reinfused. This can be introduced either before (prediluation) or after (postdiluation) the separator.

Unlike hemodialysis, which relys upon the diffusive transport of metabolites and electrolytes, hemofiltration remove solutes by predominantly a convective transport mechanism. In hemofiltration, all substances having molecular weights below the MW cutoff of the membrane are filtered at an equal rate. It can be pointed out that dialysis is favorable for the removal of the small molecules (e.g.urea); hemofiltration has superior clearance of middle molecules.

The characteristics of hemofiltration membranes are quite different from those used for conventional hemodialysis due to the very high water removal rate. The membrane used is selected for its high hydraulic permeability and retentivity characteristics. Beside these functional properties, as hemofiltration membrane must fulfill the other criteria such as non-toxicity, high blood-compatibility, high mechanical strength, etc. To date, regenerated cellulose, cellulose acetate, polyamide, polysulfone, polycarbonate, polyacrylonitrile and polymethyl methacrylate membranes with different structure and thickness, thus with different hydraulic and diffusive permeabilities, are available commercially (47-49). Mostly hollow fiber or flat-plate hemofiltration modules have been marketed by several companies. Additionally, various other membranes of different compositions and properties are in varying stages of development or undergoing clinical trials.

In conclusion, it can be said that with superior clearance of middle molecular weight substances, which are identified but unfortunately not characterized at present, hemofiltration has been given credit as an alternative of hemodialysis. However, the high cost of commercial sterile replacement solutions, together with the risk of their contamination during storage, have limited its wide spread usage.

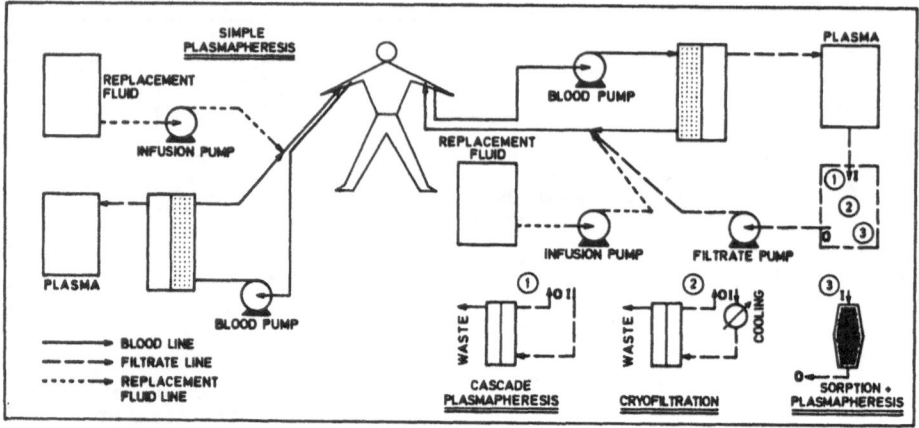

Figure 9.   Plasmapheresis.

PLASMAPHERESIS

The idea of plasma exchange has a very long history, (more than 30 years).A variety of diseases have been treated by plasma exchange. Conventionally, it has been conducted by centrifugal methods. In these methods, i.e. so-called aphresis, anticoagulated blood from the patient is pumped in a centrifuge bowl and separated into cells and plasma, the plasma is collected in a waste bag and the cells together with exchange fluid are reinfused to the patient. The main problems associated with this approach are the high cost of the plasma centrifugal separator and the need for a large quantity of blood fraction. In addition, the need for substitution of albumin and fresh plasma increase the cost and also the risk of accompanied side effects.

Membranes for plasma exchange were first utilized in 1977 (50) and this process was then coined as "plasmapheresis" is an extracorporeal treatment where blood from the patient is circulated through a membrane filter at a flow rate about 50-100 ml/min, and roughly 30 % of the whole blood is filtered (Fig. 9). The plasma separated from blood contains macromolecules (up to 2,400,000 Daltons molecular weight), and micromolecules (crystalloids). In this simple plasmaseparation the fluid phase is discarded. Due to the non-selective removal of plasma components, fresh frozen plasma with valuable proteins (e.g. albumin) is required to reinfuse. This is one of the major drawbacks of therapeutic plasmapheresis as practiced today.However,recent developments such as cryofiltration, double filtration plasmapheresis, or cascade filtration, and plasmapheresis combined with specific adsorption of the pathological plasma components has triggered this new therapeutic technique (51-54).

In cryofiltration, plasma is separated from whole blood by a membrane plasma separator. The plasma is then cooled to 2-6°C and pumped through a second membrane filter. The filtrate is returned to patient with the cell fraction. It was reported that more selective removal of pathogenic macromolecules may be achieved by this procedure, thus there is minimal need for replacement products.

In double filtration plasmapheresis, or in cascade filtration, membrane filters with different cutoffs are used in series. The plasma separated from the first filter is further treated with the second filter, and thus the pathogenic substances are removed whereas non-toxic components of the plasma are reinfused to patient. Again, by this way, the required quantity of the substitution fluid including the proteins, e.g. albumin can markedly be decreased. Use of the specific sorbents in series with membrane filters allows further improvement in respect to reduction of the pathological plasma constituents, but saving the whole plasma with albumin and other functional proteins, and thus stimulating the widespread applications of plasmapheresis.

To date a number of plasma separators utilizing membranes with improved properties, such as low or no rejection of high molecular weight proteins, without loss of filtration efficiency, have been released by several companies. In addition to most widely used porous polypropylene, the membranes made of cellulose acetate, celulose di-acetate, polymethylmethacrylate, polyethylene, polyvinylchloride, polvinylalcohol, copolymer of ethylene and vinyl alcohol, and polycarbonate are employed in commercially available plasmapheresis modules (55,56). Notice that most of these modules are in hollow fiber arrangement, some flat-plate modules are also available.

In the last seven years, a number of publications reporting succesful applications of plasmapheresis have been introduced. Despite the very high cost of the procedure, plasmapheresis is accepted as an useful tool today in the therapy of many multisystem diseases with proved or assumed pathological plasma components, e.g., antibodies, immunecomplexes, paraproteins, and toxic substances. Though a relation has not been well defined in most cases, plasmapheresis is employed with the hope that the removal of these molecules may be of therapeutic benefit. In conclusion, it is emphasized that better understanding these mechanisms, reduction of the cost of this system, and improvements in existing techniques, of course, will make the plasmapheresis more acceptable in the future.

HEMOPERFUSION

Hemoperfusion is an extracorporeal treatment method in which the blood from the patient is circulated through adsorption columns in order to remove exogeneous and endogeneous toxins from the blood (Fig. 10). Today, it is well-established procedure to treat patients who are suffering from drug intoxication (57-60). Other areas of application are still controversial but promising, such as chronic renal failure, hepatic failure and many other diseases of unknown origin, e.g., schizophrenia, psoriasis and diseases related to immunological disorders (61-64).

Activated carbons, ion exchangers, non-ionic resins, polyaldehydes, silica gel, active alumina and magnesia, aluminium gels and immunosorbents, or more complex sorbent systems containing these sorbents incorporated with antigens, antibodies, enzymes, and many other biological agents are the most widely used sorbents today.

Activated carbon is a highly porous material derived from various substances by carbonization and activation processes. Activated carbons are able to meet many of the diverse needs for adsorption, and hence have received most attention among the various adsorbents. One of the major applications in medicine is hemoperfusion cartridges in which mostly granular activated carbon is utilized.

Charcoal hemoperfusion was first demonstrated by Yatzidis in 1964 (65). In earlier applications, since blood contacts directly with charcoal in the adsorption column, inherent problems associated with this, i.e. fine particle generation, resulting in embolism to various organs, and severe depletion of platelets and leucocytes from circulating blood (or blood trauma) have been pointed out (66-71). Furthermore, sludging

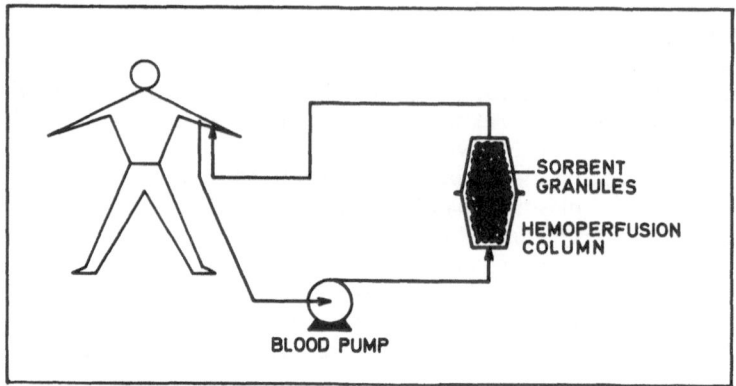

Figure 10.   Hemoperfusion.

and channeling of blood within these hemoperfusion columns which results high-pressure gradients across the column, and thus leading a high depletion of blood cells and reduces clearances, have been also noted. In order to eliminate these draw-backs,various approaches have been proposed.The most popular approach is coating,or so-called microencapsulation of sorbent granules with biocompatible semipermeable membranes, in order to prevent the occurrence of the problems associated with hemoperfusion systems, especially in long-term applications. Other configurations in which fine activated carbon powders are fixed by being sprayed onto tapes with an adhesive (72); carbon particles are entrapped in mostly Cuprophane membranes in a fiber fashion (73); or powdered charcoal is immobilized into polymer gel particles (74-78), have been pursued. Other recent developments are also given credit to prepare new types of charcoals produced by resin beads which can be used without polymeric coat (79).

The overall design of hemoperfusion devices is the first major point in the development of these systems. First of all the sorbent must be intrinsically hard, regularly shaped, easily washable and sterilizable, and must not release toxic materials. The optimization of the column and flow characteristics are other important matters to be evaluated. The shape and dimensions of the column, the flow rate and the flow type must be selected carefully in order to achieve high mass transfer rates with minimum pressure drop. The selection of the coating procedure for sorbent is of course, the most important subject in obtaining suitable systems which have high adsorptive capacity, adsorption rate and blood compatibility, and are free from fine particle generation.

Various types of polymer coatings and different coating procedures have been proposed and evaluated. In 1956, Yatzidis claimed that all side effects were eliminated by coating of charcoal with cellulose acetate without any significant change in the adsorptive capacity of charcoal (80).Rosenbaum et al., opposed the results of Yatzidis, noting severe platelet and leucocyte depletion, and charcoal emboli when cellulose acetate-coated charcoal was used (69). Andrade et al. were the first to encapsulate granular carbon with acrylic polymers (81).They concluded that Hydron Biomedical Polymer coated carbon may be suitable for use in clinical hemoperfusion applications. Fennimore and co-workers have further pursued the use of polyHEMA and developed on a commercial scale (82). The Bioengineering Unit at Strathclyde has produced a number of copolymer membranes (e.g., acrylic acid-n-butylmethacrylate,dimethylamino ethylmethacrylate-acrylonitrile,methyl methacrylate dimethyl aminoethyl methacrylate) for coating of choarcoal (83-85). Denti et al. demonstrated the spray-coating of charcoal by cellulose membranes (86). Thysell et al. used a similar approach to that of Denti in the production of a commercial hemoperfusion cartridge (87). Amano et al. developed a special petroleum pitch spherical charcoal bead and used a spray-coating method to produce collodion coated charcoal (88). This was commercialized later on. In the approach of Rostock, where charcoal was coated by the spraying of cellulose acetate in acetone (89). An ultrathin cellulose acetate coating procedure was developed by Tijssen and marketed (90). Collodion coated spherical charcoal from thermosetting resin was used recently in commercially available hemoperfusion columns (91). The most extensive, complete and well characterized study of hemoperfusion is that by Chang et al. (60,61,63,92-95). They have used nylon, collodion, heparin-benzalkonium complex collodion, albumin-collodion, cellulose acetate, radiation grafted heparin-cellulose, silicone and others. Most recently, a composite artificial kidney (CAK) which is a single unit with capillary fibers in series with 80 grams of collodion coated spherical petroleum based on their studies have been marketed (96). We have also studied the development of new coating materials and methods for hemoperfusion. Our group has tried out nylon, collodion, cellulose acetate, cellulose acetate-KOH, cellulose acetate-formamide, polyethyleneglycols and silicone coatings (91,97). Various types of polymer coatings and different coating procedures have been proposed and evaluated, many others are being studied by a number of groups. However, there is still an uncertainity about the best coating material and method. But, it seems that, today, collodion, cellulose acetate and polyHEMA are the materials of choice at market level.

MEMBRANE-MODERATED SYSTEMS AS CARRIERS OF BIOLOGICALLY ACTIVE SUBSTANCES

As discussed in the previous chapter, membrane separation technology is widely used in the treatment of solutions containing biologically active substances, such as enzymes, whole cells (microbial, plant or animal), antigens, antibodies, contraceptives and many drugs. Membranes in biotechnological and in other related industries may be employed in order to separate and isolate of macrosolutes from microsolutes. For instance, they are used to separate cells from supernatant in whole fermentation broth and to eliminate waste-disposal problems. They are nicely employed for the product recovery of valuable biological products such as hormones, antibodies, and vaccines, or for the elimination of viral, pyrogenic and immunocomplex impurities from biological solutions.

Immobilized Agents

The relatively new and rapidly growing field of biotechnology utilizes enzymes or microorganisms which are capable of producing a wide variety of antibiotics, vitamins, amino acids, hormones, etc. for several applications. Whole cells and isolated enzymes are also widely used as bioactive agents which serve as bioproducers and bioconvertors in those areas like chemical, pharmaceutical, and food industries, in

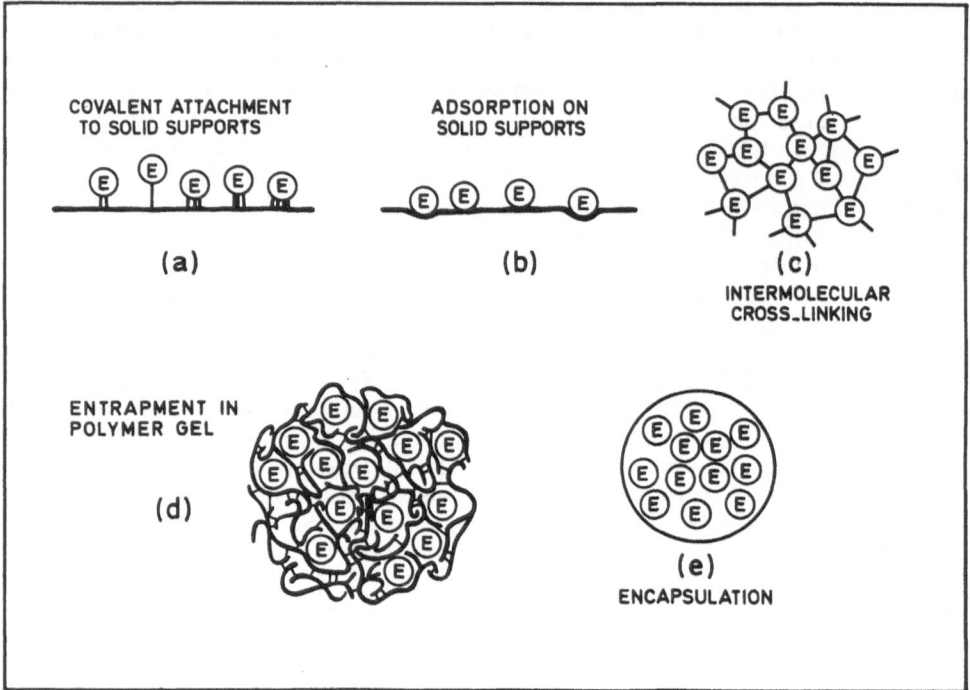

Figure 11.   Immobilization Techniques.

clinical medicine for diagnostic and therapeutic applications. There are some important drawbacks when the biologically active entities are employed in free forms. They
are not sufficiently stable under operating conditions,especially in both extremes of
temperature and pH. They are water-soluble, hence difficult to separate from substrates and products to use repeatedly. In clinical applications, when they are utilized
in free form, they usually result in immunological reactions and rapid removal and
inactivation.

Immobilization is a breakthrough to avoid the problems associated with the use
of bioactive agents in free forms. During the last decade many enzyme immobilization
techniques, which have also been adapted for immobilization of other biologically
active substances, have been elaborated (98-101), but they may be classified into the
following groups (Fig. 11).

  a. The enzymes are covalently bound to a carrier system (Fig. 11 a). A variety of
     supports have been used, such as synthetic polymers (e.g. nylons), activated
     carbon, glass, ceramics, etc. Enzymes are usually attached to the solid support
     through their amino or carboxyl groups.
  b. The enzymes are adsorbed ionically or physically to various kinds of support
     materials (Fig. 11 b). Many types of ion-exchangers and charcoals have been
     used as adsorbents.

    c. The enzymes are covalently cross-linked to each other as shown in the Figure 11 c, schematically. Attachment is obtained by using bifunctional crosslinkers like glutaraldehyde, dimethyl adipimate, etc.

    d. The enzymes are immobilized by entrapment inside the polymer gel matrices which may be in the form of membranes (Fig. 11 d).

    e. Enzymes are encapsulated with their environments within various forms of semipermeable membrane systems (Fig. 11 e).

Numerous combinations and variations of the above techniques are also possible. Membranes in these techniques are utilized as carriers or as a barrier to separate one bulk solution from another. Bioactive agents may be attached to the surface of the membrane, or entrapped within the polymeric net-work of the membrane. Today, membrane-moderated reactors (so-called bioreactors) which contain enzymes or microorganisms within the pores of the membrane matrix are considered as a novel biotechnological tools for the conduct of continuous biochemical transformations.

In addition, membranes containing bioactive substances in their matrices are showing considerable promise in the development of novel biosensors for detection and measurement of biologically important substances by means of high specificity. Various enzyme electrodes have been developed for assaying a number of substances such as urea, uric acid, glucose, amino acids, alcohol, etc. (100,102-106). In these electrodes the substances to be measured diffuse into the matrix, and react with enzymes which produce or consume the substance that is sensed by a standard electrode. Not only the enzymes, but also many other biofunctional agents such as whole cells or tissue slices containing complex enzyme systems, immunogenic materials (e.g. antibodies, antigens), etc. are also coupled to membrane carrier. These functional membranes are then installed in a conventional membrane electrode with the appropriate filling and are used in more complex biological analysis, such as immunoassays for diagnosis (107-111). It is evident that the application of membranes to the development of new and sophisticated chemical sensing and detection devices represents an exciting and promising field for innovative research and membrane-based industries over the next decade.

Enzymes or microorganisms are also entrapped into the lumen of microcapsules, nanocapsules or hollow fibers. The substrate molecules can freely permeate through the membrane and react with enzymes, or microorganisms, and the product molecules transported in the opposite direction, again freely. But, the membrane is substantially impermeable to the much higher MW species, i.e. enzymes, or microorganisms. Such arrangements utilizing hollow fiber bundles which contain enzymes or cells in the immobilized form, are already employed in bioreactors for biotechnological applications with an increasing attraction (99-101).

The process of microencapsulation was described several years ago for the production of carbonless copypapers. Numerous methods for preparing microcapsules for agricultural, pharmaceutical, medical and other biological and related applications have then been elaborated (100,101,112-114). Interfacial polycondensation and phase separation methods have been given the most credit among the others. Larger microcapsules, namely nanocapsules, have also been produced through micelle encapsulation, or similar emulsification processes. Polyamides (nylons), collodion, cellulose and derivatives, silicones, lipids with other polymers, proteins and some other polymeric materials are utilized in order to prepare micro or nanocapsules with specific membrane characteristics.

Chang was the pioneer for the immobilization of biofunctional species into micro-capsules, or by his original definition into artificial cells. Significant work has been done to extend this concept in several applications. Enzymes, cells, organelles, anti-gens, antibodies and many other bioactive agents have been entrapped into micro-capsules. Biosubstances immobilized by microencapsulation have been used in biotechnology for production of specific materials (e.g., interferon, monoclonal antibodies), in medicine for the treatment of patients suffering with renal diseases, drug overdose, liver failure, and other metabolic diseases, in enzyme replacement therapy, in the removal of immunogenic substances via specific sorbent-microcapsule systems; as artificial pancreas system, in which microcapsules containing pancreatic endocrine tissues and islets are utilized to maintain the glucose levels in diabetics; and in many other novel applications (98-101, 112-120).

Controlled Release

The application of controlled release systems, in which biologically active subs-tances are released to their environment with controllable rates has grown enor-mously in the last decade. Controlled administration of chemicals or drugs is widely publicized in the field of medicine and pharmacy, but it is also applied in other fields including agriculture, food industry, biotechnology, etc. (121-136).

Conventionally, bioactive agents are delivered to a system by periodic adminis-tration. For example, many drugs in therapeutic applications are given by periodic injection or ingestion. During this process, systemic distribution may cause of many diverse effects which are compounded by the large quantity of the drug which might be toxic to the health of cells or tissues, or the plasma level of the drug may drop to an ineffective value. By the controlled release concept of delivery, the drug concentration of plasma may be maintained effectively constant at an optimal level for prolonged periods. Additionally, specific formulations may concentrate the drug at a specific site by using targeting techniques. Sustained release systems, in some cases, could be employed to mask the taste, or odor of the drug in therapeutic applications, or to minimize the environmental side effects as in agriculture (i.e. release of pesticides, and others), or in the case of expensive agents such as pheromones administration, they offer optimal utilization, which is an economic necessity. In addition, increasing the environmental stability and compatibility of the bioactive agents by carriers are the other potential advantages of the controlled release systems.

There are a number of techniques of achieving controlled release. However, since our emphasis in this volume is on the uses of synthetic polymers in biological applica-tions, we will focus on only these type of devices here. Among the others, two types of bioagent-polymer combinations are mostly given credit, namely monolithic (or matrix) systems, and reservoir systems with rate controlling membrane, as shown in Figure 12.

In the first, bioagent is dissolved or throughly dispersed in the polymer matrix. The mixture is then treated by injection or compression molding, casting, extrusion, calendering, or by other common techniques of polymer technology, into the required geometrical shape. The active agent is released from these composites to the surround-ing environment by several mechanisms. In some cases, physically bound active agent goes out from the polymer matrix by simply diffusional mechanisms. In another category, the active agent is released as the polymeric carrier is eroded away by simply physical dissolution or by chemical degradation. The kinetic of release in the latter case is relatively complex, and constant rate of delivery, or in other terms

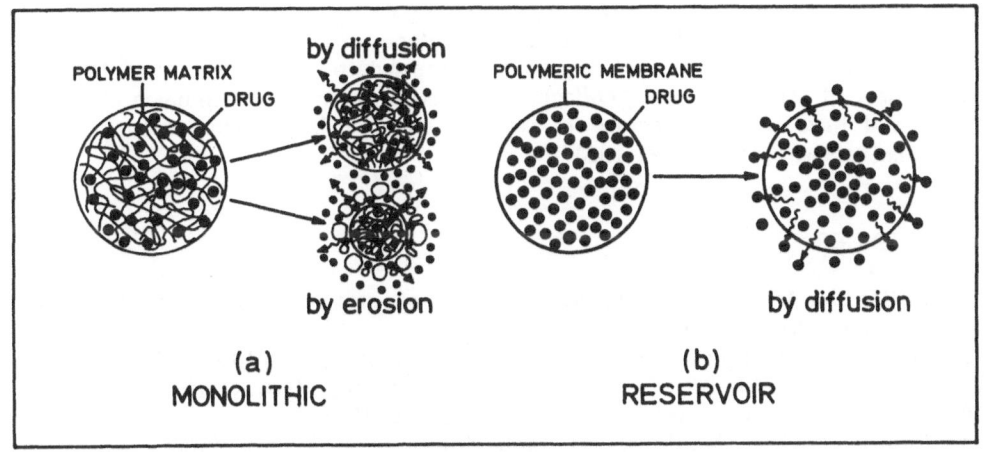

Figure 12.   Controlled Release Systems : (a) Monolithic, (b) Reservoir.

"zero order process" can hardly be achieved due to its dependence on erosion mechanism and geometry.

An important class of controlled release devices have a reservoir containing the agent to be released which is surrounded by an appropriate polymeric membrane. This device may be large (macrocapsules, i.e. 2000-3000 μm in diameter) or very small (microcapsules) capsules which are described in the previous sections of this chapter. This case, fortunately, creates a constant steady-state release rate by diffusion, the driving force of such systems is the concentration gradient of active molecules between reservoir and environment. However, this class of devices is more difficult to fabricate than the monolithic types. Many methods for microencapsulating active agents have been developed. As mentioned above, phase separation methods (e.g. aqueous or organic phase separation, meltable dispersion, spray-drying, pan coating, etc.) and interfacial condensation or addition polymerization are most widely employed among the other techniques available.

Other types of controlled-release devices, including composite devices (i.e. reservoir + monolithic), osmotic pumps, laminated structures, reservoir systems without rate-controlling membranes which utilize macroscopic devices of hollow fibers of tubes systems corporated with sorbents (i.e. ion-exchange resins), and many others, have been recognized to be wide-ranging of application and of significant value.

As mentioned previously, controlled release systems have been considered for a very wide variety of applications. Formulations for the administration of pharmaceutical, agricultural and veterinary agents have been widely accepted at commercial level. Analgesics, steroids vitamins, sedatives, hypnotics, antibiotics, antiseptics, chemotherapeutic agents, prostaglandins, enzymes, bacteria, viruses, antimicrobials, pesticides, fertilizers, herbicides, pheromones, and many other agents have been incorporated with polymeric carriers and have been successfully employed.

The list of polymers that have been used in sustained release formulations is very long. Almost all polymers available have been considered for controlled release systems. Among these, cellulosic polymers (i.e., cellulose nitrate, cellulose acetate,

156

ethylcellulose, cellulose acetate phthalate, carboxymethylcellulose, methyl cellulose), polydimethyl siloxane and other silicones, ethylene vinyl acetate copolymer, polyurethanes, polyamids, polyhydroxyethyl methacrylate and other acrylates, and copolymers of acrylates, lipids, collagen, polypetites, etc. have been given the most credit and have already emerged in commercially available membrane-moderated controlled release systems (121-136).

REFERENCES

1. Butler, J.A.V. and Katz, B., Progress in Biophysics and Biophysical Chemistry, Pergamon Press, 1959.
2. Nose, Y., The Oxygenator, The C.V. Mosby Company, Saint Luis, 1973.
3. Kolff, W.J. and Balzer, R., Trans Amer. Soc. Artif. Intern. Organs, 1:39, 1955.
4. Kolff, W.J., et al., Cleveland Clin. Quart., 23:69, 1956.
5. Clowes, G.H.A., Hopkins, A.L. and Kolobow, T., Trans. Amer. Soc. Artif. Intern. Organs, 1:23, 1955.
6. Clowes, G.H.A., Jr., Neville, W.E., Sabga, G. and Shibota, Y., Surgery, 44:220, 1958.
7. Pierce, E.C.II, Arch. Surg., 77:938, 1958.
8. Esmond, W.G. and Dibelius, N.R., Trans. Amer. Soc. Artif. Intern. Organs, 11:325, 1965.
9. Thomas, J.A., Arch. Klin. Chir., 289:286, 1958.
10. Pierce, E.C.II. and Dibelius, N.R., Trans. Amer. Soc. Artif. Intern. Organs, 14:220, 1968.
11. Esato, K. and Eiseman, B., J.Thorac. Cardiovascular Surg., 69:690, 1975.
12. Bierenbaum, H.S., Isaacson, R.B., Druin, M.L. and Plovan, S.G., Ind. Eng. Chem. Prod. Res. Develop., 13:2, 1974.
13. Gore, R.W., U.S. Patent, 3,953,566, April 27, 1976.
14. Product Information, Celgard Microporous Film, Celanese Corp., Charlotte, North Carolina, 1981.
15. Chawla, A.S., in Polymeric Biomaterials,Piskin, E., Hoffman, A.S., eds. Martinus Nijhoff Publ., The Hague, 1985. (in press)
16. Piskin, E. and Evren, V., Proc. Workshop on Design and Techniques of Extracorporeal Gas Exchange, Creteil, 1985. (in press)
17. Dawids, S.G. and Engell, H.C., Physiological and Clinical Aspects of Oxygenator Design, Elsevier, Luxemburg, 1976.
18. Kenedi, R.M., Courtney, J.M., Gaylor, J.D.S. and Gilchrist, T., Artificial Organs, The MacMillan Press Ltd., London, 1977.
19. Kolobow, T., J.Artif. Organs, 1:15, 1978.
20. Eberhart, R.C., Dengle, S.K. and Curtis, R.M., Artif. Organs, 2:19, 1978.
21. Abel, J.J., Rountree, L.G. and Turner, B.B., J.Pharm. Exp. Ther., 5:275, 1914.
22. Kolff, W.J. and Berk, H.T., ter Welle, M., van der Ley, A.J.W., van Dijk, E.C. and van Noordwijk, J., Acta Med. Scand., 117:121, 1944.
23. Scribner, B.H., Caner, J.E., Buri, R. and Quinton, W.E., Trans. Amer. Soc. Artif. Intern. Organs, 6:88, 1960.
24. Kolff, W.J., Ann. Intern. Med., 62:608, 1965.
25. Bandel, W., Chem. Z.Jahrgang, 65, 1964.
26. Ing, T.S., Daugirdas, J.T., Popli, S. and Gandhi, V.C., Int. J.Artif. Organs, 6:235, 1983.

27. Ivanovich, P., Chenoweth, D.E., Schmidt, R., Klinkmann, H., Boxer, L.A., Jacob, H.S. and Hammerschmidt, D.E., Kidney Int., 24:758, 1983.
28. Lipps, B.J., Stewart, R.D., Perkins, H.A., Holmes, G.W., McLain, E.A., Rolfs, M.R. and Oja, P.D., Trans. Amer. Soc. Artif. Intern. Organs, 13:200, 1967.
29. Babb, A.L., Popovitch, P.P., Christofer, T.G. and Scribner, B.D., Trans. Amer. Soc. Artif. Intern. Organs, 17:81, 1971.
30. Luttinger, M., Cooper, C.W., R.I., Trans. Amer. Artif. Intern. Organs, 14:5, 1968.
31. Fisher, B.S., Higley, W.S., Cantor, P.A. and Stone, W.J.R., Trans. Amer. Soc. Artif. Intern. Organs, 19:429, 1973.
32. Salyer, I.O., Ball, G.L., and Beemsterboer, G.L., in Membrane Processes in Industry and Biomedicine, Bier, M., ed., Plenum Press, New York, 1971.
33. Ota, K., Okazawa, J., Kumayaga, E., Agishi, J., Sugino, N., Mitani, N., Fugii, Y., Kimura, M., Nagao, Y., Tsukamoto, H., Tanzawa, H., Sakaj, Y., Proc. Eur. Dial. Transplant. Assoc., 12:559, 1975.
34. Lyman, D.J., Loo, B.H. and Crawfor, R.W., Biochemistry, 3:985, 1964.
35. Konstantin, P., Goehl, H. and Gullberg, C., Artif. Organs (suppl), 5:691, 1979.
36. Lyman, D.J. and Loo, B.H., J. Biomed. Mater. Res., 1:17, 1967.
37. Lyman, D.J., in Replacement of Renal Function by Dialysis, Drukker, W., Parsons, F.M., Maher, J.F., eds., Martinus Nijhoff Publ., The Hague, 1979.
38. Micheals, A., Ind. Eng. Chem., 57(10):32, 1965.
39. Bamford, C.H., Elliott, A. and Hanby, W.E., Synthetic Polypeptides, Academic Press, New York, 1956.
40. Nishihara, T., Rubin, A.L. and Stenzel, K.H., Trans. Amer. Soc. Artif. Intern. Organs, 24:662, 1978.
41. Kolff, W.J. and Watschinger, B., J.Lab. Clin. Med., 47:969, 1956.
42. Kiil, F., Acta Clin. Scand. Suppl., 253:142, 1960.
43. Gieger, A., J. Physiol., (London), 71:111, 1931.
44. Skeggs, L.T., Leonards, J.R. and Kahn, J.R., Lab. Invest., 1:488, 1952.
45. Henderson, L.W., J.Clin. Invest., 45:950, 1966.
46. Quellhorst, E., Rieger, J., Doht, B., Beckmann, H., Jacob, I., Kraft, B., Mietzsch, G. and Scheler, F., Proc. EDTA, 12:314, 1976.
47. Holland, F.F., Klein, E., Wendt, R.P. and Eberle, K., Trans. Amer. Soc. Artif. Organs, 14:662, 1978.
48. Henne, W., Duenweg, G. and Gullberg, C.A., Contr. Nephrol., 32:20, 1982.
49. Gohl, H., Konstantin, P. and Gullberg, C.A., Contr. Nephrol., 32:20, 1982.
50. Inoue, N., Yamazaki, Z., Oda, T., Sugiura, M., Wada, T., Fuijsani, Y., Hayano, F., Trans. Amer. Soc. Artif. Intern. Organs, 23:698, 1977.
51. Samtleben, W., Blumenstein, M., Liebl, L. and Gurland, H.J., Trans. Amer. Soc. Artif. Intern. Organs, 26:12, 1980.
52. Agishi, T., Kaneko, I., Hasua, Y., et. al., Trans. Amer. Soc. Artif. Int. Organs, 26:406, 1980.
53. Malchesky, P.S., Asanuma, Y. and Blumenstein, M., Mitt. Klin. Nephrologie, 10:44, 1981.
54. Gurland, H.J., Lysaght, M.J. and Samtleben, in The Past, Present and Future of Artificial Organs, Piskin, E. and Chang, T.M.S., eds., Meteksan, Ankara, 1983.
55. Henne, W., Gerlach, K., Tretzal, J. and Pelger. M., Membrane Technology for Plasmapheresis, presented, Int. Workship on Plasma Separation and Plasma Fractionation, Rottach-Egern, March, 1983.
56. Nose, Y., Matchesky, P.S. and Smith, J.W., Plasmapheresis, ISAO Press, Cleveland, 1983.

158

57. Vale, J.A., Ress, A.J., Widdop, B., Br.Med.J.1:5, 1975.
58. Rosenbaum, J.I., Kramer, M.S., Raja, R., Arch. Intern. Med., 136:236, 1976.
59. Winchester, J.F., Gelfand, M.C., Knepshield, J.H., Schreiner, G.E., Trans. Am. Soc. Artif. Intern. Organs., 23:762, 1977.
60. Chang, T.M.S., Clin, Toxicol., 17:529, 1980.
61. Chang, T.M.S., Kidney Int., 7:387, 1975.
62. Williams, R., Murray-Lyon, I.M., eds., Artificial Liver Support, Pitman Medical, London, 1975.
63. Chang, T.M.S., Artif. Organs, 2:359, 1978.
64. Gilchrist, T., in Hemoperfusion, V. Bonomini., and T.M.S. Chang., eds., pp.285, Karger, Basel, 1982.
65. Yatzidis, H., Proc. Eur. Dial. Transplant. Assoc., 1:83, 1964.
66. Dunea, G., Kolff, W.J. Trans. Am. Artif. Intern. Organs, 11:178, 1965.
67. Hagstam, K.E., Larsson, L.E., Thysell, H., Acta Med. Scand., 180:593, 1966.
68. Demyttenaere, M.H., Maher, J.F., Sacheiner, G.E., Trans. Am. Soc. Artif. Intern. Organs, 13:19, 1967.
69. Rosenbaum, J.L., Ronquillo, E., Arguyres, S.N., J.Albert Einstein Med. Cnt., 16:67, 1968.
70. Dutton, R.C., Dedrick, R.L., Bull, B.S., Thromb. Diath. Haem., 21:367, 1969.
71. Barakat, T.C., Mac Phee, I.W., Brit. J.Surg., 57:580, 1970.
72. Hill, J.B., Palaia, F.L., Horres, C.R., in Artificial Organs, R.M. Kenedi, J.M., Courtney, et al, eds., pp. 123, London, McMillian Press Ltd., 1977.
73. Gurland, H., Castro, L.A., Hillebrand, G., Schmidt, B., in Hemoperfusion., S. Sideman., T.M.S. Chang., eds., pp.105, Washington, Hemisphere, 1980.
74. Ozdural, A.R., Mann, H., Byrne, T., Piskin, E., Life Support Systems (Suppl.), pp.55, 1982.
75. Ozdural, A.R., Mann, H., Byrne, T., Piskin, E., in Hemoperfusion and Artificial Organs, E. Piskin., T.M.S. Chang., eds., Ankara, Artif. Organs Soc., 1982.
76. Piskin, E., Kiremitci, M., Arca, E., Piskin, K., Evren, V., Mutlu, M., in Proc. Int. Sym. Hemoperfusion and Artificial Organs, Tianjin, 1983.
77. Kiremitci, M., Piskin, E., Life Support Systems (Suppl.), pp.398, 1984.
78. Kiremitci, M., Piskin, E., Int. J. Artif. Organs, 1985.(in press)
79. Piskin, E., In Proc. 6th, Int. Sym. on Hemoperfusion and Blood Detoxification, Mexico 1985. (in press)
80. Yatzidis, H., Paper presented at Cleveland Clinic, Cleveland, Ohio, 1966.
81. Andrade, J.D., Van Wagenen, R., Chen. C., Kopp, K., Kolff, W.J., A critical review, Proc.Eur.Dial. Transplant. Ass., 9:210, 1972.
82. Fennimore, J., Watson, P.A., Munro, G.D., Kolthammer, J., Proc. Eur. Soc. Artif. Organs, 1:90, 1974.
83. Courtney, J.M., Gilchrist, T., Walker, J.M., Edwards, R.O., 10th Int.Conf.Med. Biol.Eng., Dresden, 10:133, 1973.
84. Courtney, J.M., Gilchrist, T., Hood, R.G., Townsend, W.B.A. Proc.Eur.Soc. Artif.Organs, 2:210, 1975.
85. Gilchrist, T., Jonsson, E., Martin, A.M., Naucler, L., Cameron , A., Courtney, J.M., in Artificial Liver Support, R.Williams. and I.M. Morray-Lyon., eds., pp.319-329, Pitman Medical, London, 1975.
86. Denti, E., Lubox M.P., Tessore, V., I. Biomed, Mater. Res., 9:143, 1975.
87. Thysell, H., Lindholm, T., Heinegard, D.,Henriksson, H., Nylen, U., Svensson, T., Bergkvist, G., Gullberg, C.A., Proc.Eur.Soc. Artif. Organs, 2:212, 1976.

88. Amano, I., Kano, H., Saito, A., Manji, T., Yamamota, Y., Iwatsuki, W., Takahiri, H., Ohta, K., Maeda, K., Proc. Eur. Dial. Transplant. Assoc., 13:262, 1976.
89. Schmidt, R., Falkenhagen, D., Holtz, M., Osten, B., Kroger, E., Glasel, E., Gott schall, S., Ahrend, K.F., Bremer, H., Tiess, D., Klinkmann, H., Dt. Gesund. Wes., 32:45, 1977.
90. Tijsen, J., Bantjes, A., van Doorn, A.W.J., Feijen, J., van Dijk, B., Vonk, C.R., Dijkhuis, I.C., Artif. Organs, 3:11, 1979.
91. Piskin, E., in The Past, Present and Future of Artificial Organs, E. Piskin and T.M.S. Chang., eds., pp. 152, Meteksan, Ankara. 1983.
92. Chang, T.M.S., ed., Artificial kidney, artificial liver, and artificial cells, Plenum Press, New York, 1978.
93. Sideman, S., Chang, T.M.S., eds., Hemoperfusion : Kidney and liver support and detoxification, Part I, Hemisphere, Washington, 1980.
94. Bonomini, V., Chang, T.M.S., eds., Hemoperfusion, S. Karger, Basel, 1982.
95. Piskin, E., Chang, T.M.S., eds., Hemoperfusion and Artificial Organs, Artif. Organs Soc., in Turkey, Ankara, 1982.
96. Chang, T.M.S., Barre, P., Kuruvilla, S., Messier, D., Man, N.K., Trans.Am.Soc. Artif.Intern.Organs, 1982. (in press)
97. Piskin, E.,Proc. 5th Int. Symp.on Hemoperfusion and Artificial Organs, Tianjin, 1983. (in press)
98. Zaborsky, D.R., Immobilized Enzymes, CRC Press, Cleveland, 1973.
99. Thomas, D. and Kernevez, J.P., Analysis of Control of Immobilized Enzyme Systems, North-Holland, Amsterdam, 1976.
100. Chang, T.M.S., Biomedical Applications of Immobilized Enzyme and Proteins, Vols. I and II, Plenum Press, New York, 1976.
101. Mattiason, B., Immobilized Cells and Organelles, CRC Press, Boca Raton, Florida, 1983.
102. Guilbault, C.G. and Montalvo, Jr., J.G., J. Amer. Chem. Soc., 91: 2164, 1969.
103. Rechnitz, G.A., Chem. Eng. News, 27:29, 1975.
104. Rawls, R.L., Chem. Eng. News, 5:19, 1976.
105. Hirose, S., Hayashi, M., Tamura, N., Suzuki, S. and Karube, I., J. Molecular Catalysis, 6:251, 1979.
106. Arnold, M.A. and Rechnitz, G.A., Anal. Chem., 52:1170, 1980.
107. Solsky, R.L. and Rechnitz, G.A., Science, 204:1308, 1979.
108. Solsky, R.L. and Rechnitz, G.A., Anal. Chim. Acta, 123:135, 1981.
109. Rechnitz, G.A., Science, 214:287, 1981.
110. Cheung, P.W., et al., Theory, Design and Biomedical Applications of Solid State Chemical Sensors, CRC Press, Boca Raton, Florida, 1978.
111. Sevier, E.D., et al., Clin. Chem., 27:1797, 1981.
112. Chang, T.M.S., Artificial Cells, Charles C. Thomas, Springfield, Illinois, 1972.
113. Gutcho, M.H., Microcapsules and Other Capsules, Noyas Data Corp., Park Ridge, New Jersey, 1979.
114. Lim, F., Biomedical Applications of Microencapsulation, CRC Press, Boca Raton, Florida, 1980.
115. Mosbach, K., Methods in Enzymology-Immobilized Enzymes, Academic Press, New York, 1976.
116. Lim, F. and Sun, A.M., Science, 210:908, 1980.
117. Micheals, A.S., Desalination, 35:329, 1980.
118. Chang, T.M.S., in The Past, Present and Future of Artificial Organs, E. Piskin and T.M.S. Chang, eds., Meteksan, Ankara, 1983.

119. Rupp, R.G., Proc. Amer. Chem. Soc., Academic Press, 1985.
120. Goosen, M.F.A., O'Shea, G.M., Gharapetian, H.M., Chou, S. and Sun, A.M., Biotech. and Bioeng., 27:146, 1985.
121. Tanguary, A.C. and Lacey, R.E., Controlled Release of Biologically Active Agents, Plenum Press, New York, 1974.
122. Colbert, J.C., Controlled Action Drug Forms, Noyes Data Corp., Park Ridge, New Jersey, 1974.
123. Cardarelli, N., Controlled Release Pesticide Formulations, CRC Press, Boca Raton, Florida, 1976.
124. Paul, D.R. and Harris, F.W., Controlled Release Polymeric Formulations, ACS Symp. Ser. 33, American Chemical Society, Washington, D.C., 1976.
125. Scher, H.B, Controlled Release Pesticides, ACS Symp. Ser. 53, American Chemical Society, Washington, D.C., 1977.
126. Robinson, J.R., Sustained and Controlled Release Drug Delivery Systems, Marcel Dekker, New York, 1978.
127. Kostelnik, R.J., Polymeric Delivery Systems, Gordon and Breach Science Publishers, New York, 1978.
128. Kydonieus, A.F., Controlled Release Technologies: Methods, Theory and Applications, Vols. I and II, CRC Press, Boca Raton, Florida, 1980.
129. Baker, R., Controlled Release of Bioactive Materials, Academic Press, New York, 1980.
130. Johnson, J.C., Sustained Release Medications, Noyes Data Corp., Park Ridge, New Jersey, 1980.
131. Chandrasekaran, S.K., Controlled Release Systems, AIChE Symp. Ser. No. 206, 77, 1981.
132. Lewis, D.H., Controlled Release of Pesticides and Pharmaceuticals, Plenum Press, New York, 1981.
133. Urquhart, J., Controlled-Release Pharmaceuticals, American Pharmaceutical Association, Washington, D.C., 1981.
134. Bruck, S.D., Controlled Drug Delivery, Vols. I and II, CRC Press, Boca Raton, Florida, 1983.
135. Langer, R.S. and Wise, D.L., Medical Applications of Controlled Release, Vols. I and II, CRC Press, Boca Raton, Florida, 1984.
136. Wise, D.L., Biopolymeric Controlled Release Systems, Vols. I and II, CRC Press, Boca Raton, Florida, 1984.

BIOPOLYMERS IN CONTROLLED RELEASE SYSTEMS

R. Langer

Massachusetts Institute of Technology, Department of Applied Biological Sciences, Cambridge, Massachussets, USA

INTRODUCTION

In a controlled release system a bioactive agent is incorporated into a carrier, generally a polymeric material. The rate of release of the substance is determined by the properties of the polymer itself and is only weakly dependent on environmental factors (such as the pH of bodily fluids). Controlled release systems are capable of delivering substances slowly and continuously for up to several years.

These controlled release systems are a new development that evolved out of a need to prolong and better control drug administration. The significance of such systems can be appreciated by considering typical drug levels resulting from conventional drug formulations (tablets, injections). In most cases, drug levels reach a maximum and then fall to a minimum, at which point repeated administration becomes necessary. However, if the maximum and minimum drug concentrations fall above or below the toxic level or minimum effective levels, respectively, alternating periods of toxicity or inefficacy can result. This is particularly problematic if the toxic and minimum effective levels are close together. The goal of a controlled release system is to maintain the drug concentration between these two levels from a single dosage form. A controlled release system should release drug continuously in a fixed, predetermined pattern for a desired time period. Ideally, this should result in a uniform drug concentration as a function of time, require smaller dosages, and cause fewer side effects.

In order for the drug to be taken up by the desired site of the body, several events must occur. The drug must first be released from the device, it must then diffuse from the surface of the device to the surrounding bloodstream, and eventually it must be transported to its target. Ideally, the first of these steps should be rate-limiting so that release is totally dependent on the device itself and not on the surrounding environment.

Early efforts to prolong release involved the use of slowly dissolving coatings, complexes of drugs with salts or ion-exchange resins, suspensions, emulsions, or compressed tablets. These systems were considered sustained release formulations and served to prolong the length of time before the drug concentrations in bodily fluids fell below the minimum effective level. However, such methods did not generally permit long-term release (greater than one day) and were subject to variations in release rates as a function of environmental conditions, Controlled release formulations were first used in the agricultural industries for low molecular weight fertilizers, pesticides and antifoulants in the 1950s (1). In the 1960s these approaches were extended into the medical field (2,3). By the mid-1970s, controlled release formulations for large molecular weight drugs (e.g., polypeptides) were designed (4). In this article we review biopolymers as they relate to controlled drug delivery systems.

TYPES OF POLYMER SYSTEMS

Polymers release drugs by four general mechanisms: diffusion, chemical control, solvent activation, and magnetism (5,6).

The most common mechanism is diffusion, whereby the drug migrates from its initial position in the polymer to the polymer's outer surface and then to the body. Two types of diffusion controlled systems have been developed: the reservoir and the matrix. In the reservoir system, a core of drug is surrounded by a polymer film, whereas in the matrix system, the drug is uniformly distributed through a polymer.

In chemically controlled systems, release is accomplished either by biodegradation of the polymer or by chemical cleavage of the drug from a polymer backbone on which the drug had been bound as a pendent group.

Solvent activation involves either a swelling or osmotic mechanism. For swelling-controlled systems, the drug is locked into place by surrounding molecular chains of polymer; on exposure to environmental fluid, the outer polymer region begins to swell, allowing the drug to diffuse outward. In an osmotic system, water permeates a drug-polymer matrix due to osmotic pressure, which causes pores to form or open and thereby facilities drug release. Alternatively, a laser drilled hole can be made in a non-porous semipermeable membrane surrounding a core of drug. Water penetrates through the membrane by osmosis and pushes drug out of the laser drilled hole.

In magnetically controlled systems, drug and magnetic beads are distributed within a solid polymer matrix. Upon exposure to environmental fluid, the drug is released in a fashion typical of a diffusion-controlled system. However, the drug is released at a much higher rate in the presence of an oscillating magnetic field, presumably because the drug is "squeezed" out through pores in the matrix.

Release rates from polymeric systems can be controlled by the choice of the polymer and the design of the system (e.g., thickness and shape). The advantage of having systems with different release mechanisms is that each can accomplish different goals. For example, reservoir systems are able to produce near-constant release rates, whereas matrix systems are inexpensive to manufacture. Chemically controlled systems result in elimination of the polymer, whereas solvent-activated systems have release rates independent of the pH of bodily fluids. Although magnetic systems are at an experimental stage of development, they offer the opportunity of increasing or externally controlling release rates.

POLYMERS FOR CONTROLLED RELEASE FORMULATIONS

Numerous polymers have been used in the design of drug release systems. Non-biodegradable matrix and reservoir devices can be prepared from hydrophilic and hydrophobic polymers. Polymers based on monomers connected by labile backbone bonds are generally used as biodegradable polymers.

Hydrophilic Polymers

A variety of reservoir and matrix devices are prepared from swollen crosslinked hydrophilic polymers (hydrogels) (7). Most successful devices of this kind are based on poly (2-hydroxyethyl methacrylate) (PHEMA) and related polymers although hydrophilic homopolymers of (poly vinyl 1-2-pyrrolidone) (PNVP), poly (vinyl alcohol) (PVA) and copolymers thereof have been tested with considerable success.

PHEMA swollen systems are made by crosslinking of hydroxyethylmethacrylate (HEMA) in the presence or absence of water, using varying amounts of crosslinking agents such as ethylene glycol dimethacrylate (EGDMA) or tetraethylene glycol dimethacrylate (TEGDMA) (8). Cross-linking is followed by swelling in distilled water or saline up to thermodynamic equilibrium usually at 37°C. Crosslinked copolymers of HEMA and methoxyethyl methacrylate (MEMA) and methoxy ethoxyethyl methacrylate (MEEMA) have also been investigated (9). Copolymers of HEMA with methylmethacrylate (MMA) lead to poorly swollen hydrogels which have been reported to give an almost zero-order release of low molecular weight solutes for long periods of time (10). Numerous other copolymers of HEMA with various vinyl monomers are also reviewed in several papers (11,12).

Poly (vinly alcohol) hydrogels are usually prepared by chemical or irradiation cross linking of aqueous solution of PVA. The polymer is produced by hydrolysis of poly (vinyl acetate) and related poly (vinyl esters). Copolymers of PNVP with PVA, pure PNVP and polyacrylamide are additional hydrogels which have been used as successful drug release systems (13, 14).

Hydrophobic polymers

Hydrophobic polymers are usually available as uncrosslinked matrices of membranes prepared by compression of powdered polymer or by dissolution in and evaporation of a non-toxic solvent.

Polydimethyl siloxanes (PDMS) are available in medical grades (under the name Silastic, Dow Corning) either in a crosslinked homopolymer network form or as copolymers with small amounts of other silicon-containing monomers. Their preparation and properties are described in standard references (15).

Ethylene-vinyl acetate (EVA) copolymers are prepared by emulsion copolymerization of ethylene and vinyl acetate. They are soluble in organic solvents and they can be used to prepare films or rods of dimensional stability and good mechanical strength (16).

Biodegradable Polymers

The most commonly used biodegradable polymers for drug delivery systems are poly (lactic acid), poly (glycolic acid) and their copolymers. They are prepared by polyesterification of lactic or glycolic acid at 120°C, or via cyclic monomers (17).

Other biodegradable polymers which have been used for controlled drug delivery systems include polymers based on caprolactone (18) various copolymers of amino acids (19), poly (alkyl cyanoacrylates) (20), polyanhydrides (21) and polyortho-esters (22).

Drug release from bioerodible matrix devices can be controlled by either diffusion or eroison. If erosion of the matrix is much slower than diffusion, the release kinetics are essentially those of a diffusion controlled matrix system. If, however, the drug is immobilized in the matrix so that diffusional release is minimal compared to erosion, the rate of drug release will be erosion controlled. Physically, there are two general erosion mechanisms-heterogeneous and homogeneous erosion. Heterogeneous erosion occurs when degradation takes place only at the surface of a polymer matrix (surface erosion), whereas homogeneous erosion is the result of degradation occurring through the polymer matrix. Heterogeneous erosion is much more desirable because: (a) It can lead to zero-order drug release provided diffusional release of the drug is minimal and the overall surface area of the device remains constant; (b) release rate is independent of the chemical and physical properties of the drug; (c) release rate can be varied simply by varying drug loading, making the device easy to design; and (d) mechanical integrity is maintained because erosion is confined to the matrix surface. Hydrophobic polymers are more likely to erode heterogeneously since water is excluded. Since hydrophilic polymers absorb water, homogeneous erosion will be favored. The only polymers known to display hydrolytically controlled surface erosion and where the polymers break down to monomers are polyorthoesters when certain additives are included (22) and polyanhydrides (21).

APPLICATIONS

Ocular Disease

The first controlled - release polymer system to be used clinically was the Ocusert[R] a reservoir system designed to improve therapy for glaucoma, one of the world's leading causes of blindness. The conventional treatment for this disease was for the patient to use eyedrops containing pilocarpine (which reduces intraocular pressure) four times a day. These eyedrops often caused side effects, and patient compliance was sometimes poor. The Ocusert[R] is a diffusion controlled reservoir system composed of ethylene-vinyl acetate copolymer which delivers 20 or 40 µg/h pilocarpine continuously over one week. The implant is placed in the lower eyelid's conjuctival cul-de-sac, where it floats in the tear film. Advantages of the Ocusert[R] include; (a) control of intraocular pressure with less total amount of drug, resulting in fewer side effects; (b) convenience of once a week application; (c) enhancement of patient compliance; and (d) assurance of round the clock medication (23). Despite these advantages, the Ocusert[R] has not achieved widespread use, initially because of the expense and poor acceptance by older patients who were reluctant to adjust to this system and more recently because of the introduction of drugs that require only two applications per day.

A second ocular system, known as the Lacrisert[R] (hydroxypropyl cellulose) was recently introduced for use in artifical tears. This system is a biodegradable polymer rod, which is inserted with a special device beneath the tarsus of the lower eyelid. The rod slowly dissolves over a one-day period, providing continuous lubrication and tearfilm stability to the eye (24).

Contraception

The use of polymers to deliver contraceptive steroids has been one of the most widely studied applications of controlled release (25). Four types of systems have generally been studied; (a) Subdermal reservoir implants composed of non-biodegradable polymers, particularly silicone rubber, and capable of release times of over five years; (b) subdermal implants composed of biodegradable polymers; (c) steroid-releasing reservoir intrauterine devices (IUDs), such as the Progestasert[R], a diffusion controlled reservoir system composed of ethylene-vinyl acetate copolymer, which contains a three-day supply (38 mg) of the amount of progesterone normally taken orally, but which, since it delivers progesterone to its target locally at a rate of approximately 65 µg/d, lasts for ever one year (26); and (d) vaginal rings, generally silicone coated, which are reservoir systems used for six months, with a schedule of three weeks of implantation followed by one week of withdrawal to allow for bleeding.

Immunization

Conventional methods for immunizing both animals and humans generally require multiple injections and often cause tissue irritation. In some cases, as in the treatment of allergies, shots have to be given weekly over several years.

A recent study considered the possibility that controlled-release polymers might provide a simple, safe, and effective means of immunization by acting as a series of continuous minishots. Small (0.3 mm^3) injectable pellets, composed of matrix systems of ethylene vinyl acetate copolymer, containing 100 µg of different test antigens, were positioned subcutaneously in mice. The immune response stimulated by sustained antigen delivery was compared to the conventional method of immunizing animals-i.e. two injections of antigen in complete Freunds's adjuvant (Freund's adjuvant is an oil in water suspension containing bacteria to stimulate the immune response). The results indicate that the immune response induced by antigen in polymer is comparable or superior to that induced by the same dose of antigen using the conventional technique. In addition, a single polymer pellet caused a sustained immune response for six months. No tissue irritation was observed with the controlled release system (27).

Anticoagulation

Polymeric systems are being developed to release either the anticoagulant, heparin, alone or heparin in conjunction with prostaglandins (28). The goal of these studies is to develop biomaterials that do not induce clot formation when exposed to blood and to use controlled release to add agents that would prevent platelet damage.

Cancer

Controlled release polymers have also been used to treat certain forms of cancer. For example, silicone pellets releasing ethyl estradiol for over a year have been used in several hundred patients with prostate cancer (29).

Diabetes

Insulin-dependent diabetics normally require insulin injections once or twice daily. Besides being inconvenient, this schedule of insulin administration results in peaks and valleys in blood glucose levels. It is possible that poor control of blood glucose may be responsible, in part, for diabetic complications, such as blindness and heart and kidney disease. Over the past few years, studies in humans have shown that excellent control of blood glucose can be achieved using large pumps that infuse insulin at a constant rate, but are capable of increasing the rate before meals.

Implantable polymeric drug delivery systems may also be useful in maintaining normal glycemia in diabetics and provide useful ways of miniaturizing pumps; because they contain no moving parts and because powdered drug is used in the polymer, 100 fold higher levels of insulin can be loaded per unit volume. Small subcutaneous polymer implants composed of matrices of ethylene vinyl acetate copolymer containing insulin have been used to control blood glucose levels in diabetic rats for one month (30).

Dentistry

One application being studied, is the use of a reservoir device composed of hydroxyethyl methacrylate-methyl methacrylate copolymer that can be attached to a tooth and can release fluoride at rate of 0.02 to 1 mg/d for 30 to 180 days to establish higher and more constant levels of fluoride within the oral cavity (10). These devices are attached to the buccal surface of the upper first molar using direct-bonding cement.

Another dental application is the delivery of tetracycline for periodontal disease. Tetracycline (300 μg) has been incorporated into reservoirs composed of hollow fibers of 0.25 mm in diameter. When placed into the periodontal pocket, these fibers produced a reduction in bacterial numbers, particularly spirochetes, and a reduction in the clinical signs of gingivitis. Furthermore, because the fibers were placed next to the target area, treatment was accomplished with less than one thousandth of the normal systemic dose (31).

Transdermal Systems

Transdermal delivery involves placing a polymeric system containing a contact adhesive on the skin. For a drug to diffuse through the skin into the systemic circulation, the drug must traverse a number of skin layers. The principle resistance occurs in the top layer, the stratum corneum, which is composed primarily of keratin and lipids. For a drug to have high skin permeability, it must have good water solubility, a low molecular weight and a high oil/water partition coefficient. Transdermal delivery is best suited to drugs that are administered in small doses and that have a high degree of skin permeability.

One advantage of transdermal delivery is that it reduces the problem of first-pass metabolism. Thus, drugs that cannot be taken orally because they are rapidly degraded may be considered candidates for transdermal delivery. Transdermal systems also provide an easy method for localizing the drug, and they are easy to apply and remove (compared to inserts and implants). There may, however, be a significant lag time (two to six hours) before the drug concentration in the systemic circulation reaches a steady state, due to the slow diffusion of the drug from the skin surface to the blood vessels (32). Thus, transdermal delivery may be more desirable for chronic rather than acute treatments.

Several transdermal systems have recently been introduced clinically. One of these is the Transderm-Scop^R, a diffusion controlled reservoir system that contains 1.5 mg scopolamine and delivers 0.5 mg at a constant rate over three days for treatment of motion sickness. It is a diffusion controlled reservoir system with a rate controlling microporous polypropylene membrane. Tight control of serum scopolamine concentration prevents adverse effects, such as tachycardia and hallucination, associated with other scopolamine dosage forms.

For the same bioavailibility profile to result between identical transdermal dosage forms, it is essential that the skin be capable of absorbing the drug at a much faster rate than the rate of drug release from the device (i.e. the device must be rate limiting). For this reason, it is desirable to place the device where the stratum corneum is thin, such as behind the ear, so that the drug can be absorbed at a rate considerably greater than that of its passage through the rate-controlling membrane.

Several transdermal nitroglycerin systems have been developed for the treatment of angina. Since nitroglycerin is subject to a significant first-pass effect when taken orally and because nitroglycerin has high skin permeability, transdermal skin pastes have been used successfully. However, such pastes are neither dependable nor convenient; thus, attention has been devoted to developing controlled-release dosage forms. Three such systems are being used clinically in the United States: (a) The Transderm Nitro, which works on the same principle as the scopolamine device described above; (b) the Nitro-Dur, a matrix system, and (c) the Nitrodisc, which is a microsealed silicone system (a type of reservoir system). Devices range from 5 to 20 cm^2 in surface area and release from 2.5 to 10 mg/d.

A transdermal system has also been used recently to deliver clonidine to hypertensive patients for seven days (33). Other transdermal systems for drugs such as estradiol are under investigation.

Other Applications

Controlled release formulations may be applied to other clinical areas, including the release of narcotic antagonists, antibiotics, interferons, anesthetics, antiarrhymics, and antimalarial drugs. Significant veterinary applications include the delivery of insect-growth regulators to livestock to prevent infection; the delivery of antiparisitic drugs, nutrients, or growth regulators; and the delivery of the active agents in flea and tick collars.

FUTURE PROSPECTS

Although controlled release systems have already significantly improved the delivery of some existing drugs, these systems will play an even greater role in future drug development. First, investigational drugs that may have been toxic when given by conventional means can be given more safely in controlled release dosage forms. Second, since many of the new drugs being developed (such as polypeptides, macromolecules, or vaccines) are rapidly destroyed by the body, the use of controlled release systems may be critical to prolonging their biological lifetimes.

Another important area being studied is the targeting of drugs to specific cells or organs. In some studies, drugs have been encapsulated in liposomes or coupled to polymers, antibodies, DNA or peptides. These systems can be designed to enable certain cells (such as cancer cells) to take up the drug more easily than others (an

168

approach that could greatly minimize systemic toxicity). The potential of such approaches to improve the way medicines are administered should have considerable impact on the future of drug therapy.

ACKNOWLEDGEMENTS

This work was supported by NIH grant GM 26698.

REFERENCES

1. Lurt, O.R., J. Aqric. Food Chem. 19:797, 1971.
2. Folkman, J. and Long, D.M., J. Surg. Res., 4:139, 1964.
3. Desai, S.J., Simonelli, A.P., and Higuchi, W.I., J. Pharm. Sci., 54:1459, 1964.
4. Langer, R. and Folkman, J., Nature, 263:797, 1976.
5. Langer, R., Chem. Eng. Commun., 6:1, 1980.
6. Langer, R.S., and Peppas, N.A., Biomaterials, 2:201, 1981.
7. Ratner, B.D. and Hoffman, A.S., in Hydrogels for Medical and Related Applications, J.D. Andrade, ed., pp.1, Amer. Chem. Soc. Symp. Ser. 31, ACS, Washington, 1976.
8. Gregonis, D.E., Chen, C.M. and Andrade, J.D., in Hydrogels for Medical and Related Applications, J.D. Andrade, ed., pp. 88, Amer. Chem. Soc. Symp. Ser. 31, ACS Washington, 1976.
9. Rabek, J.F., Experimental Methods in Polymer Chemistry, J.Wiley, New York, 1980.
10. Cowsar, D.R., Tarwater, O.R. and Tanquary, A.C., in: Hydrogels for Medical and Related Applications, J.D. Andrade, ed., pp. 180, ACS, Washington, 1976.
11. Pedley, D.G., Skelly, P.J. and Tighe, B.J., Brit. Polym. J., 12:99, 1980.
12. Kost, J., Langer, in Hydrogels in Medicine and Pharmacy, N.A. Peppas, ed., Vol. II, CRC Press, Boca Raton, FL, 1985.
13. Graham, N.B., Brit. Polym. J., 10:260, 1978.
14. Davis, B.K., Proc. Nat. Acad. Sci, 71:3120, 1974.
15. Thames, S.F. and Bufkin, B.G., in Applied Polymer Science J.K. Graver and R.W. Tess, eds., pp. 748, ACS, Washington, 1975.
16. Salyer, I.D. and Kenyon, A.S., J. Poly. Sci., 9:3083, 1971.
17. Wise, D.L., Fellman, T.D. Sanderson, J.E. and Wentworth, R.L., in: Biology and Medicine, G. Gregoriadis, ed., pp. 237, Academic Press, London, 1979.
18. Pitt, C.G., Jeffcoat, A.G. Zweidinger, R.A. and Schindler, A., J. Biomed. Mater. Res. 13:497, 1979.
19. Sidman, K.R., Schwope, A.D., Steber, W.D., Rudolph, S.E. and Poulin, S.B., J.Memb. Sci., 7:277, 1980.
20. Couvreur, P., in Emploi des Polymeres dans L'Elaboration de Nouvelles Formes Medicamentouses, P. Bur., E. Doelker, and P. Pasquier, eds., pp. 102, University of Geneva, 1980.
21. Rosen, H., Changes, J., Wnek, G., Linhardt, R., and Langer, R. Biomaterials, 4:131, 1983.
22. Heller, J., Penhale, D.W.H., Helwing, R.F., Fritzinger, B.K. and Baker, R.W., AICHE Symp. Ser., 206:28, 1981.

23. Stewart, R.H., Novak, S., Ann Ophthalmol, 10:325, 1978.
24. Lamberts, D.W., Langston, D.P., Chu, W. Ophthalmology, 85:794, 1978.
25. Segal, S., J. Clin. Therapeutics, 155, 1982.
26. Pharriss, B.B., J. Reprod. Med., 20:155, 1978.
27. Preis, I. and Langer, J., Immunol Methods, 28:193, 1979.
28. Ebert, C., McRea, J., Kim S.W., in Controlled Release of Bioactive Materials, R. Baker., ed., pp. 107, New York, Academic Press, 1980.
29. Frick, J. and Kincl, F.A., in Medical Applications of Controlled Release, R. Langer, and D.Wise, eds., Boca Raton, FL, CRC Press, 1984.
30. Creque, H.M., Langer, R., Folkman, J., Diabetes, 29:37, 1980.
31. Goodson, J.M., Haffajee, A., Socranski, S., J. Clin. Periodontal 6:83, 1979.
32. Chandrasekaran, S.K., Bayne, W., Shaw, J.E., J. Pharm. Sci, 67:1370, 1978.
33. Mroczek, W.J., Ulriych, M., Yoder, S., Clin. Pharmcol. Ther 31:252, 1982.

HYDROGELS IN CONTROLLED DRUG DELIVERY

N.B. Graham

University of Strathclyde, Department of Pure and Applied Chemistry, Glasgow, Scotland

INTRODUCTION

Hydrogels are water-insoluble but water-swellable polymers made by a variety of chemical methods utilizing both natural and synthetic polymer backbones. They can be prepared in a wide-variety of physical forms such as foams, films, sheets, beads, powders, tubes and blocks. Thermoplastic and thermosetting forms are known and they present a very versatile class of materials capable of considerable development. The natural hydrogel material gelatin has been used in pharmaceutical formulation for more than a century and is well known in the form of soft or hard-gelatin capsules. The modern synthetic hydrogel polymers have a broad capability for specific synthetic design and the skills of polymer scientists in tailor-making the polymers and devices utilizing them will lead to a considerably expanded use of these reproducible materials in the future. This introductory presentation will be restricted to these synthetic hydrogels.

THE NEED FOR HYDROGELS IN CONTROLLING DRUG DELIVERY

From the point of view of discussion of their permeability, polymers in general, but hydrogels in particular, can be broadly classified by the presence or absence of the following structural features (a) crystallites (b) amorphous glass (c) amorphous rubber and (d) water-swollen rubber. Only highly ordered polymers contain crystallites but all polymers contain some proportion of disordered amorphous molecular structures which in many cases comprises the entire material. A linear polymer which contains both crystalline and amorphous regions will have two thermal transitions on heating across a wide range of temperature. Thus at some temperature which can be as low as -100°C a glass transition temperature (T_g) is observed as the transition of the physical nature of the material from glassy and rigid to a soft rubber which may even flow. For partially crystalline polymers the materials will not flow until the crystalline melting temperature (T_m) is attained when the materials soften further and may become liquid. This formation of a liquid with no retention of dimensional stability is undesirable in most drug delivery applications and can be prevented by building in flow restraining structures at the molecular level. The permeability of polymers for a given species would in general terms be many decades larger for the rubber state of a polymer than for the crystalline or glassy states. Because of low permeability it is quite exceptional to find glassy polymers used for controlled drug delivery though one major exception is in commercial use for the delivery of antibiotics from a polymeric glass over several months. Polymeric glasses normally only allow release of microgram quantities per day from devices suitable for implantation or oral use. Polymeric rubbers on the other hand, having both higher mobility of the molecular chains than glasses and also a larger proportion of molecular sized holes (so called free volume) into which diffusing molecules can jump, exhibit much higher permeabilities. From conventional implant or oral tablet sized device they can often release milligram quantities of drug per day up a maximum or around 20mg/d typical of rubbers such as silicones or ethylene/vinylacetate copolymers. Such rates of release in these hydrophobic membranes are only obtained in favorable circumstances usually with hydrophobic drugs such as steroids which are reasonably soluble in the membrane and the many hydrophilic drugs and salts could not reach even these low levels and certainly not the often desired levels of hundreds of milligrams per day. This is where hydrogels come into their own as when swollen with water they can provide fluxes of drug many decades higher than the rubbery hydrophobic membranes and matrices and are indicated as the material of choice in many controlled release applications. The controlled and sustained release of hundreds of milligrams per day becomes possible with their utilization.

THE CHEMICAL NATURE OF HYDROGELS

Hydrogels are made from polymers which are water-soluble, by the introduction of an interaction at a molecular level which prevents their dissolution in water, but not the absorption of water by the polymer, to provide a swollen but insoluble structure with dimensional integrity. This is done by covalent crosslinking, entanglement crosslinking, strong interactions or by submicron size phase separation. The water-soluble backbones typically used in the preparation of hydrogels are presented in Table I. The many materials of natural origin such as protein, cellulose and starch derivatives commonly used in conventional pharmacy have been omitted.

THE FORMATION OF HYDROGELS BASED ON POLY (ETHYLENE OXIDE)

This is the only material which provides partially crystalline hydrogels and is the mainstay of work in the author's laboratory. It serves as an example of the four mechanisms by which insoluble hydrogels may be prepared. Poly (ethylene glycols) or poly (ethylene oxides) referred to as PEG or PEO are made in three broad groups of materials all made by the polymerization of ethylene oxide (1). These are (a) low molecular weight materials ($M_n < 1500$) which are liquid at ambient temperature (b) moderate molecular weight materials ($M_n : 2000-20,000$) which are solid and crystalline at ambient temperature and (c) very high molecular weight crystalline polymers ($M_n$ca 10^6-10^7). Classes (a) and (b) can be crosslinked by reacting the hydroxyl groups present on each end of their chains with a polyfunctional isocyanate

Table I. Synthetic Neutral Polymers that are Water Soluble at Ambient Temperatures.

NAME	ABBREVIATION	POLYMER STRUCTURAL UNIT
POLY (ETHYLENE OXIDE)	PEO	
POLY (ETHYLENE GLYCOL)	PEG	$-CH_2-CH_2-O-$
POLY (OXY ETHYLENE)	POE	
POLY (VINYL ALCOHOL)	PVA	$-CH_2-\underset{\underset{OH}{\vert}}{CH}-$
POLY (VINYL METHYL ETHER)	PVME	$-CH_2-\underset{\underset{O-CH_3}{\vert}}{CH}-$
POLY (VINYL FORMAL)	PVF	$-CH_2-\underset{\underset{O}{\vert}}{CH}-CH_2-\underset{\underset{O}{\vert}}{CH}-$ with CH_2 bridging
POLY (VINYL METHOXY ACETAL)	PVMA	$-CH_2-\underset{\underset{O}{\vert}}{CH}-CH_2-\underset{\underset{O}{\vert}}{CH}-$ with $\underset{\underset{O-CH_3}{\vert}}{CH}$ bridging
POLY (VINYL ETHYL ETHER)	PVEE	$-CH_2-\underset{\underset{O-CH_2-CH_3}{\vert}}{CH}-$
POLY (2-HYDROXY ETHYL METHACRYLATE) / POLY (ETHYLENE GLYCOL MONO METHACRYLATE)	PHEMA	$-CH_2-\underset{\underset{CO.OCH_2-CH_2-OH}{\vert}}{\overset{\overset{CH_3}{\vert}}{C}}-$

Table I. Cont.

NAME	ABBREVIATION	POLYMER STRUCTURAL UNIT
POLY (2-HYDROXY PROPYL METHACRYLATE) POLY (PROPYLENE GLYCOL MONO METHACRYLATE)	PHPMA	$-CH_2-\underset{\underset{CO.OCH_2-C-OH}{|}}{\overset{\overset{CH_3}{|}}{C}}-$ CH_3
POLY (ACRYLAMIDE)	PAAm	$-CH_2-\underset{\underset{CONH_2}{|}}{CH}-$
POLY (METHACRYLAMIDE)	PMAAm	$-CH_2-\underset{\underset{CONH_2}{|}}{\overset{\overset{CH_3}{|}}{C}}-$
POLY (N-METHYLOLACRYLAMIDE)	PNMAAm	$-CH_2-\underset{\underset{CONH-CH_2OH}{|}}{CH}-$
POLY (N-METHYLOLMETHACRYLAMIDE)	PNMMAAm	$-CH_2-\underset{\underset{CONH-CH_2OH}{|}}{\overset{\overset{CH_3}{|}}{C}}-$
POLY (VINYL PYRROLIDONE) POLY (N-1-VINYL PYRROLID-2-ONE)	PVP	$-CH_2-CH-$
POLY (VINYL METHYLOXAZOLIDONE) POLY (N (3)-VINYL-5-METHYL-OXAZOLID-2-ONE)	PVMO	$-CH_2-CH-$

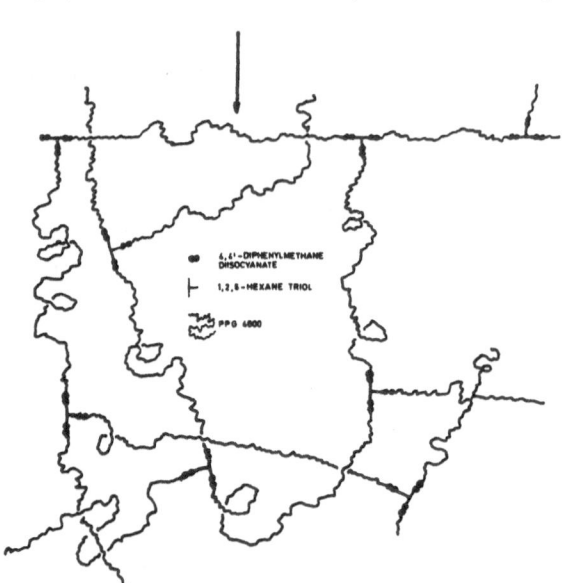

Figure 1. The Reaction of PEG 4000 with a Triol and a Diisocyanate to Form a Crosslinked Water-Insoluble but Swellable Hydrogel.

and including a polyol of functionality greater than two in the formulation. This is illustrated above in Figure 1 in which typically the crosslinking reaction is that of a hydroxyl with an isocyanate. This proceeds slowly at room temperature or more rapidly at elevated temperatures such as 100°C. A typical mixture would comprise a diisocyanate (e.g., 4,4'-diphenylmethane diisocyanate) a triol (e.g., 1, 2, 6-hexane triol) and a poly (ethylene glycol) of molecular weight from 400 to 20,000 in a weight ratio providing one hydroxyl for each isocyanate group present. An amine or transition metal catalyst is usually included. The preparation and some physical properties of such materials have been described by Graham (2) and the toxic nature of the isocyanates used in the preparation should be noted. These are not present in the final polyurethane product but the isocyanates are so reactive that their removal by reaction by water is quite simple. By these reactions monolithic blocks and sheets of materials can be obtained. The use of poly (ethylene glycols) of number average molecular weight (M_n) over 3000 provide partially crystalline hydrogels which surprisingly can provide constant drug delivery from monolithic devices (3,4) which because of the crystallinity have a high level of dry strength and reasonably high water swollen strengths and will be discussed later.

Though they are not convenient for the manufacture of controlled drug delivery devices it has been shown (39) that dilute solutions of very high molecular weight poly (ethylene oxides) (M_n 3×10^6) could be crosslinked by γ-irradiation to provide a water-insoluble but highly swellable sheet material suitable for a sheet wound dressing. A similar material has been commercialized. In this case the irradiation causes reaction between poly (ethylene oxide) chains to provide covalent junctions (crosslinks) between them. There is a concurrent chain-scission occuring and the overall process is quite complex.

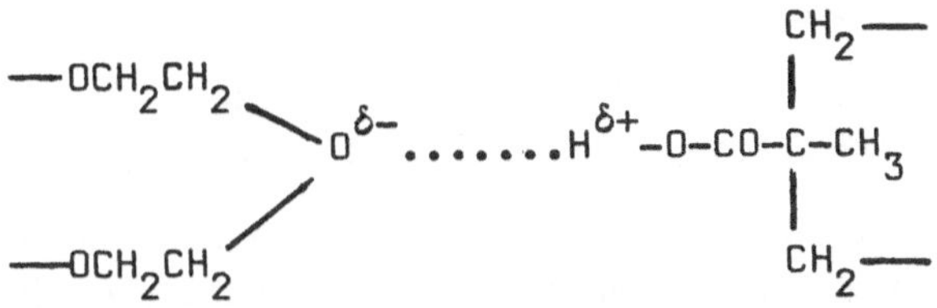

Figure 2.   Hydrogen Bonds Between Carboxyl Groups and Ether Groups Responsible for Gel Formation in Poly (ethylene oxide) Poly (methacrylic acid) Mixtures.

A means of making high molecular weight polymers insoluble by introducing a proportion of a multifunctional polymerizable monomer has been utilized in the crosslinking of poly (vinyl chloride) and in "curing" ethylene/propylene rubbers. The same technique of entanglement crosslinking has been patented for the crosslinking of very high molecular weight polyethylene oxides using divinylbenzene (5) and a free radical generating initiating system for its polymerisation. This technique does not appear to have been widely used in practice.

The ether groups of poly (ethylene oxide) are weakly basic and will interact with carboxylic groups to a sufficient degree that water-insoluble hydrogels are formed on mixing with poly (acrylic) or poly (methacrylic) acids. These are formed as a result of association by hydrogen bonds as shown in Figure 2. The water insoluble gels so produced become water soluble on neutralization with sodium hydroxide or the addition of acetic acid. These gels have been recently reviewed (6) and are from part of a large class of such interacting systems.

THE FORMATION OF HYDROGELS BASED ON VINLY OR ACRYLIC MONOMERS

Monomers containing double bonds are polymerised readily in the presence of free radicals derived from a variety of initiators. The polymerization may be by utilizing the monomer alone or in a mixture with solvent, in the case of hydrogel formation this is commonly water. Typical polymer structures formed in this way are shown in Table I but poly (vinly alcohol) is not made directly as the monomer vinyl alcohol does not exist. Instead it is made by hydrolysis of poly (vinyl acetate) which is itself made from vinyl acetate. Polymers such as poly (hydroxyethyl methacrylate) (PHEMA) are water insoluble but swell with water to a significant degree, poly (hydroxyethylmethacrylate) itself swells up to 40% and can be used in hydrogel applications without added crosslinking agent but it is in fact very difficult to obtain the hydroxyethyl methacrylate monomer completely free from glycol dimethacrylate impurity and so it is difficult to obtain such systems which are not crosslinked. It is common practice when making hydrogels from the water soluble polymers in Table I to incorporate up to 5 molar percent of crosslinking monomers such as glycol dimethacrylate $CH_2=C(CH_3) - COOCH_2CH_2OCOC(CH_3)=CH_2$. Frequently, copolymers incorporating a monomer giving a very water-soluble polymer such as polyacrylamide or poly (vinyl pyrrolidone) with a low water solubility polymer producing monomer such as PHEMA are made. The largest commercialization of such systems has been in the field of contact lenses where the first soft contact lenses were made from PHEMA and more recently long-wear lenses have been made from copolymers of up to five monomers (7,8).

HYDROGELS SENSITIVE TO ACIDS OF BASES

Advantages of synthetic hydrogels include the ease with which new compositions can be made to provide answers to particular problems. In certain circumstances it is desired to have a largely impermeable unswollen polymer in the acid pH of the human stomach but a highly permeable or soluble coating at the approximately neutral pH of the duodenum (9). In delivery of drugs to cattle the reverse is often the case where the protective impermeable coating is required at the neutral pH of the rumen but a rapid release at the acid pH of the abomassum (10). Such acid and base responsive polymers which are readily synthesisable are given in Table II and III.

These three groups of monomers used to form the polymers in Table I, II and III may be combined together to form copolymers in almost any ratio and thus a very large variety of materials becomes available for the solution of specific drug delivery problems. However the chemical picture presented is only a small part of the definition of reproducible polymeric hydrogels. Polymers are complex species and their physical nature must be understood and defined.

THE PHYSICAL NATURE OF POLYMERS

Polymers are in general complex mixtures of molecules and rarely if ever a single entity. They are therefore rather difficult to characterize precisely. The first most important characteristic is the size of the molecules being considered. This, for individual molecules, is defined by a precise figure, the molecular weight (11). The term molecular weight for a synthetic polymer though often carelessly used, frequently has no precise meaning. All polymer molecular weights are average values and it is only possible to determine a molecular weight average, the nature of which must be specified. Different types of average are obtained from different techniques utilised for the determination.

Two common averages are the weight (M_w) and number (M_n) average determined by e.g., light scattering and osmometry respectively. The weight average molecular weight can be many times higher (e.g., 10x) than the number average and the ratio of the two is often used to represent the molecular weight distributions. Values of M_w/M_n of close to unity indicate very narrow molecular weight distributions while high values, e.g., 10 would indicate wide molecular weight distributions. Gel Permeation Chromatography is extensively used to provide information on molecular weight distribution directly as represented in Figure 3.

As the molecular weight distribution can have an effect on important physical properties such as processing characteristics and diffusion coefficients it is important to be aware of its nature. The properties of a polymer can also be altered by its thermal or other prehistory as well as its molecular make-up. This change in properties is caused by modifications to the physical macromolecular structure and these molecular scale structures must be understood and their time dependence known if the properties are to be predictable. In some cases the polymer properties can be changed remarkably merely by casting films from different solvents. Some styrene-butadiene ABA block copolymers can give either a brittle solid or a rubber from the identical material (12).

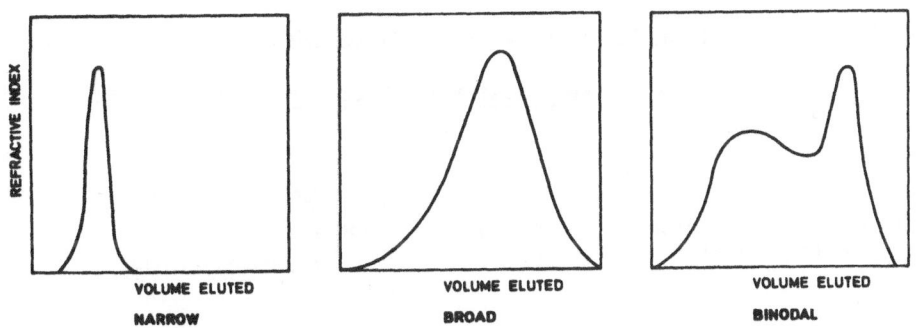

Figure 3. Gel Permeation Chromatography Plots for Narrow, Broad and Binodal Molecular Weight Distribution.

Table II. Synthetic Acidic Polymers Soluble in Water with or without Neutralization.

NAME	ABBREVIATION	POLYMER STRUCTURAL UNIT
POLY (ACRYLIC ACID)	PAA	$-CH_2-CH-$ $\quad\quad\ \ $ COOH
POLY (METHACRYLIC ACID)	PMAA	CH_3 $-CH_3-CH-$ $\quad\quad\ \ $ COOH
POLY (MALEIC ANHYDRIDE COPOLYMERS)	PMalA	$-CH_2-CH-CH-CH-$ $\quad\quad\ X\ \ CO\ \ CO$ $\quad\quad\quad\quad\ \ O$
POLY (MALEIC ACID HALF-ESTERS)		$-CH_2-CH-CH-CH-$ $\quad\quad\ X\ \ COOH\ COOR$
POLY (SODIUM STYRENE SULPHONATE)	PSSS	$-CH-CH-$ SO_3Na

Table III. Synthetic Basic Polymers Soluble in Water with or without Neutralization.

N A M E	ABBREVIATION	POLYMER STRUCTURAL UNIT
POLY(DIMETHIL AMINO ETHYL METHACRYLATE)	PDMAEM	$-CH_2-\underset{\underset{CO.OCH_2CH_2-N(CH_3)_2}{\vert}}{\overset{\overset{CH_3}{\vert}}{C}}-$ n
POLY (2-VINYL PYRIDINE)	P 2 VP	$-CH_2-CH-$
POLY (4-VINYL PYRIDINE)	P 4 VP	$-CH_2-CH-$
POLY (4-VINYL PYRIDINE-N-OXIDE)	P 4 VPNO	$-CH_2-CH-$
NYLON FROM N,Nᴵ-BIS(3-AMINOPROPYL) PIPERAZINE AND 1,10-DICARBOXY n-DECENE UNIT		$-NH(CH_2)_3\,N\diamondsuit N(CH_2)_{10}NHCO(CH_2)_3CO-$

CHANGE IN PROPERTIES WITH MOLECULAR WEIGHT
THE PHYSICAL STATES OF POLYMERS

Polymers exist in whole or in part in the three distinct states mentioned earlier. These are the glassy state, (13) the rubbery state (14) and the crystalline state (15). In the glassy state polymers are hard, rigid and often brittle. There is a low level of molecular movement and the rate of diffusion of large molecules is very low. So low that very active chemical species such as radicals attached to polymers may be stabilized at room temperature and do not rapidly destroy themselves by diffusion

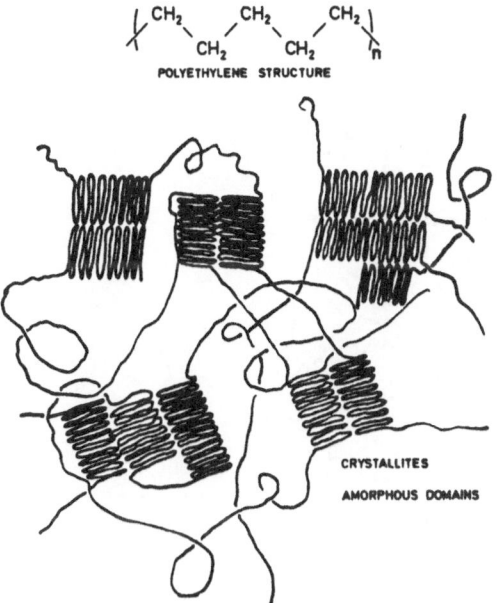

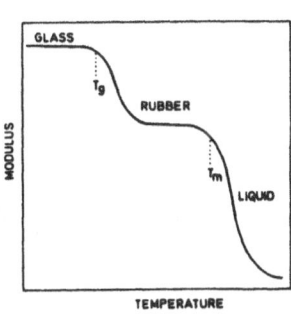

Figure 4. Modulus - Temperature Plot Showing T_g and T_m for a Thermoplastic Polymer.

Figure 5. Poly (ethylene) Showing the Regular Structure which Allows Ready Crystallization to Occur as Shown in the Schematic Two Dimensional Representation of Crystallites and Amorphous Domains. Note One Molecule Passes Through Number of Crystallites Thus Preventing Flow of the Material.

together followed by combination. On heating at a defined rate a glassy solid changes to a more flexible rubbery solid over a given small temperature range as shown diagrammatically by the change in modulus in Figure 4. Above the so-called glass transition temperature the polymer is in the rubbery state and, if not constrained by some molecular interaction or bonding, will exhibit fluid flow. The fluid flow is prevented in many useful plastics by the presence of phase separation, crystallites or cross-linking. Crystallites can form in polymers when long sequences of the polymer chain have a stereoregular structure. The simplest example of this is poly (ethylene) as shown in Figure 5. The close alignment of the chains to provide a fringed micellar type of crystallite set into amorphous polymer is shown. Polymer chemists often use the very approximate relationship that $T_g = 2/3 . T_m$ in degrees Kelvin is the temperature at which the crystallites melt. The main point to take from this equation is that $T_m > T_g$ and as polymers are never 100% crystalline such polymers above their T_g contain rubbery portions bound together with varying proportions of crystalline domains through which many chains pass. It is perhaps not too difficult to see how the macromolecular structures can vary with the thermal prehistory of such systems. In the case of poly (ethylene oxide) hydrogels in which the poly (ethylene oxide) units are particularly suitable for alignment to form crystals Graham (16) has shown that structures frozen into the polymer during its manufacture are relaxed during its first swelling in water.

Cross-linking involves the formation of a covalent bond between adjacent chains as illustrated in two dimensions in Figure 6 and typical crosslinking agents for vinyl polymers are given in Table IV. In general both cross-linking and crystallinity reduce the mobility of polymer chains and as a result reduce diffusion.

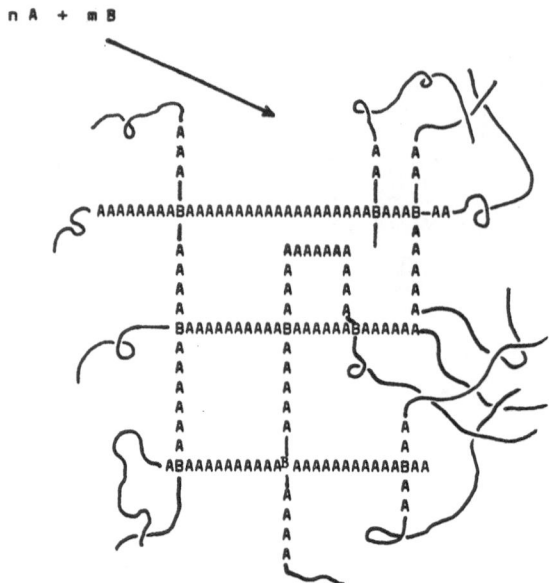

Figure 6. Two Dimensional Representation of the Formation of Crosslinked Structure by Copolymerization of Difunctional A (Hydroxyethyl - Hydroxethylmethacrylate $-CH_2= C (CH_3)$ $COOCH_2CH_2OH$) with Tetrafunctional B (Glycol dimethacrylate $CH_2= C (CH_3) COOCH_2 OCOC (CH_3)= CH_2$)

Table IV. Typical Crosslinking Agents for Hydrogels.

$CH_2 = C (CH_3)CONHCH_2NHCOC (CH_3) = CH_2$
Methylene bismethacrylamide

$CH_2 = C (CH_3)COO (CH_2CH_2)_nOCOC (CH_3) = CH_2$
Ethylene glycol (and polyethyleneglycol) dimethacrylates

Polymers can be made which comprise long sequences of two or more different polymers. Such polymers are called block or graft copolymers (17) and are illustrated in Figure 7 and Figure 8. As high molecular weight chains rarely dissolve in each other such block or graft copolymers form a mixture of domains in which polymer separation has occurred and the units of each species have aggregated. When one type of these separate domains is glassy or crystalline while the other is rubbery, the effect is to prevent flow of the chains and hence the bulk polymer. The separated domains can have a variety of structures as spheres, rods or sheets.

Cross-linking whether of a physical or chemical bonded nature has an important contribution to make to considerations of diffusion quite apart from its contribution to preventing fluid flow and allowing a polymer to be used as a membrane controlling diffusion. This contribution is the ability of a cross-linked system to swell with appropriate solvents which can be used both to charge the hydrogel with a drug solution and to control the permeability.

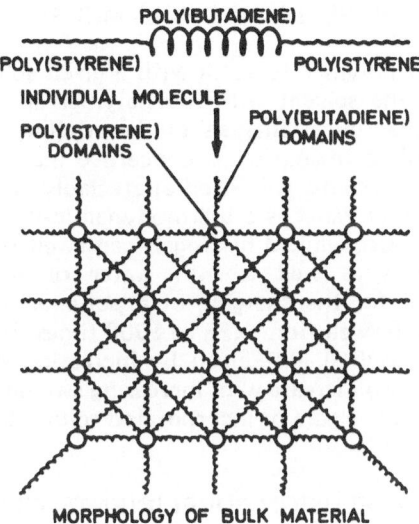

Figure 7. Schematic Two Dimensional Representation of the Morphology of a Styrene / Butadiene/ Styrene ABA Block Copolymer of Mn= 40,000.

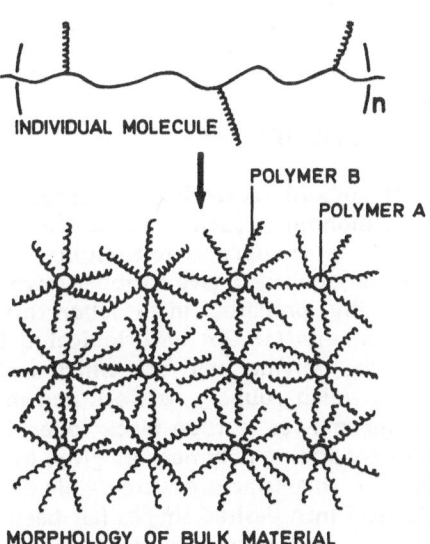

Figure 8. Schematic Two Dimensional Representation of the Morphology of a Hypothetical Graft Copolymer Containing Two Mutually Incompatible Segments.

THE SWELLING OF CROSS—LINKED POLYMERS

The ability of a polymer to swell with a given solvent is governed by the free energy of mixing of the solvent with the polymer and by the density of the cross-linking (18). The theoretical analysis of the swelling is complex and will not be discussed here. As this contribution is concerned mainly with hydrogel systems we can assume that such systems will swell appreciably with water, but this is not the same thing as saying that water is a thermodynamically good swelling solvent as this is often not the case. Crosslinked hydrogels can swell to a considerable degree with many organic solvents as well as with water or water solvent mixtures. This is particularly important for the charging of a polymer matrix with a drug solution. Typically hydrogels can swell from 1.25 to 1000 times their dry weight.

The degree of swelling is reduced by increasing the cross-linking density. As diffusion coefficients also increase with increasing swelling this can be used as a means of controlling the rate of release of incorporated solute drugs.

RELATIONSHIP OF DIFFUSION COEFFICIENTS TO PHYSICAL STATE OF THE POLYMER

The density of a polymer, indeed any particular material, will usually decrease in the order crystalline state, glassy state, rubbery state. This change in density is related to the molecular holes or free volume present in each state. This free volume increases from the lowest in the crystalline state to the highest in the rubbery state. As the free volume represents the holes into which diffusing molecules jump as they move down a concentration (or chemical potential) gradient, it is easy to postulate in general terms how diffusion coefficients increase as one goes from the crystalline to the glassy and then to the rubbery state.

PHASE SEPARATION IN HYDROGELS

By far the largest amount of work on hydrogels has been done on polymers made from hydrophilic monomers such as those shown in Tables I—IV. These can be polymerized in the presence of appropriate amounts of crosslinking agent, as listed in Table IV in water or water/solvent to give a rubbery swollen hydrogel capsule. Though such products are readily prepared in a laboratory they are often quite weak mechanically. Various patents (19,20) have indicated that it is highly desirable to incorporate units into the polymer network which will phase separate. These small domains reinforce the swollen rubbery network and improve its physical properties in much the same manner as carbon black does in rubber formulation. Some examples of such phase separating polymers are given in Figure 9.

The necessity to manufacture cross-linked devices, which cannot subsequently be reformed into desired shapes has been overcome by I.C.I (21) who have patented the use of poly (ethylene oxide) block copolymers for use particularly illustrated in Figure 10 and combine both the domain separated reinforcing principle and the desirable attribute of reformability by heating or dissolution of the polymers.

TOUGHENED HYDROGELS

		% MONOMER BY WEIGTH				
HEMA	$CH_2=CMeCOOCH_2CH_2OH$	98.5"	88.4	71	89	33
MACROMER (ADIPRENE L-167 + HEMA)	$CH_2=CMeCOO-[1-O(CH_2CH_2CH_2CH_2O)_{20}]1-OCOCMe=CH_2$	-	11.6	29	-	-
MACROMER (POLYMEG 2000 + ISOPHORONE DIISOCYANATE + HEMA)	$CH_2=CMeCOO-[1-O(CH_2CH_2CH_2CH_2O)_{28}]1-OCOCMe=CH_2$	-	-	-	11	22
NVP	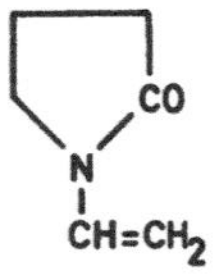 (N-vinyl pyrrolidone structure) CO—N—CH=CH_2	-	-	-	-	45
DEGREE OF SWELLING WITH WATER (%)		45	52	22	47	96
DRY TENSILE STRENGTH (psi)		2320	4560	4670	5910	6620
DRY ELONGATION (%)		15	41	89	50	67
WET TENSILE STRENGTH (psi)		69	185	490	120	85
WET ELONGATION (%)		83	99	113	120	60

- REMAINDER IS GLYCOL DIMETHACRYLATE CROSSLINKING AGENT

From British Patent 1,511,563 to CIBA-GEIGY (1978)

Figure 9. Hydrogel Compositions in Which Phase Separation on a Microscopic Scale is Believed to Exist.

1. $HO+CH_2-CH_2-O)_n H$ POLYETHYLENEGLYCOL OF MW 4000

2. 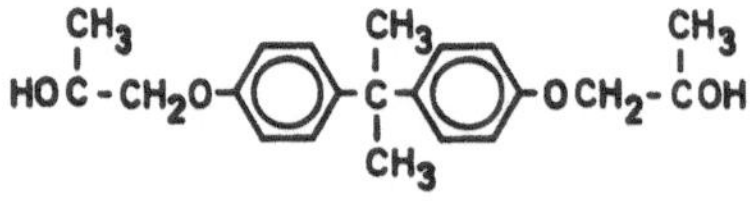 $HO\overset{CH_3}{\underset{CH_3}{C}}-CH_2O-\bigcirc-\overset{CH_3}{\underset{CH_3}{C}}-\bigcirc-OCH_2-\overset{CH_3}{C}OH$ 1,1'-ISOPROPYLIDENE-BIS-P-PHENOXY DIPROPANOL-2

3. 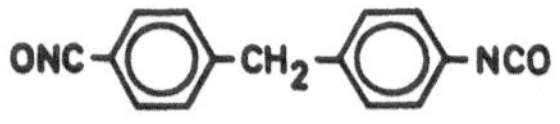 $ONC-\bigcirc-CH_2-\bigcirc-NCO$ 4,4'-DIPHENYL METHANE DI-ISOCYANATE

	MONOMER COMPOSITION		
	A	B	C
1	51	40	60
2	28	14.1	15
3	23	12.5	15
% BY WEIGHT HYDROPHILIC BLOCK	50	60	67
% BY WEIGHT HYDROPHILIC BLOCK	50	40	33
EQUILIBRIUM SWELLING WITH WATER AT 37°C AS PARTS PER INITIAL 100	100	150	210

Polymer 1 was cast from solution in tetrahydrofuron + water + fluprosterol sodium + sodium carbonate to provide films of 0.02 cm thickness after subsequent pressing at 110°C under pressure. These were placed around a silicone tube of diameter 0.4 cm and length 0.7 cm. This contained 12 g of fluprostanol sodium, 70-90% of the medicament was released in 24 hours in vivo (rats).

Fildes, F.J.T. and Hutchinson, F.G. German App. 2,755,505 (1977).

Figure 10. Thermoplastic Block Copolymer Elastomeric Hydrogels in which Microscopic Phase Separation is Believed to Exist.

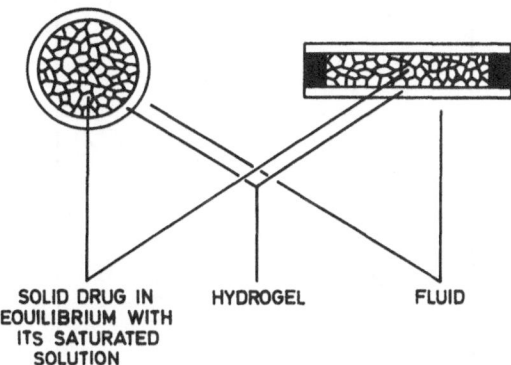

SOLID DRUG IN
EQUILIBRIUM WITH
ITS SATURATED
SOLUTION　　　　HYDROGEL　　　　FLUID

Figure 11. Envelope Configurations of Hydrogel Devices Which Should Provide Zero Order
　　　　　　Release.

The hydrogel permeability is governed to a considerable degree by the water content. High permeation rates are obtained, from water-soluble drugs, in gels with higher water contents. This can be varied by the choice of polymer and cross-linking density.

FORMS OF HYDROGEL DEVICES

Hydrogel dosage forms can be used in either the fully swollen state or in a dried condition. The hydrogel can also be used as a coating to provide a more complicated sandwich or envelope structure which would be expected to provide constant, or zero order (22) rates of release in vitro. This is illustrated in Figure 11.

PREDICTION OF THE RELEASE PROFILE FOR PRESWOLLEN DRUG —CONTAINING HYDROGELS

White and Dorian (23), Davis (24) and Langer and Folkman (25) studied the factors governing the release of a wide variety of biologically active materials from preswollen cylinders of hydrogels. The molecular weights of the materials studied covered a wide range (148—150,000). Davis studied the following six materials both in vitro and in vivo; rabbit immunoglobulin (M.W. 150,000); bovine serum albumin (M.W. 67,000); luteinizing hormone (M.W. 33,000); insulin (M.W. 36,000); prostaglandins F_2 (M.W. 345); and I (Nal. M.W. 125). The release of these materials from cross-linked gels of both poly (acrylamide) and poly (vinylpyrrolidone) were studied and the diffusion coefficients calculated from the theoretical equation governing release from such systems. The degree of swelling by its influence on permeability can be used to control the period of release but it is clear that it must be accurately reproduced if variable samples are not to be obtained.

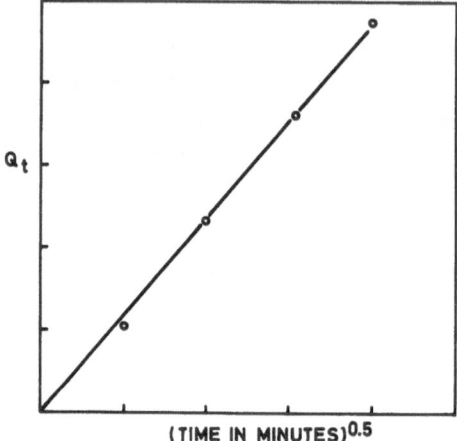

(TIME IN MINUTES)$^{0.5}$

Figure 12. The Release of Phenergan at 37°C from a Fully Swollen Device. Fractional Release at Plotted Against the Square Root of Time.

In general and fully confirmed by Davis the diffusion coefficients for the materials diffusing in water tend to decrease as the molecular weight of the materials increases. High molecular weight permeants show a much greater sensitivity to increase in the polymer content of the gels. Davis did not find any difference between the results with the two different polymers and concluded that the nature of the polymer was not a very important variable in the highly water-swollen release characteristics. He deduced the following empirical expression allowing the diffusion coefficient of any water soluble drug in any hydrogel to be estimated,

$$D_p = D_o \exp\left[-(0.05 + 10^{-6}M)\, P\right]$$

where D_o is the diffusion coefficient for the solute in pure solvent. D_p is the diffusion coefficient of the solute in the swollen polymer gel containing $P\%$ (by weight) of polymer. M is the solute molecular weight.

This diffusion coefficient can be used to estimate the release profile of any desired preswollen hydrogel device for which the mathematical analysis for the particular geometry is available. The profile of release should be largely independent of the chemical nature of the hydrogel.

The equations for a thin film, cylinders and spheres containing dissolved solute during the first part of the contained drug-release are given in Figure 12. Combining the equation for a thin film for a given polymer, solute and dimensions

$$\frac{Q_t}{Q_\infty} = 4\left(\frac{D_p t}{\pi L^2}\right)^{0.5} \qquad \text{for } \frac{M_t}{M_\infty} \leqslant 0.6$$

with the Davis equation above we get

$$\frac{Q_t}{Q_\infty} = 4\left[\frac{D_o \exp -(0.05 + 10^{-6}M)\, P\; t}{\pi L^2}\right]^{0.5} = Kt^{0.5}$$

where Q_t and Q_∞ are the masses of initial solute released at times t and infinity and L is the thickness of the film or slab.

The D_p estimated from the known composition, and using the information from the Davis paper, can be checked for a thin slab configuration by studying solute release from the hydrogel into a large volume of solvent which approximates to an infinite sink. Under such conditions a plot of (Q_t/Q_∞) against $t^{0.5}$ should be a straight line of early slope $(16 D/\pi L^2)^{0.5}$ from which D can be readily calculated. As a useful preliminary calculation the time for one half release (valid for a slab) may be calculated. Thus taking a value for D_o of 75×10^{-7} $cm^2 sec^{-1}$ for prostaglanding F_2 (M.W. 354) in 10mM phosphate-buffered saline, pH7.2 at 37°C we can calculate the value of D_p in a typical hydrogel swollen with 60% of water and containing 40% of polymer.

$$D_p = 75 \times 10^{-7} \exp[-(0.05 + 10^{-6}.354)\,40]$$

$$= 10^{-6} cm^2 sec^{-1}$$

By using the equation for a slab and a value of $(Q_t/Q_\infty) = 0.5$ we can calculate table of the thickness L required for various half-release times as $L = 8[D_p t_{1/2}/\pi]^{0.5}$. These are gives in Table V.

Table V. Illustration of How the Diffusion Coefficient of Prostaglandin F_2 Varies with the % Polymer Content P of a Water Swollen Hydrogel and How the Half-Life for Release Rates to Swollen Thickness Varies for Various P values.

P%	Estimated D in $cm^2 sec^{-1}$ $(\times 10^7)$	L in cm					
5	58.32	1.52	2.15	2.69	3.32	4.70	5.76
10	45.33	1.29	1.82	2.23	2.82	3.99	4.89
20	27.40	1.00	1.41	1.74	2.20	3.11	3.80
40	10.00	0.61	0.86	1.05	1.33	1.88	2.30
60	3.66	0.37	0.52	0.63	0.80	1.13	1.39
80	1.34	0.22	0.31	0.38	0.49	0.69	0.84
$t_{1/2}$ in hours		5	10	15	24	28	72

COMPARISON WITH A CYLINDER

Taking $D_p = 10^{-6} cm^2 sec^{-1}$, t = 15 hours and r = 0.5 (1.05 cm)

$$\text{then} = \frac{Q_t}{Q_\infty} = 4[\frac{10^{-6}.15.3600}{\pi.0.525^2}]^{0.5} - [\frac{10^{-6}.15.3600}{0.525^2}] = 0.80$$

Thus a cylinder releases much more rapidly than an infinite slab of thickness equivalent to the cylinder diameter.

By control of the proportion of polymer in the hydrogel and the thickness of the slab or diameter of the cylinder it is possible to obtain drug release over periods from hours to days. This release is not, however, at a constant rate.

UNSWOLLEN HYDROGELS

The calculations above indicate that highly swollen hydrogels have to be moderately large devices with swollen diameters or thicknesses of 0.5 cm if release of contained low molecular weight species are to be prolonged for 24 hours or more. There is some advantage to be gained by commencing with predried devices which swell during use. This type of device has a changing diffusion coefficient with time and the analysis of the kinetics of release is much more complex. Some analysis of this complex situation has been reported by Good (26) for diffusion out of poly (2—hydroxyethylmethacrylate) sheets containing tripelenamine hydrochloride and more recently by both Peppas (27) and Lee (28).

The release characteristics can in special circumstances approximate zero order (constant rate of release). Graham and McNeill have recently reported constant delivery monoliths for prostaglandin E_2 utilizing swelling crystalline rubbery hydrogels (4).

Akkapeddi (29, 30) has reported studies on dried hydrogel cylinders which he successfully used to induce abortions in rabbits using the swellable cylinder as a cervical dilator which released a prostaglandin concurrently.

CLINICAL EXAMPLES OF THE USE OF HYDROGELS

The previous part of this presentation has dealt with general considerations and some elementary theory. Hydrogels are now in a period of expansion of clinical use. Thus soft contact lense applications of both short and longer-wear varieties are now well established. The use of hydrogel dressings for wounds, ulcers and burns is also quite extensive and novel products in the form of powder, water-swollen gels or sheets are now in a period of rapid increase in number and presumeably also total market size. The clinical use of hydrogels in controlled drug delivery is in its infancy and will develop rapidly over the next decade. The following examples serve to illustrate and consolidate the earlier discussion.

HYDROGEL FOAMS FOR CONTRACEPTION

Polymer and materials scientists for the greater part concentrate their research onto the design of systems releasing drugs over months or over years while the main interest of the pharmaceutical industry is usually up to only a few days. The use of a hydrogel contraceptive sponge has recently been described (31). This device takes the form of a cervical foam cap containing a gram of spermicide (Nonoxynol—9) which is released over a few days and can provide an effective contraceptive action over this period of time. Extensive clinical evaluation of this device has been undertaken and the product has been on sale in the USA since 1983. It provides an example of a crude but effective use of hydrogels for short term local delivery.

PROSTAGLANDIN STABILIZATION AND DELIVERY

Using a mixture of moderate molecular weight poly (ethylene glycols) around 8000 with polyols and diisocyanates results in a polymerization which forms partially crystalline crosslinked hydrogels which are tough and leathery rather than brittle or rubbery. They can thus be cut readily to precise thickness slices, if desired, after forming from the reacting liquid mix into any desired shape. They can also be quite conveniently converted to powders of particle size between 100 and 1000 μm.

Tests of compatibility with growing mouse fibroblast cultures have not given any indication of any undesirable interaction and it has been shown on limited testing that these materials do not appear to support bacterial growth. USP extraction and feeding studies in rats have also been completed without any evidence of toxicity or undesireable reaction. They can be sterilized by means of ethylene oxide.

These hydrogels find particular use with many families of chemicals which have been found over the past few decades to have a very marked physiological effect in minute quantities. Thus, for example, many steroids and prostaglandins are active in daily doses of micrograms. The body protects itself agains its own very active species such as prostaglandin E_2 (PGE_2) by rapidly destroying them, e.g., in one passage through the lungs. The biological half-life of PGE_2 is thus very short and this is true of most naturally occurring prostaglandins. Pharmaceutical chemists have typically and expertly responded to solve this problem by devising novel prostaglandins with a longer in vivo lifetime. Though many such modified prostaglandins (33) are now known a quite different approach could have been used. This would have been to stabilize the natural prostaglandins and deliver them in a continuous and controlled manner into the body. This is the basis of intravenous utilisation of prostaglandins E_2 and F_2 in parturition and the evaluation of prostacyclin (PGI_2) in the treatment of Raynaud's disease (34). Until recently this type of therapy has been limited as intravenous therapy is of restricted use because of its very nature. The prospect for the use of prostaglandins in more conventional pharmaceutical formulations has now been opened up by the discovery that at least some of these unstable materials are stabilized for more than a year at 4 ^{O}C and for at least six months at room temperature when incorporated into a urethane crosslinked poly (ethylene oxide) hydrogel (35). Crosslinked starch hydrogels have also been shown to provide an extended shelf-life of one year for PGE_2 incorporated therein (36). These hydrogels thus provide promise of prostaglandins stabilised as powders which could, in principle, be used as oral dosage forms. The poly (ethylene oxide) hydrogels can be made in any size or shape and release of the prostaglandin over 24 hours is a quite reasonable expectation. In addition these crystalline, high swelling urethane crosslinked poly (ethylene oxide) hydrogels not only are capable of chemically stabilizing and prolonging the release of PGE_2 but also in many cases providing quite constant rates of release for the first ca. 40—50% of the contained drug (4).

MONOLITHIC VAGINAL PESSARIES FOR CERVICAL RIPENING

As mentioned earlier hydrogels which are partially crystalline tough leathery materials capable of swelling highly in both water and organic solvents such as chloroform can be made from grades of poly (ethylene glycols) of molecular weight of over 4000 by crosslinking them with a diisocyanate and a triol such as 1,2,6-hexanetriol. These polymers will swell easily to 5 times their volume in aqueous or organic solu-

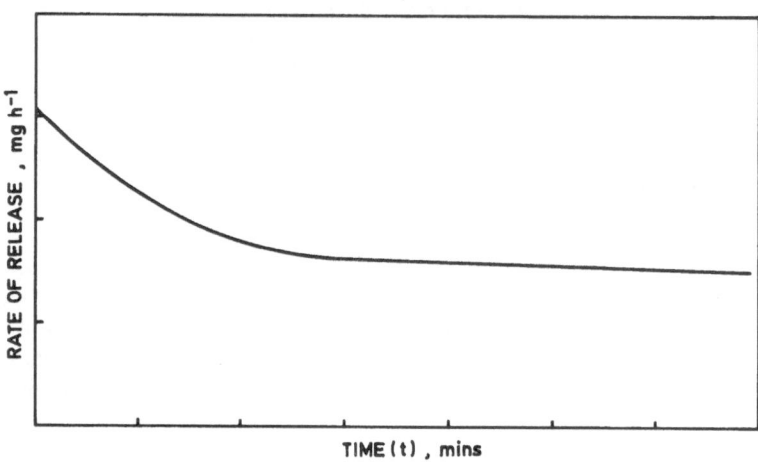

Figure 13. Phenergan Release from a Dry Slice of a Poly (ethylene glycol) Based Hydrogel into 0.1 N HCl at 37°C.

tions of drugs (2) and it is usually quite a straightforward matter to incorporate at least 20% of the dry polymer weight as drug. In the fully swollen state the monoliths of swollen polymer act much like any other swollen hydrogel and release approximately half of the contained drug according to the well known standard diffusion equations. The release of Phenergan^{TM} from a swollen device at 37°C is shown in Figure 12. The expected straight line plot of fraction of contained drug released against (time)$^{0.5}$ was obtained. The apparent diffusion coefficient of the phenergan in the swollen hydrogel can be readily calculated from the slope of this plot. When the slab device is tried under vacuum and the release of phenergan was again studied at 37°C the very surprising result was found that a constant rate of release occurred for approximately the first 30% of the contained drug as shown in Figure 13 where the absolute release is now plotted directly against time and not (time)$^{0.5}$. This unusual feature of these crystalline polymers in providing very good profiles of release from dried down flat slabs has proved very useful in the formulations of pessaries for the vaginal delivery of prostaglandin E_2(4) which is also stabilized into a distributable dosage form as mentioned earlier. The fractional release plotted against time for an optimised dry hydrogel pessary containing 10 mg PGE_2 is given in Figure 14. The release rate in this case is constant and is very acceptable. The half-life of 6.8 hours was predetermined by the thickness of the device, it having been found that the half-life for drug release of the dry devices at constant total drug delivery was proportional to the square of the thickness. Mr. M.P. Embrey has used these pessaries in the induction of labor in over 200 patients who at full term suffered from varying degrees of 'unripened cervix'. Some of the results have been published (37) and clearly demonstrated that a beneficial effect on cervical ripening, shortening and easing labour and a significant reduction in the need for caesarian sections when compared with delivery without the use of PGE_2 was obtained. It has also been found that the swelling of the devices in vivo is slower that in vitro and this will necessarily produce a somewhat slower release in vivo than shown by the in vitro results.

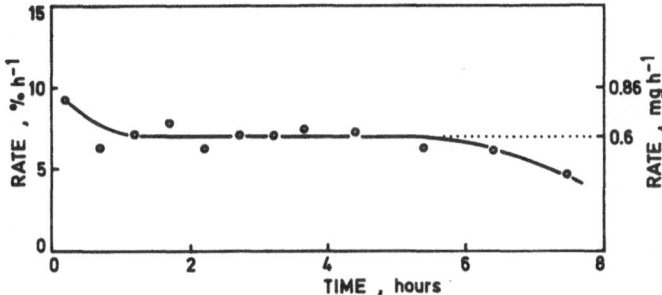

Figure 14. Prostaglandin E_2 Release from a Dry Slice of Crosslinked PEO 8400 Hydrogel into Water at 37°C. Half Life $t_{1/2}$= 7.2 h, Total Initial Content PGE_2= 8.6 mg. "Uniform" Rate = 0.6 mgh^{-1}.

MONOLITHIC RECTAL PESSARIES FOR ANALGESIA

Prolonged and precisely programmed delivery can be achieved by a designed rectal pessary based on the urethane crosslinked poly (ethylene oxide) hydrogels (28). The rectal route of delivery has many advantages and disadvantages some of which are listed below.

RECTAL DRUG ADMINISTRATION

Advantages
    Not dependent on gastric emptying
    Unaffected by nausea and vomiting
    Administration may be discontinued.
    May avoid some hepatic first pass metabolism
    Metabolism of drug by gut wall may be reduced
Disadvantages
    Patient acceptability
    Variable inter—individual absorption
    Administration interrupted by defecation.

A device to release morphine at a constant rate for at least 10 hours was designed in our laboratories. An initial charging surge of 10mg was requested by the clinicians Prof. G. Smith and Dr. C.D. Hanning of the Leicester Royal Infirmary. This was provided by a hollow cylindrical shape corresponding to a rolled up slab configuration. It was first charged uniformly with an aqueous solution of morphine hydrochloride and then dried before receiving extra charging doses on the interior and exterior to provide the surge and later the uniform release. The success of this technique can be seen from the in vitro release shown as rate of release against time in

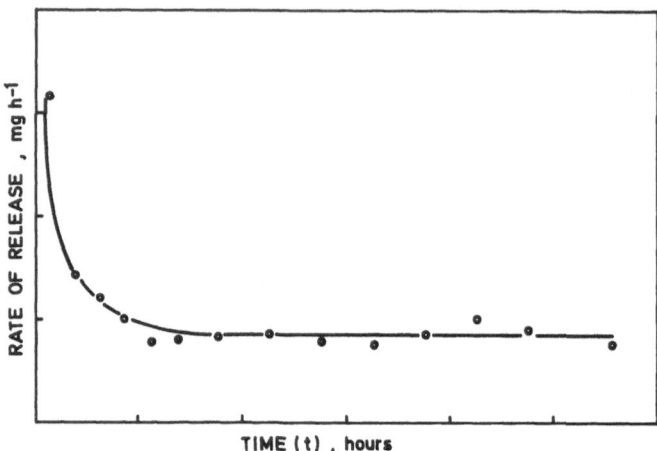

Figure 15. The Release of Morphine Hydrochloride from a Concentration Profiled Rectal Pessary at 37°C. The Polymer is a Crosslinked Crystalline - Rubbery Poly (ethylene glycol).

Figure 15. In vivo results again showed that the rate of swelling of blank devices was slower than in vitro and somewhat lower rates of drug release would therefore be expected. The blood plasma levels of morphine determined in four subjects clearly showed that steady release over 12 hours was obtained but with considerable patient to patient variability. This type of delivery clearly has the potential to provide overnight and programmed drug delivery with a peak of drug being delivered in the early morning if required. As this is not a currently available therapy but could be useful, in a number of conditions, e.g., asthma, hypertension and rheumatism, these systems are being further devoleped.

THE FUTURE

An exposition as short as this one cannot be comprehensive. Many aspects have been omitted or dealt with very briefly such as pH enzyme and vibration responsive systems, sub-microscopic domains, colloidal forms of hydrogels, microporous systems and microencapsulation. Each of these areas is likely to form a significant part of the future clinical applications for hydrogels and indeed some such systems are currently being evaluated in animals or humans. The clinical prospects for hydrogels are most promising and it will be a great surprise and disappointment to the author if a significant number of new therapies do not arise from their utilization.

REFERENCES

1. Bailey, F.E. and Koleske, J.V., eds., Poly (ethylene oxide). Academic Press, 1976.
2. Graham, N.B., Nwachuku, N.E. and Walsh, D.J., Polymer, 23: 1345, 1982.
3. Graham, N.B. and McNeill, M.E., Biomaterials, 5:27, 1984.
4. Graham, N.B. and McNeill, M.E., J.Controlled Release, 2, 1984 (in press).
5. Lundberg, R.D., Crosslinked Polyethers. Canadian Patent 756190, 1967.
6. Interactions Between Macromolecules in Solution in Advances in Polymer Science No. 45. Springer Verlag, 1982.
7. Tighe, B.J., Contact Lens Materials. Chapter 13 in Contact Lenses. A Textbook for Practitioner and Student., Eds., J. Stone and A.J. Philips. Butterworths, 1981.
8. Peppas, N.A., Contact Lenses as Biomedical Polymers. Chapter 2 in Extended Wear Contact Lenses., Ed., J. Hartstein. C.V. Moskylo., St. Louis, 1982.
9. Improvements in or Relating to Sustained-release Medicaments. Czechoslovak Academy of Science. British Patent, 1,135,966, 1967.
10. Fildes, F.J.T., Compositions, British Patent, 1,440,217, 1976.
11. Vollmert, B., ed., Polymer Chemistry. Springer Verlag, 1973.
12. Allport, D.C. and Jones, W.H., eds., Block Copolymers. Applied Science Publishers, 1973.
13. Howard, R.N., ed., Physics of Glassy Polymers. Applied Science Publishers, 1973.
14. Treloar, L.R.G. The Physics of Rubber Elasticity, Clarendon Press, 1958.
15. Billmeyer, F.W., Textbook of Polymer Science, Wiley, 1962.
16. Graham, N.B. and McNeill, M.E., in Artificial Organs., Eds., J.P.Paul, J.M. Courtney, J.D.F. Gaylor, T. Gilchrist and B.J.A. Andrews. Macmillan Press 1984 (in press).
17. Cerease, J.R., ed., Block and Graft Copolymerization, Vols 1 and 2. Wiley, 1973 and 1976.
18. Walsh, D.J., Plastics and Rubber: Materials and Applications, February: 17,1976.
19. Graham, N.B., Ellams, C and Hutchison, F.G., Ger. Offen. 2,312,973, 1973.
20. British Patent, 1,511,563.
21. Fildes, F.J.T. and Hutchinson, F.G., Release Medium for Biologically Active Substances. U.K. Patent, 1,551,620, 1979.
22. Lee, P.I., Cold Water-insoluble Polyvinylalcohol Pouch for the Controlled Release of Active Ingredients. U.S. Patent 4,340,491, 1982.
23. White, M.L. and Dorion, G.H., J. Polym. Sci., 55:731, 1961.
24. Davis, B.K., Proc. Nat. Acad. Sci. USA, 71: 3120, 1974.
25. Langer, R. and Folkman, J.M., Polymer Delivery Systems, pp. 175—196, R.J. Kostelink, Gordon and Breach Science Publishers Inc., 1978.
26. Good, W.R., Diffusion of Water-soluble Drugs from Initially Dry Hydrogels, loc.cit., pp. 139—156.
27. Korsmeyer, R.W. andPeppas, N.A., in Controlled Release Delivery Systems. Eds. T.J. Roseman and S.Z. Mansdorf, Dekker, New York, p. 77, 1983.
28. Lee, P.I., J.Membrane Sci., 7:225, 1980.
29. Balin, H., Halpern, B.D., Davis, R.H., Akkapeddi, M.I. and Kyriazis, B.A., J. Reproductive Med., 13:208, 1974.
30. Akkapeddi, M.K., Halpern, B.D., Davis, R.H. and Balin, H., in Controlled Release of Biologically Active Agents, A.C. Tanquary and R.E. Lacery., eds., Advances in Experimental Medicine and Biology Vol. 47, pp. 165—76, Plenium, 1974.

31. Taylor, R.N., Jr, Goldsmith, A., Beklkovic, B., Stanojlovic, B., and McCahn, M.F., in Vaginal Contraception: New Developments, pp. 119—127., Eds., Zatuchin Harper and Row, Hagerstown, 1979.
32. Vorhaner, B.W., in Bifluid Mechanics, Vol. 2. pp. 93—124, Eds. D.J. Schnick, Plenium, New York, 1980.
33. Bergstrom, S., Angew. Chem. Int. Ed. Engl., 22' 858, 1983.
34. Belch, J.J.F., Newman, P., Drury, J.D., Capell, H., Leiberman, P., Jones, W.B., Forbes, C.D. and Prestice, C.R.M., Thrombosis and Haemostasis, 45, Part 111: 255, 1981.
35. Embrey, M.P., New Prostaglandin Delivery Systems, Chapter in Voluntary Interuption of Pregnancy., Eds, Toppozade, M., Byggerman, M. and Haffez, E.S.E., M.T.P. Press, Lancaster, 1984.
36. Harris, A. and Stenberg, P., Pharmacy International, May: 113, 1981.
37. Embrey, M.P., Graham, N.B., and McNeill, M.E., BMJ, 281:901, 1980.
38. Hanning, C.D., Smith., G., McNeill, M.E. and Graham, N.B., Proc. Anaesthetic Research Soc., pp. 2—3, 1982.
39. King, P.A., Novel Dressing and Use Thereof. U.S. Patent 3,149,006, 1968.

CONTROLLED DRUG DELIVERY WITH COLLOIDAL POLYMERIC SYSTEMS

R. Gurny

University of Geneva, School of Pharmacy, Geneva, Switzerland

INTRODUCTION

A great variety of pharmaceutical preparations are submicroscopic dispersions, such as nanoparticles (1), nanocapsules (2), liposomes (3), macromolecular complexes (4) and the so-called latex formulations (5). Chiefly, because of their submicroscopic particle size, these systems offer a great many interesting applications, not only in the field of medicine but also in agricultural, veterinary and industrial applications. To justify their name, the so called colloidal systems are limited to the size range from a few nanometers up to one micron. In medicine, these types of preparations may be used for parenteral administration, as sustained release injections or for the delivery of an active compound to a specific organ or target site in the body. An ideal colloidal carrier system would transport the drug, entrapped, bound, encapsulated or dissolved in or on the carrier, to its desired site of action and then release the active ingredient at a suitable rate. The system would be non toxic and able to decompose in vivo if injected. At the same time it would have good storage stability.

In the last few years, a new type of system for parenteral and ophthalmic use has been described (6,7) and successfully tested in animals, the so-called pseudolatices.

Vanderhoff and co-worker (8) developed one of the basic technologies to prepare these colloidal dispersions from already formed polymers.

Most of the latex formulations are produced by the mechanism of emulsion polymerization (9). This technique requires that the initiator create radicals in the aqueous medium which are captured in the micelles formed by an emulsifier. These micelles are swollen by the diffusing monomer. The polymerization process takes place within the swollen micelles and as the monomer is consumed it is replaced by diffusion of additional quantities of the monomer from the outer phase. There are still two major problems in using this type or pharmaceutical carrier (10), (a) the lack of biodegradation of most of the polymers and (b) the possibility of occurrence of toxic reaction (i.e. inflammation, carcinogenesis). The main source of the reverse reaction is the low molecular weight residuals (mainly monomers) in the final product. To ensure the safety of these polymeric preparations for in vivo use, the final product must be free of residual monomers. For this reason, as long as ten years ago, a limit of 500 ppm (11) was set as the acceptable level of unreacted acrylamide in filters, for example.

The disadvantages mentioned and the impossibility of obtaining latex systems by emulsion polymerization, e.g. epoxy resins, polyurethanes, polyesters, ethylcellulose and elastomers such as cispolyisoprene, led directly to a new technology, the so-called pseudo-latices. These latices commonly have slightly poorer stability than dispersions prepared by emulsion polymerization because the particles are somewhat larger. Three distinct techniques may be mentioned:

(a) Self-emulsification, the one commercial technique that can produce comparable particle sizes, is limited in application because the systems are rather water-sensitive,
(b) Phase inversion,
(c) Solution emulsification.

The latter method involves dissolving the polymer in a volatile solvent, dispersing the organic phase in water, emulsifying by a conventional method and finally removing the solvent by steam stripping.

Recent research (12) suggests the possibility of using mixed emulsifying systems, e.g. laurylsulfate-cetylalcohol, hexadecyltrimethyl ammonium bromidedecetylalcohol or a steric stabilizer such as polyoxyethylene. The active ingredient is usually added in the organic phase during preparation of the latex or is adsorbed onto the surface of the particles once the latex is formed.

Figure 1 shows the main differences between the two methods for preparing latex systems. The one on the left is a typical emulsion polymerization, the one on the right is a dispersion of an already formed polymer in water, called pseudolatex by some polymer chemists.

In general, the three main categories of latex products may be distinguished according to their origins (13):

(a) Natural latices which occur as the metabolic products of various plants and trees;
(b) Synthetic latices prepared directly from their corresponding monomers by the process of emulsion polymerization;
(c) Artificial latices (Pseudolatices) prepared by dispersion of bulk polymers already formed in aqueous media.

POSSIBILITIES FOR THE PREPARATION OF COLLOIDAL PARTICLES FOR DRUG CARRIERS

Emulsion Polymerization Using Organic and Aqueous Continuous Phase

The basic method is already mentioned in Figure 1. E.g. polyacrylic nanoparticles are modifications or special cases of emulsion polymerization. The most widely accepted theory by Harkins (15) is explained in Figure 2.

The preparation of nanoparticules can be carried out by two different methods (14):

(a) Using a continuous organic phase
(b) Using a continuous aqueous phase.

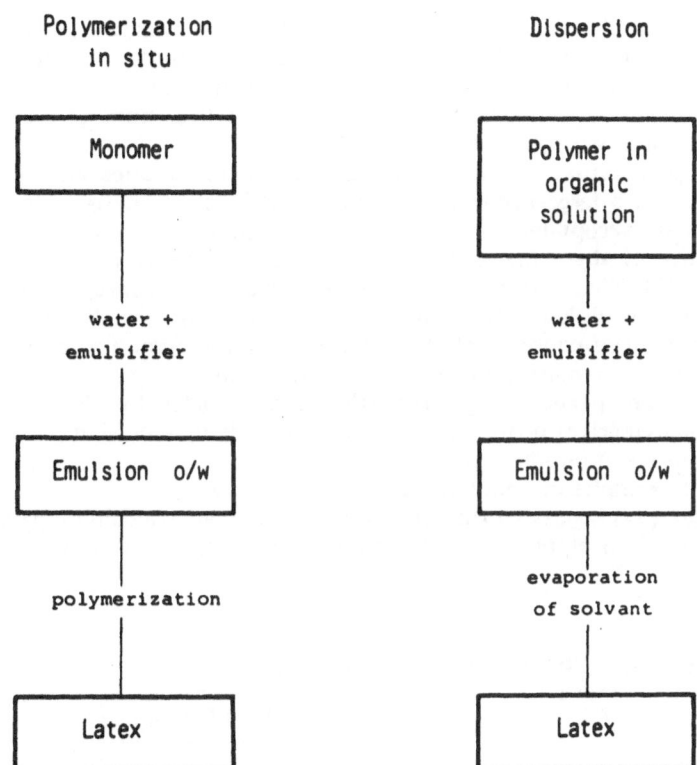

Figure 1. Methods of Latex Preparation.

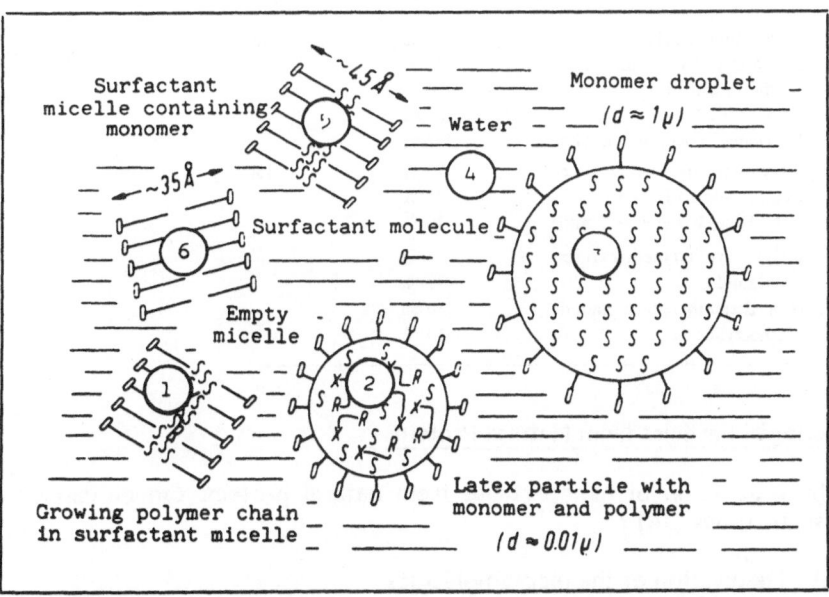

Figure 2. Mechanism of Emulsion Polymerization: According to the HARKINS Theory (15).

For the first case a large number of articles are available (14-20). Furthermore, by incorporation of dextran into these polyacrylamide polymer chains one can obtain biodegradable particles (21). An interesting feature is that these polyacryl dextran particles are metabolized in vitro by rat liver homogenates and eliminated in-vivo after intraperitoneal injection into mice.

The preparation of nanoparticles using a continuous aqueous phase is also investigated in a large number of studies (22) involving detergents. Although a few detergents are acceptable for use in parenteral administration, it is desirable to avoid the presence of these materials in injectables because of their effects on biological materials (30). These effects can either be enhanced or depressed or can even lead to inactivation of biologically active material like antigens. Kreuter and coworkers (32, 33) produced nanoparticles by emulsifier-free polymerization initiated by γ-irradiation or by peroxodisulfate combined with heating.

Copolymer particles have recently been reported by Rembaum (34-36). The author copolymerizes different acrylic compounds by emulsion polymerization using chemical means or γ-radiation.

Some examples of copolymers are given in Table I.

Margel (37) suggested the preparation of polyglutaraldehyde particles by alcohol polycondensation at pH > 7. The mechanism of the polycondensation is shown in Figure 3.

Table I. Acrylic Copolymer Nanoparticles (35).

Composition		Diameter [nm]
Methyl methacrylate	53 %	40
2-Hydroxyethyl methacrylate	30 %	
Methacrylic acid	10 %	
Ethyleneglycol dimethacrylate	7 %	
Methyl methacrylate	33 %	80
2-Hydroxyethyl methacrylate	25 %	
Methacrylic acid	10 %	
Acrylamide	25 %	
Ethyleneglycol dimethacrylate	7 %	
2-Hydroxyethyl methacrylate	70 %	150
Methacrylic acid	20 %	
N,N'-Bismethyleneacrylamide	10 %	
2-Hydroxyethyl methacrylate	30 %	60
Acrylamide	30 %	
N,N'-Bismethyleneacrylamide	30 %	
Methacrylic acid	10 %	

Colloidal Particles from Natural Proteins

The production of nanoparticles from natural proteins can be carried out by two basic methods (14) :

(a) Desolvation of the macromolecules
(b) Denaturation at high temperature.

$$\underset{\displaystyle CHO-(CH_2)_3-CHO}{} + \underset{\displaystyle CH_2-(CH_2)_2-CHO}{\overset{\displaystyle CHO}{\overset{|}{}}} \rightarrow$$

$$\underset{\displaystyle CHO-(CH_2)_3-CH-CH-(CH_2)_2-CHO}{\overset{\displaystyle OH \quad CHO}{\overset{|\qquad |}{}}} \rightarrow$$

$$\underset{\displaystyle CHO-(CH_2)_3-CH=C-(CH_2)_2-CHO}{\overset{\displaystyle CHO}{\overset{|}{}}} + H_2O \quad \frac{+[CHO_2(CH_2)_3]_{x-1}}{-[H_2O]_{x-1}}$$

$$\underset{\displaystyle CHO-(CH_2)_3-[CH=C-(CH_2)_2]_x-CHO}{\overset{\displaystyle CHO}{\overset{|}{}}}$$

Figure 3. Polycondensation of Glutaraldehyde (37).

Desolvation

Macromolecules can be desolvated by charge changes, pH changes or by the addition of a desolvating agent causing the salting out phenomenon. Bungenberg (38) already observed the formation of coacervate. After a certain degree of desolvation, the molecules begin to aggregate and phase separation occurs. The formation of these coiled macromolecules can be observed by turbidity measurements (39).

The production of human albumin nanoparticles was successfully carried out with this technique by Marcy (40).

Denaturation at High Temperature

The denaturation of protein at high temperatures is another possibility for producing albumin nanoparticles. Kramer (41) and Scheffel (42) used this technique successfully to produce a carrier for drugs.

PRACTICAL USE OF SOME COLLOIDAL SYSTEMS

Drug Targeting

We are still confronted with the problem of drug action specificity. The problem is how to bring molecules into intimate contact with a specific target site. With some new systems, it seems possible to give a partially satisfactory answer. By means of nanoparticles coated with monoclonal antibodies it is possible to direct cytotoxic agents to tumor cells. It is now known (43) that liposomes lose much of their phospholipid content to plasma high density lipoprotein and that entrapped drugs are also too rapidly released in the blood stream. Polyalkylcyanoacrylates are more stable than liposomes in biological fluids and have a prolonged shelf life.

These biodegradable polymeric nanoparticles are obtained by emulsion polymerization following an anionic initiation mechanism. A freeze-fracture study shows a solid porous structure (Figure 4) of the particles which can adsorb efficiently different kinds of drugs.

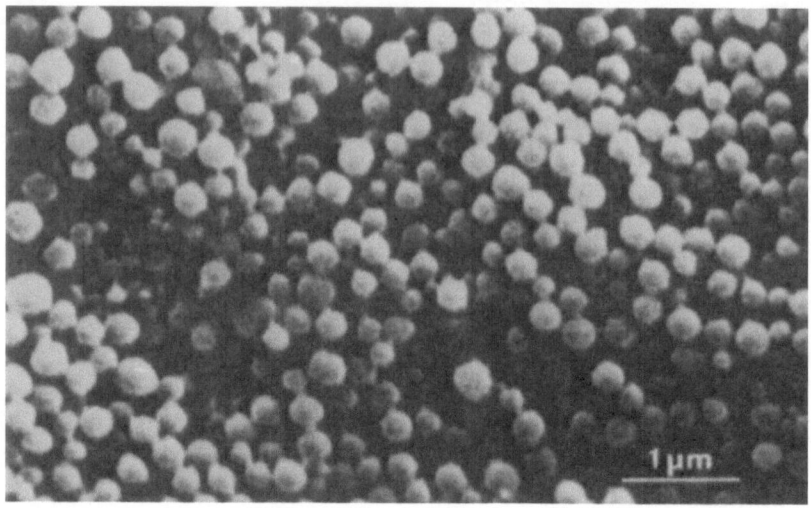

Figure 4.　Scanning-electron Microscopy of Polyisobutylcyanoacrylate Nanoparticles (43).

The most interesting characteristic of these nanoparticles is that they are more or less quickly degraded, depending on the length of their alkyl chain (44). The particles undergo an enzymatic ester hydrolysis on the side-chain, producing a primary alcohol and a water-soluble polycyanoacrylic acid. To a lesser extent there can be observed a chain-scission producing cyanoacetic acid and formaldehyde. Couvreur (44) says the use of these nanoparticles as carriers for dactinomycin considerably increases its anticancer activity. Furthermore the toxicity of doxorubicine by linkage to nanoparticles is significantly reduced. However an excessive accumulation of the carrier at some places is shown by whole body radiography (Figure 5).

The liver acts as a reservoir for nanoparticles. For this reason Couvreur (44) considers the exciting idea of guiding nanoparticles with the aid of monoclonal antibodies.

Two designs of coupling of monoclonal antibodies to nanoparticles may be considered:
  — without using a spacer molecule
  — using protein A as a spacer.
Figure 6 shows the possible concept.

The specific interaction between monoclonal antibody-coated carriers and antigenic tumor cells has been confirmed in vitro.

By using a spacer molecule it was shown that it is possible to have good reactivity of the immunoreactive portions pointing outside the carrier.

Controlled Release of Hormones with Pseudolatices

The first experimental pseudolatex for parenteral use was prepared by a direct emulsification technique (45). Poly d, l latic acid ($\overline{M}_W$=62,400) was used as the drug carrier and (4-^{14}C) testosterone was employed as the model drug. The drug was molecularly dispersed in the latex particles. A nonionic surfactant (poloxamer) was used

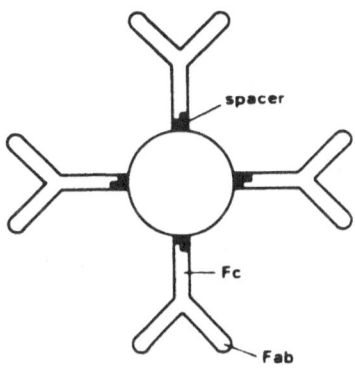

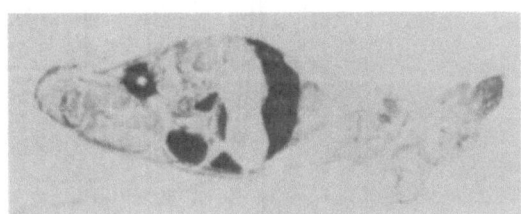

Figure 5. Whole Body Autoradiography of a Mouse 4h after Intravenous Administration of
^{14}C-polyisobutylcyanoacrylates Nanoparticles (2.5 μ Ci).

Figure 6. Representation of Monoclonal Antibodies Coating Nanoparticles with the Aid of Protein
A as Spacer Molecule.

in the latex preparation. The apparent average particle size was determined by laser
spectroscopy and was found to be in the range of 0.4 μm with a polydispersity index
of 3, i.e. an essentially mono-sized system. The final latex was prepared in order to
have solid content of 40 % wt/wt corresponding to an apparent Brookfield viscosity
of 128 cps at 20°C.

The in-vitro release of drug from such colloidal systems was determined by
the authors (45) by dialysis. For comparison, a reference formulation with peanut
oil was tested.

An interesting foreign-body histopathologic evaluation of the latex system
was carried out by injecting 0.2 ml into the anterior thigh muscle of white Sprague
Dawley rats (6). Studies were carried out in 2 phases (a) short term (4 days) and
(b) long term (1 to 4 months). Sections of the anterior thigh muscle with the injection site were collected, processed and stained. As usual after an injection, some
multinucleated giant cells and myofibers showing evidence of attempted regeneration
were found 7 days postinjection (PI). On PI day 28, lesions were smaller than those
found earlier. Except for a reduction in size, lesions on PI day 56 were identical with
those seen earlier.

Figure 7 shows the results of the drug release studies carried out on an average
of 6 rats for each formulation tested. The rapid release of the drug from the oil
solution seen in vitro obviously occured in-vivo as well. The much slower release of
the entrapped drug in the PLA latex is seen in the in-vivo study. While the drug
containing PLA latex does not produce an ideal release profile in-vivo (showing
a peak before the plateau) it does demonstrate its ability to produce a protracted
nearly steady state blood level from day 4 through day 14.

This study demonstrates that a biodegradable polymer may be prepared as a
colloidal system which appears to have a certain shelf-life stability at room temperature. Drug entrapment in a latex system at the molecular level, as shown by X ray
diffraction (15), however, does show an initial and usually undesirable burst of drug

202

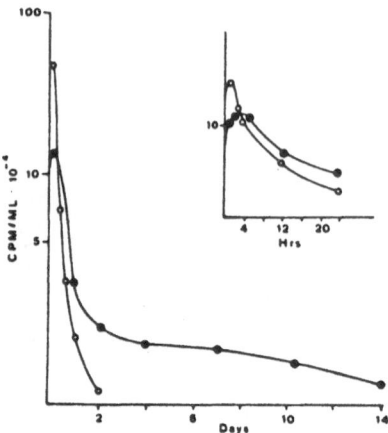

Figure 7.   In Vivo Release Tested in Six Animals.

release. As currently developed, it releases the drug more rapidly than do implants formulated with similar polymers (16-23).

Colloidal Carrier for the Ocular Route

Frequent dosage is probably the major reason for non-compliance with prescribed schedules of administration. Moreover, especially in the case of ocular therapy, the pre-corneal disposition factors for all ocular drugs increase the difficulty of preparing an acceptable controlled-release formulation. Unlike most systemic therapies, the major portion of a topically instilled drug leaves the absorption site (cornea) unabsorbed. This occurs because of tear dilution and a washout phenomenon (60,61). While drugs in saline solutions are commonly used in ophthalmic practice, solutions with viscosities of 1 to 50 cps are used in order to improve comfort or lubrication and also to achieve a slight prolongation in action. In recent years, different types of ocular therapeutic systems have been extensively tested and improved:

    (a)   Reservoir type systems
    (b)   Soluble or insoluble inserts
    (c)   Emulsions
    (d)   Liposomes
    (e)   Implantable pumps
    (f)   Colloidal formulations

Among these new types of delivery systems are submicroscopic dispersions for ophthalmic use which have been tested in animals and man in recent years (58,59, 62-64). The authors call these new systems latices and pseudolatices or emulsions, and have reported promising results in ocular therapy.

In pharmaceutics, most of the researchers make no distinction between latices and pseudolatices, since the final products have the same characteristics. However, in the first case, the dispersion is prepared by the well known technique of emulsion polymerization, while the second is a typical mechanical dispersion of already existing polymer particles. Two possible means for incorporation of the active ingredient are feasible:

(a)   Incorporation during manufacture of the latex or
(b)   Adsorption on the surface once the latex is prepared.

Ticho et al. (63) worked on an aqueous polymer emulsion to be used as pilocarpine releasing eye drops for the treatment of glaucoma. The active ingredient is chemically bound to the polymer.

Such a system, containing 3.4 % pilocarpine as a polymeric salt has been evaluated in numerous studies. (59,62-67)

The in-vitro release patterns of such systems (62) were studied by determining the amount of pilocarpine liberated from a dialysis bag containing the latex (pilocarpine base or aqueous solutions of pilocarpine hydrochloride). The release medium was an agitated isotonic saline solution (pH 7.1) maintained at 37°C. The results, summarized in Figure 8, indicate that the release time of 80% of the active ingredient from the polymeric salt is 6 hours against 1 hour for the corresponding solutions.

Figure 9 shows the average diurnal intraocular pressures (IOP) of nine eyes on the third day of pilocarpine treatment with the emulsion in comparison with a 4% solution of pilocarpine. The latex system (emulsion) had a lower level of pilocarpine (3.4%   wt/vol) and showed less fluctuation than the corresponding solution (4% wt/vol). Data concerning the volunteer subjects treated show a reduction of 5.25 mm Hg in the average diurnal value.

Throughout a one year study only one patient out of thirty with open angle glaucoma complained of a local sensitivity reaction. The very promising results collected over a period of 8 to 12 months are given in Figure 10. Out of fifteen patients studied, 87% had an IOP value of less than 24 mm Hg throughout all measurements and no patient showed progression of field loss.

In another large study involving more than thirty patients the comparative evaluation of the polymeric system and a pilocarpine solution against no treatment is shown in Figure 11. The partial results of the extensive study showed that over 80% of the eyes treated with a long acting system (Piloplex[R] 11) had a lower mean IOP value than the control group treated with an aqueous solution of pilocarpine (2% solution).Again the diurnal IOP value of the group treated with the polymeric salt was significantly lower ($p < 0.005$) than the one treated with the solution, by 2.32 mm Hg 67.6 % of the eyes treated with the new therapeutic system were under control (IOP   values $\leqslant$ 20 mm Hg), whereas only 45.2% were under control with the ordinary pilocarpine treatment.

There were no objective signs of damage and specifically, neither corneal abrasion nor intraocular inflammatory signs were present.

The first report on a latex system for ocular delivery with variable viscosity in relation to the pH was in 1980 (64). Since then, various papers (58, 68-70) have been published on the preparation of these formulations and their use for the controlled release of drugs in the eye.

These drug delivery systems are based on cellulose acetate hydrogen phtalate (CAP) used widely in the pharmaceutical industry. The cellulose derivative in the latex starts to dissolve at a pH of about 5.0 and will form a gel within seconds after application.

204

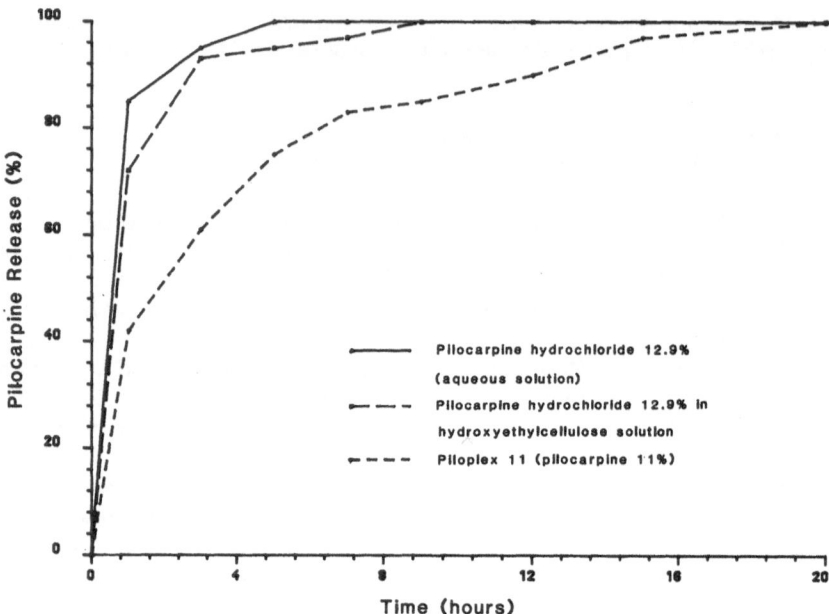

Figure 8. In Vitro Release of Pilocarpine from a Polymeric Salt (Piloplex) and Pilocarpine Hydro-chloride Solution, from a Dialysis Bag. The Medium was an Agitated Isotonic Saline Solution (pH 7.1), Maintained at 37°C. The Active Ingredient was Determined Spectro-photometrically.

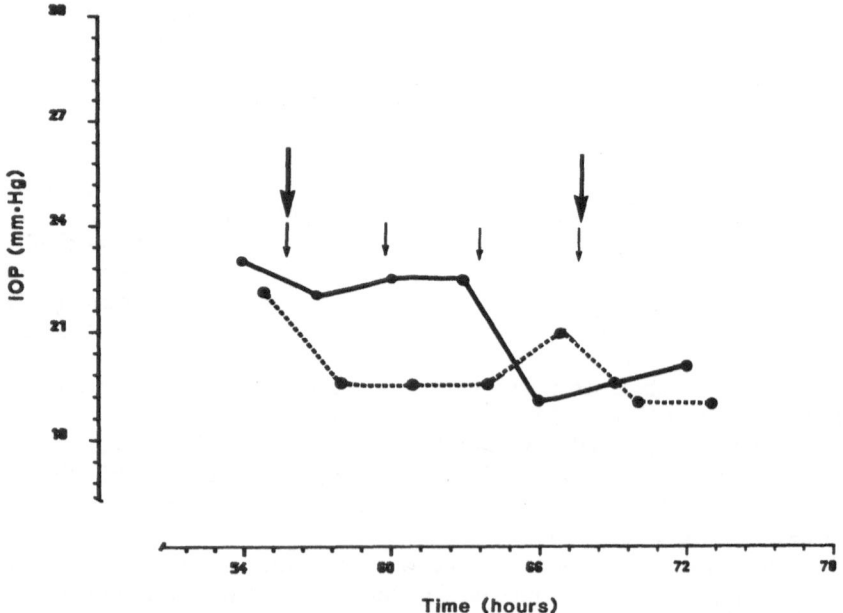

Figure 9. Average Diurnal IOP Curves of 9 Eyes on the 3rd Day of Pilocarpine Hydrochloride 4% Treatment: —, and on the 3rd Day of Polymer Emulsion (Piloplex[R] 3.4) Treatment: ..., Time of Pilocarpine Solution Application: ↓, Time of Emulsion Application: ↓. (63).

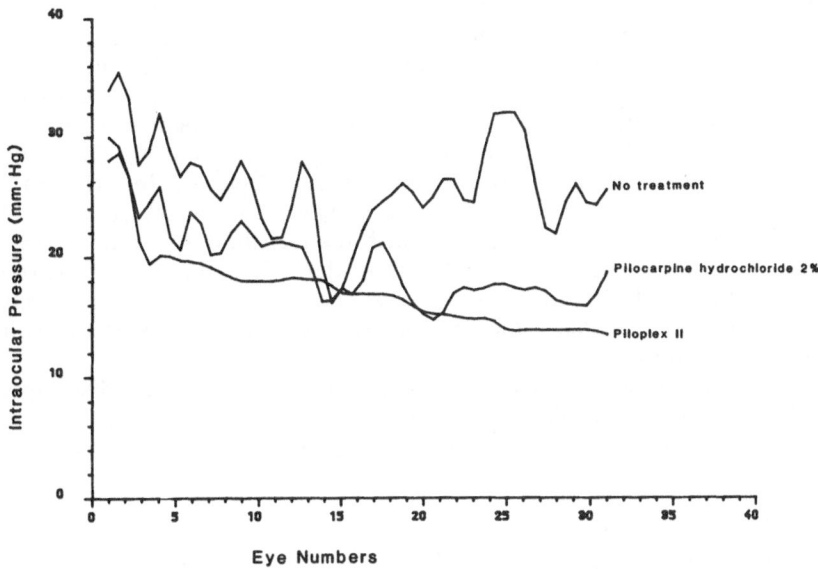

Figure 10. Average Morning IOP Curve of the 30 Eyes Studied during Medication with Pilocarpine Hydrochloride, 4 Times Daily Followed by Piloplex[R] Treatment Twice Daily (62).

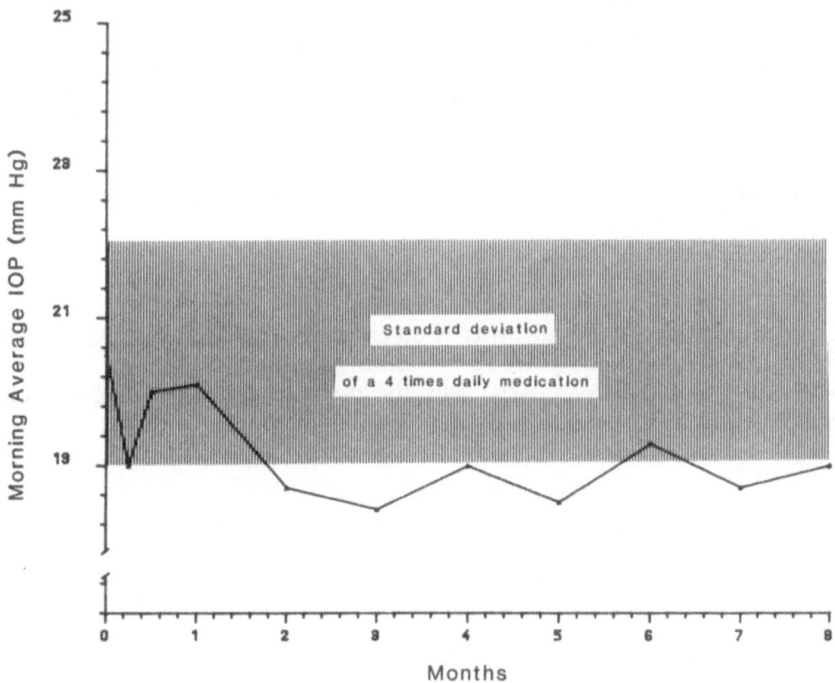

Figure 11. Average Diurnal IOP Values of 31 Eyes in 3 Different Periods (63).

The CAP latices containing the active compound (pilocarpine) adsorbed partially onto the surface of the colloidal polymeric beads of the dispersions have a pH of 4.5 and show Brookfield viscosities between 50 and 200 cps. The particular behavior of these latices is to coagulate as soon as they are applied in the cul-de-sac, since the lacrimal fluid has a pH of 7.2. The gel thus formed from the latex has a Brookfield viscosity of several ten-fold above the initial viscosity. The gelified form cannot be washed out by the lacrimal fluid. Figure 12 gives a close view of the coagulation process in pictures taken with a scanning electron microscope. Within a few seconds after contact of the preparation with the tear fluid, which has a pH 2.8 units above the one of the preparation, the surface of the polymeric beads starts to dissolve.

The long-acting latices, once coagulated, have no effect on visual acuity. The relative miotic response over time of these new therapeutic systems in comparison to solutions is given in Figure 13.

The delivery device contains 30 % wt/vol polymer and the active ingredient at the level of 4% wt/vol. Table II gives the area under the curve (AUC) time to peak (t_{max}), the maximum relative response intensity of miosis (RI_{max}), and the duration at half the maximum response ($\Delta_{1/2}$).

Table II. Average Pharmacokinetic Values of Miosis in Six Rabbits after Instillation of a Solution and a Latex.

Parameter	Latex System	Solution
Active Ingredient % (wt/vol)	4	4
Polymer content % (wt/vol)	30	—
AUC (% min)	5214 (1040)	3396 (835)
RI_{max} (%)	27.4 (1.5)	27.3 (1.5)
t_{max}	60 (-)	30 (-)
$\Delta_{1/2}$ (min)	198 (12)	132 (18)

( ) Standard deviation

The comparative values for other drug concentrations are plotted in Figures 14 and 15 for ordinary solutions as well as colloidal dispersions.

The correlation between AUC and the drug concentration shows clearly the interesting features of these new systems.

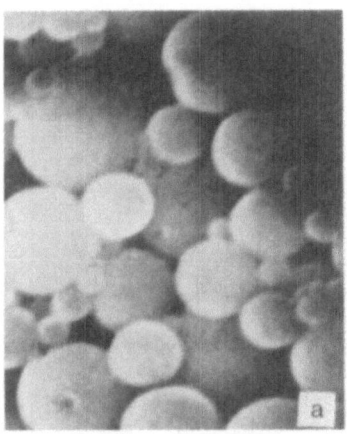 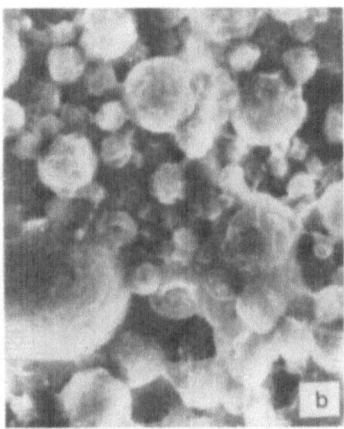

Figure 12. Transformation of a Latex into a Gel Due to pH Change. a. Stable Latex. b. Beginning of Coalescence and Gelification (68).

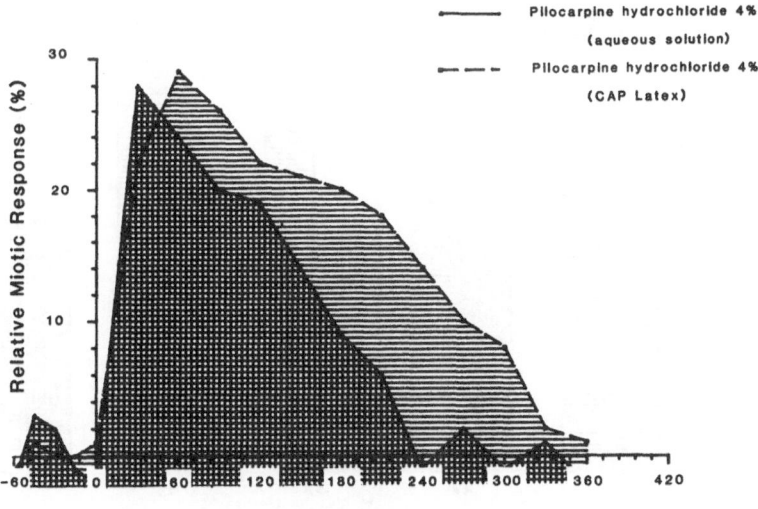

Figure 13. Comparison of the Miotic Response to two Dosage Forms. Solution of Pilocarpine. HCl (4%) and Latex CAP with Pilocarpine. HCl (4%).

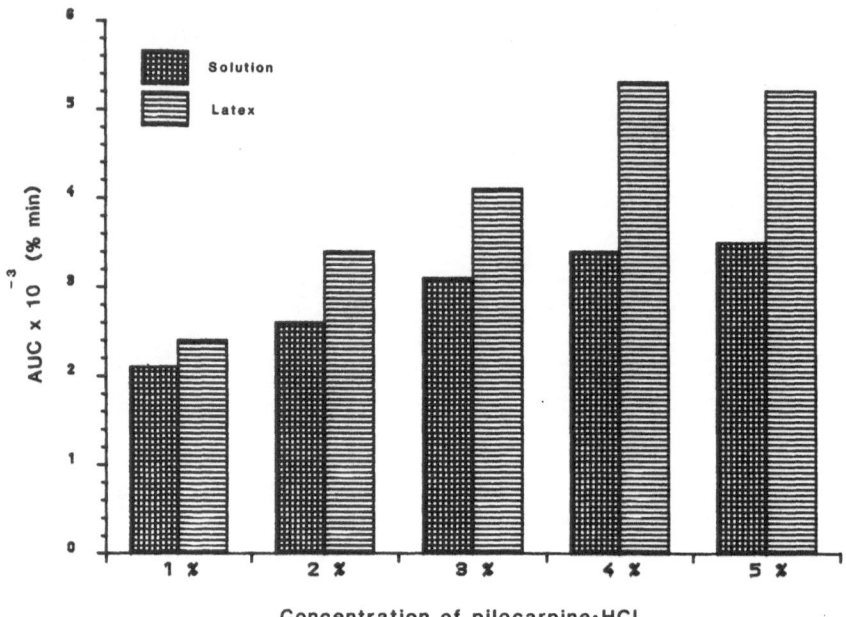

Figure 14. Comparison of the AUC Values between Ordinary Solutions of Pilocarpine HCl and Latices Containing between 1 and 5% pds/vol of Active.

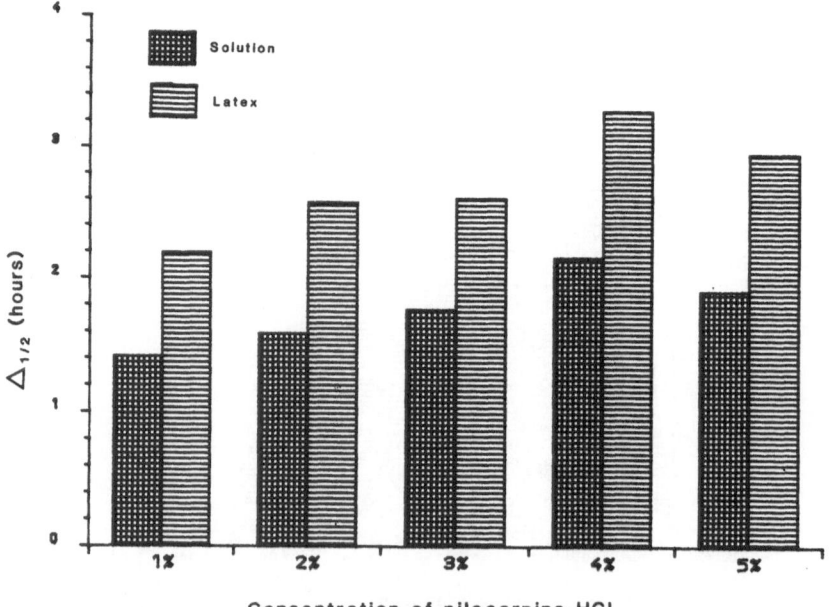

Figure 15. Comparison of the $\Delta_{1/2}$ Values between Solutions and Latices Containing 1 to 5% wt/vol of Pilocarpine|HCl.

REFERENCES

1. Pharmaceutical Society of Victoria and Speiser, P., Austr. Prov., Patent PB. 8951/74, 1974.
2. Birrenbach, G., Ph.D. thesis 5071, ETH, Zurich, 1973.
3. Papahadjopoulos, D., Ann. N.Y. Acad. Sci., 300, 1978.
4. Zolle, I., Rhodes, B.A. and Wagner, H.N., Intern. J. Appl. Rad. and Isotop., 21:155, 1970.
5. Gurny, R., Pharm. Acta Helv., 56:130, 1981.
6. Gurny, R., Peppas, N.A., Harrington, D.D. and Banker, G.S., Drug Dev. Ind. Pharm., 7:1, 1981.
7. Ticho, U., Blumenthal, U., Louis, S., Gal, A., Blanc, I. and Mazor, Z.W., Ann. Ophtalmol., 11:555, 1979.
8. Vanderhoff, J.W., El-Asser, M.S. and Ungelstad, J., U.S. Patent 4,177,177, 1979.
9. Smith, W.V. and Ewart, R.H., J. Chem. Phys., 16:592, 1949.
10. Gester, R.M., Garvin, P.J., Klamer, B., Robinson, R.U., Gibson, W.R., Wheeler, F.C. and Carlson, R.G., Bull. Patent. Drug Assoc., 27:101, 1973.
11. Derrick, A.P., Introduction to Practical Polymer Flocculation, Royal Austr. Chem. Institut, Melbourn, 1973.
12. Banker, G.S., U.S. Patent 152, 872, 1980.
13. Advances in Emulsion Polymerization and Latex Technology 10th Annual Short Course, Lehigh University, Bethlehem, P.A., 1979.
14. Kreuter, J., Pharm. Acta Helv., 58:196, 1983.
15. Harkins, W.D., J. Am. Chem. Soc., 69:1428, 1947.
16. Birrenbach, G. and Speiser, P.P., J. Pharm. Sci., 65:1763, 1976.
17. Ekman, B. and Sjoholm, I., J. Pharm. Sci. 67:693, 1978.
18. Ljungstedt, I., Ekman, B. and Sjoholm, I., Biochem. J., 170:161, 1978.
19. Ekman, B., Lofter, C. and Sjoholm, I., Biochem. J., 15:5115, 1976.
20. Kopf, H., Joshi, R.K., Soliva, M. and Speiser, P., Pharm. Ind., 39:993, 1977.
21. Edman, P., Ekman, B. and Sjoholm, I., J. Pharm. Sci., 69:838, 1980.
22. Juhlin, L., Acta Dermato-Vener, 26:131, 1956.
23. Juhlin, L., Acta Physiol. Scand., 47:365, 1959.
24. Juhlin, L., Acta Physiol. Scand., 48:78, 1960.
25. Schoenberg, M.D., Gilman, P.A., Mumaw, V.R. and Moore, R.D., Brit. J. Exp. Pathol., 42:486, 1961.
26. Gesler, R.M., Garvin, P.J., Klamer, B., Robinson, R.U., Thompson, C.R., Gibson, W.R., Wheeler, F.C. and Carlson, R.G., Bull. Parenteral Drug Assoc., 27:101, 1973.
27. Couvreur, P., Kante, B., Roland, M., Bauduin, P. and Speiser, P., J. Pharm. Pharmacol., 31:331, 1979.
28. Couvreur, P., Kante, B., Roland, M. and Speiser, P., J. Pharm. Sci., 68:1521, 1979.
29. Couvreur, P., Kante, B., Lenaerts, V., Scaileur, V., Roland, M. and Speiser, P., J. Pharm. Sci., 69:199, 1980.
30. Bohme, H. and Hartke, K., in: Europaisches Arzneibuch, Band III, Kommentar, Wissenschaftl. Verlagsgesellsch., Stuttgart Govi-Verlag, Frankfurt, pp. 707, 1979.
31. Gall, D., in: International Symposium on Adjuvants on Immunity, Symp. Series Immunobiol. Standard., Vol. VI, pp.49, Karger, Basel and New York, 1967.
32. Kreuter, J. and Speiser, P.P., J. Pharm. Sci., 65:1624, 1976.

33. Kreuter, J. and Zehnder, H.J., Effects, 35:161, 1978.
34. Rembaum, A., Yen, S.P.S., Cheong, E., Wallace, S., Molday, R.S., Gordon, I.L. and Dreyer, W.J., Macromolecules, 9:328, 1976.
35. Rembaum, A., Yen, S.P.S. and Molday, R.S., Macromol. Sci.-Chem. 13:603, 1979.
36. Rembaum, A., Pure Appl. Chem., 52:1275, 1980.
37. Margel, S., Zisblatt, S. and Rembaum, A., J. Immunol. Meth., 28:341, 1979.
38. Bungenberg de Jong, H.G. and Kruyt, H.R., Proc. Koninkl. Akad. Wetensch., 32:849, 1929.
39. Marty, J.J., Oppenheim, R.C. and Speiser, P., Pharm. Acta Helv., 53:17, 1978.
40. Marty, J.J. and Oppenheim, R.C., J. Pharm. Sci., 6:65, 1977.
41. Kramer, P.A., J. J. Pharm. Sci., 63:1646, 1974.
42. Scheffel, U., Rhodes, B.A., Natarajan, T.K. and Wagner, H.N.Jr., J. Nucl. Med., 13:498, 1972.
43. Couvreur, P., in: Topics in Pharmaceutical Sciences, D.D. Breimer, ed., pp. 305, Elsevier, 1983.
44. Couvreur, P., Kante, B., Rowland, M. and Speiser, P., J. Pharm. Sci., 68:1521, 1979.
45. Gurny, R., Gonzalez, M.A., Banker, G.S. and Kildsig, D.O., Drug Dev. Ind. Pharm., 5:437, 1979.
46. Mason, N., Thies, C. and Cicero, T.J., J. Pharm. Sci., 65: 847, 1976.
47. Woodland, J.H.R., Yolles, S., Blake, D.A., Helrick, M. and Meyers, F.J., J. Med. Chem., 16:897, 1973.
48. Yolles, S., U.S. Patent 3,887,699, 1975.
49. Jackanicz, T.R., Nash, H.A., Wise, D.L. and Gregory, J.B., Contraception, 8:227, 1973.
50. Yolles, S., Leafe, T.D. and Meyer, F.J., J. Pharm. Sci., 64:115, 1975.
51. Yolles, S., Leafe, T.D., Woodland, J.H.R. and Meyer, F.J., J. Pharm. Sci., 64:348, 1975.
52. Renning, R.H., Malspeis, L., Frank, S. and Notari, R.E., Natl. Inst. Drug Abuse Res. Mongr. Ser., 4:43, 1976.
53. Thies, C., Natl. Inst. Drug Abuse Res. Mongr. Ser., 4:19, 1976.
54. Steinke, G., in: Ophthalmica, Wissenschaftliche Verlagsgesellschaft mbH, 1:20, Stuttgart, 1975.
55. Trueblood, J.H., Rossomondo, R.M., Carlton, W.H., Arch. Ophthalmol., 93:127, 1975.
56. Adler, C.A., Maurice, D.M., Patterson, M.E., Exp. Eye Res., 11:34, 1971.
57. Heilmann, K., in: Therapeutic Systems, G. Thieme Publishers, Stuttgart, 1977.
58. Gurny, R., Pharm. Acta Helv., 56:130, 1981.
59. Mazor, Z., Ticho, U., Rehany, U. and Rose, L., Brit. J. Ophthal., 63:48, 1979.
60. Chrai, S.S., Makoid, M.A., Eriksen, S.P. and Robinson, J.R., J. Pharm. Sci., 63:333, 1974.
61. Chrai, S.S., Patton, T.F., Mehta, A. and Robinson, J.R., J. Pharm. Sci., 62:1112, 1973.
62. Ticho, U., Blumenthal, M., Zonis, S., Gal, A., Blank, I. and Mazor, Z.W., Br. J. Ophthalmol., 63:45, 1979.
63. Ticho, U., Blumenthal, M., Zonis, S., Gal, A., Blank, I. and Mazor, Z.W., Annal. Ophthal., 11:555, 1979.
64. Gurny, R., and Taylor, D., in: Proc. Int. Symp. of the British Pharmaceutical Technology Conference, M.H. Rubinstein, ed., London, 1980.

65. Mazor, Z., Kazan, R., Kain, N., Ladkani, D., Ross, M. and Weiner, B., Int. Symp. on Glaucoma, Jerusalem, 1983.
66. Bonomi, L., Perfetti, S., Belluci, R. and Massa, F., Boll. Oculistica, 60:909, 1981.
67. Robinson, J.R. and Li, V.H.K., Int. Symp. on Glaucoma, Jerusalem, 1983.
68. Gurny, R., in: Topics in Pharmaceutical Sciences, D.D. Breimer, and P. Speiser, eds., pp. 227, Elsevier, Amsterdam, New York, Oxford, 1983.
69. Gurny, R., in: Systemes therapeutiques nouveaux et experimentaux, F. Puisieux, X. Rowland and P. Buri, eds.,Technique et Documentation, Paris. (in press)
70. Boye, T., Gurny, R. and Buri, P., in: Int. Symp. on Biopharmaceutics and Pharmacokinetics, Salamanca, 1981.

BIOADHESIVE INTRAORAL RELEASE SYSTEMS

R. Gurny

University of Geneva, School of Pharmacy, Geneva, Switzerland

INTRODUCTION

Adhesion (1) to tissue may be affected by (a) physical or mechanical bonds; (b) secondary chemical bonds and/or (c) primary, ionic or covalent chemical bonds. Physical or mechanical bonds are obtained by deposition and inclusion of the adhesive material in the crevices of the substrate. Under these conditions the surface roughness of the substrate may be important in the overall process. Merill (2) has discussed microscopic characteristics of surface roughness in tissues. Roughness may be defined at the molecular or microscopic level. Obviously, only highly fluid products or suspensions that can be incorporated in the size of anomalies of these substrates can be considered successful adhesive systems (3). A rough surface may be defined by the ratio of maximum depth, d, to maximum width, h. This aspect ratio may be considered as describing an insignificant roughness for adhesive purposes when it has values of $d/h < 1/20$.

Secondary chemical bonds contributing to bioadhesive characteristics include hydrogen bonding and van der Waals attactions. These forces are related to the chemical structure since, for example, hydrophilic polymers would create an interaction favorable to adhesion due to hydrogen bonding (4). Secondary chemical bonds are important for bioadhesion in oral applications. Types of surface chemical groups that would contribute to this type of adhesion include hydroxyls, carboxyls, amines and amides.

Primary chemical bonds refer to bonds created by chemical reaction of groups. This is hardly the case with bioadhesive formulations for the intraoral applications under consideration here, and they will not be discussed further.

BIOADHESION AND DEGREE OF SWELLING

The swelling state of the polymer contributes to its bioadhesive behavior (4,7). However, the general idea that increased swelling contributes to stronger bioadhesive bonds is not correct. Researchers have found for example, in studies with hydro-collaids (more specifically Orabase[R]) that although the wet adhesive strength (mea-sured as stress at break) which developed as the hydrocolloid components absorbed water increased with increasing degrees of swelling (or hydration), excessive water content led to an abrupt drop in adhesive strength. This is clearly an indication of disentanglement at the hydrocolloid/tissue interface due to low concentration of the active components, if one accepts the diffusion theories of adhesion of Bueche et al. (9) and Voyutskii (10), according to which bioadhesion is a result of interpenetration of polymer chains through the bioadhesive interface to the substrate.

One must now examine the characteristics of wet adhesion, the type of adhe-sion observed with the present oral formulations.

SWELLING TIME

The swelling time is important for assessment of adhesiveness. Studies have shown (4) that shortly after the beginning of swelling, adhesion does occur, but that the bond formed is not very strong. Clearly, at the molecular level, neither the neces-sary hydrogen bonds have been totally created nor the potential interpenetration of the macromolecular chains of the adhesive and the substrate (in the range of 150-200Å) has been achieved.

This effect can be easily quantified by examining the dimensionless Fourier time, τ and performing some order-of-magnitude calculations (11,12). The Fourier number is defined as

$$\tau = Dt / \ell^2$$

For an order of magnitude analysis, one lets $\tau = 1$, which gives the following propor-tionality relation

$$\ell \sim \sqrt{Dt}$$

If the interface between adhesive and substrate is at the early stage of swelling (hydration), a macromolecular chain from the adhesive would interpenetrate the "first layer" of the substrate with a diffusion coefficient of a macromolecular chain through a macromolecular system of low "solvent" content (10).Then, in 15 minutes, an interpenetration depth of 30 Å will have been obtained. However, for a system which has already swollen considerably in 15 minutes, one should expect a diffusion coefficient of about 10^{-11} cm^2/sec, typical of diffusion of large macromolecules through a concentrated, entangled macromolecular solution (13). Then the pene-tration length will be much higher, of the order of 9500 Å. Therefore interpene-tration would have occurred in 15 minutes.

MOLECULAR WEIGHT OF BIOADHESIVE

There have been reports (14) that adhesive strength increases as the molecular weight of the adhesive polymer increases up to 100,000 and that beyond this level there is not much effect. Although a critical length of the molecules is necessary to produce the interpenetrating layer and molecular entanglements between the bio-

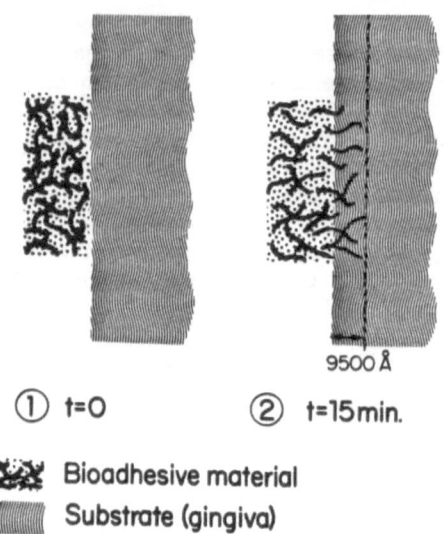

9500 Å

① t=0   ② t=15min.

Bioadhesive material
Substrate (gingiva)

Figure 1.   Model of Interpenetration of Hydrocolloids into the Gingiva (1).

adhesive and the substrate, one must also consider the size and configuration of the adhesive macromolecules that interpenetrate. Thus for example, with polyethylene oxide (4), adhesive strength increases even up to molecular weights of 4,000,000 since this polymer is known to contain molecules of highly linear configurations, which actually would contribute to the increase of the penetration depth. Dextrans of molecular weights as high as 19,500,000 have been reported (4) to have bioadhesive strength similar to those with a molecular weight of 200,000. There, due to the coiled conformation (a) many of the adhesive-active groups are "shielded" inside the coils and do not actively participate in the adhesion process; and (b) due to the coiling, one may find intramolecular hydrogen bonds which are ineffective, rather than interfacial intramolecular hydrogen bonds which are effective.

CONCENTRATION OF ACTIVE POLYMER

There seems to exist an effective concentration for best bioadhesive strength. In a concentrated solution, the coiled molecules become solvent-poor, the macromolecules approach the dimensions of the unperturbed state, and available chain length for interfacial penetration decreases significantly. It has also been pointed out (16) that excessive crosslinking of the polymer adhesive does not contribute to bioadhesion for the same reasons.

The aforementioned parameters have been taken into consideration during the development, formulation and testing of the present bioadhesives.

SOFT TISSUE ADHESIVES AND TREATMENT OF THE ORAL CAVITY

Attempts to treat oral mucus in cases of paradontoses, aphthae and lesions by trauma have been hampered by difficulties in maintaining the medication at the site of application. An ideal bioadhesive drug release system should be easy to apply to the mucus and withstand salivation, tongue movement and swallowing for a period of time, usually hours. In terms of physical and mechanical behavior, these two conditions translate into avoiding an excessive degree of swelling and withstanding shear and tensile loads.

More than thirty years ago, Rothner and coworkers (11) reported for the first time the use of sodium carboxymethylcellulose (NaCMC) in petrolatum as a vehicle for the local use of penicillin, which could provide longer contact at the site of application. In addition, a large number of vegetable gums and animal proteins can produce an adhesive paste when moistened or hydrated by water. The first registered products of this sort were Orahesive[R] powder and Orabase[R], the latter consisting of very finely ground pectin (partially methoxylated polygalacturonic acid), gelatin and NaCMC in a polyethylene/mineral oil gel base (12,13). Early clinical experience with both adhesives indicated that a powder type product would be better. Unfortunately, application of this system on the mucus creates considerable technical problems. Another approach has been the use of NaCMC dispersed in various polymers such as polyisobutylene, rolled into sheets, and laminated to form polyethylene films (14). This type of bandage adheres to either wet or dry surfaces. The adhesion to a dry surface occurs through a mechanism similar to those for pressure-sensitive adhesives because of the polyisobutylene contained.

There are several experimental techniques for determination of the adhesive bond strength. Salter (15) claimed that it was difficult to assess the adhesive bond strength by a simple test and implied that it was virtually impossible to reproduce the exact conditions of the in situ mode of application and adhesion. Therefore, most of the techniques used up to now have been devised as efforts to compare performance rather than to measure the absolute adhesive bond strength of hydrated hydrocolloids.

In general, Chen and coworkers (14) determined the following list of hydrocolloids which can be used for adhesives (Table I).

The properties of the same colloids related to wet adhesion are molecular characteristics and are influenced by water dispersibility. Table II shows the molecular weight of some selected polymers and the in vivo screening of adhesion. Among the van der Waals forces, hydrogen bonding appears to play a major role in wet adhesion. Compounds with good adhesion usually have a molecular weight $> 150\ 000$.

Beside the hydrocolloids, the adhesives most investigated and tested are cyanoacrylates which are used in a large number of different situations (14).

The first available cyanoacrylate, the methylester from Eastman 910^{TM} became a well-known glue. Wounds glued with cyanoacrylates appear to be held more firmly when higher homologues of cyanoacrylates are employed. (Table III).

Biodegradability occurs rather rapidly for the homologous methyl (Fig. 2).

However, long-term implants of these polymers have been reported to be carcinogenic. For this reason, only experimental formulations have been used. Precautions are advocated in the use of cyanoacrylate glue to avoid the formation of impermeable films. Dispensing the adhesive by a microaerosol produces a porous film as the Freon[R] escapes and easier biodegradation and drainage will result.

Recent publications again suggest using hydrocolloids. Typical ointments that have been developed in this way are based on polyacrylate (Carbopol[R])/calcium carbonate/liquid paraffin suspension or suspensions of sodium carboxymethylcellulose, pectin in polyethylene-paraffin base (Orabase[R]). In some cases, polymethylmethacrylate (Eudispert[R]) is an interesting candidate as it is a polymer with lipophilic methyl groups and hydrophilic carboxyl and ester groups. Both of these functional

Table I. Polymers with Adhesive Properties.

Adhesiveness	**High**	Amylopectin Carboxymethylcellulose, sodium Hydroxyethylcellulose
	Medium	Acrylates Gelatin Guar gum Karaya gum Tragacanth
	Low	Agar agar Alginic acid Carboxymethylcellulose, calcium Dextran Methylcellulose Pectin Polyethylen glycol Polyvinylpyrrolidone

Table II. Relation between Molecular Weight of Hydrocolloids and In-Vivo Adhesiveness (14).

Hydrocolloid	Molecular Weight	Relative Time of Adhesion
Amylopectin	300,000 - 800,000	+++
Carboxymethylcellulose, sodium	158,000	+++
Guar gum	200,000	+++
Hydroxyethylcellulose	150,000	+ +
Karaya	9,500,000	+ +
Dextran	30,000	+

Table III. Average Spreadability and Polymerization Times for Cyanoacrylates (17).

H_2O (pH 7.1)

Monomer	Spreadability (cm)	Polymerization (time in sec)
Methyl	20	10
Ethyl	14.5	10
n-Propyl	10	10
n-Butyl	18	10
n-Amyl	16	15
n-Hexyl	16	64
n-Heptyl	20	300
n-Octyl	18	300

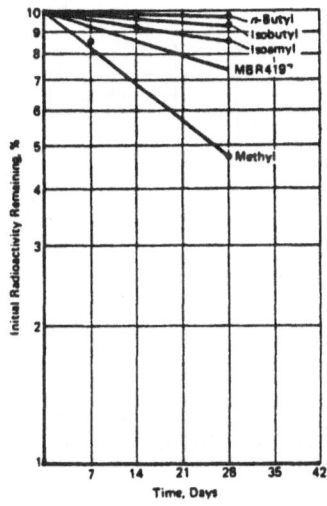

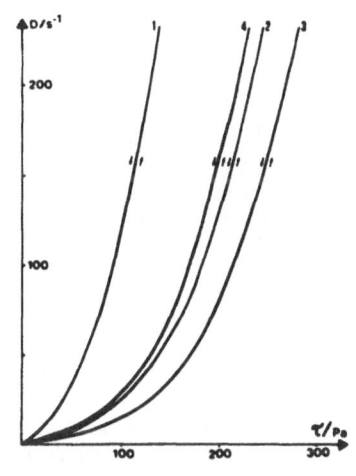

(1) Neutralized with $Na_2B_4O_7$ (2) NaOH

(3) Triethanolamine (4) Diisopropanolamine

Figure 2. In Vivo Degradation Rates for Cyanoacrylates (18).

Figure 3. Flow Curves of 5% Polymethylmethacrylate (20).

groups are well known to be essential for a mucosal adhesive ointment. The adhesiveness and viscosity can easily be varied by different degrees of neutralization. Figure 2 gives the flow curves of gels containing 5% polymethylmethacrylate neutralized with different agents.

Very recently, experimental efforts by Gurny and coworkers (1) were made on adhesive systems based on sodium carboxymethylcellulose and hydrolyzed gelatin in a polyethylene gel (Orabase[R]) with a local anesthetic. The gels, with various compositions (cellulose/gelatin), were hydrated with artificial saliva. One of the important variables is the time of release of a given amount of bioactive agent. This can be controlled by the degree of swelling of the formulation. However, the authors also determined the adhesive bond strength of these systems. Figure 4 gives a diagram of the cell for determination of the adhesive bond strength.

The mechanical properties of the biomaterials prepared were determined in the novel tensile cell described earlier (1), and conclusions about the adhesive bond strength attained were drawn from a comparative study of all pastes. Figure 4 shows a typical plot of the stress (in MPa) as a function of elongation (in μm) for a non-hydrated formulation prepared with 12% NaCMC. Initially, there is an increase of stress in proportion to strain, up to a yield point where further extension does not create additional stress. This phenomenon is associated with slippage of the macromolecular chains of the formulation, leading eventually to separation of the biomedical paste between the two plates. In all mechanical tests, the available surface area for adhesion was 9.788 cm^2. The initial modulus from Figure 4 was determined as 1.24 MPa, which is of course higher than the value of the same formulation in artificial saliva.

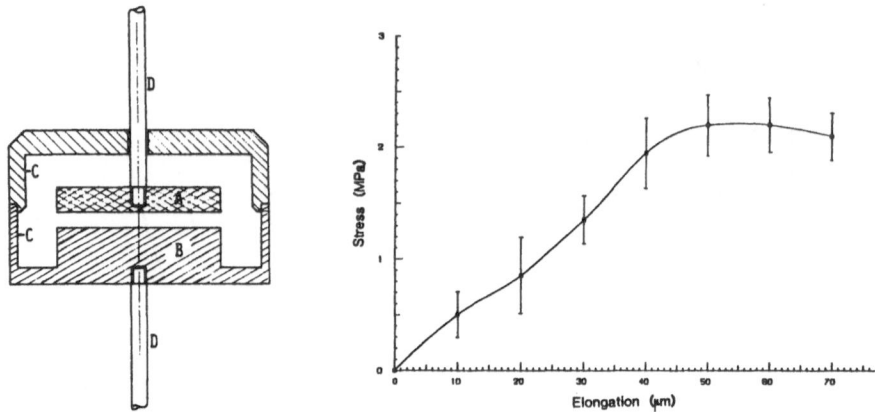

Figure 4.   Schematic Diagram of the Cell for Determination of the Adhesive Bond Strength. Major Components Include a Movable Disk (A), a Lower Supporting Disk (B), Cell Enclosures (C), and Metallic Connecting Bars (D) (1).

Figure 5.   Stress as a Function of Elongation for a Controlled Release Formulation in the Non-Hydrated State, Containing 12 wt% NaCMC, 22 wt% Hydrolyzed Gelatin and 66 wt% Polyethylene Gel. Initial Disk Separation of 2 mm. The results are the Average of three Experiements ± sd (1).

Since sodium carboxymethylcellulose is the main bioadhesive component of the formulation, several additional studies of its effect on the mechanical properties were undertaken. For example, after mixing the preparation with equal amounts of artificial saliva for 120 minutes, the initial elastic modulus was determined for all formulations. This modulus is plotted against the NaCMC concentration in Figure 5. It can be seen that as the NaCMC concentration increases, the modulus reaches a maximum which is characteristic of the optimum NaCMC concentration for best bioadhesion. As the amount of NaCMC increases beyond this value, either because of shielding of active groups in the coiled molecules or because of macromolecular slippage, the molecules of NaCMC are not as effective in the bioadhesive process.

These studies indicate that selection is very important in these systems. It must be noted that all studies were of a comparative nature, since the results compare the effectiveness of various formulations.

Controlled-release experiments were performed in a dissolution cell especially constructed for this purpose. The cell consisted of a cylindrical 50-ml chamber filled with artificial saliva (1) which was thermostated at $37.0 \pm 0.5°$ C and equipped with an impeller at an agitation rate of 30 rpm. The bioadhesive product was placed in a petri-dish of diameter 20 mm located in the bottom of the cell and the impeller was lowered to 1 cm from the upper surface of the bioadhesive sample.

The quantity release per surface area of each active component, was measured as a function of time.

The effect of NaCMC concentration on the controlled release of febuverine is shown in Figure 6 where we plot the amount of drug released after 120 minutes at $37.0 \pm 0.5°$C, normalized per unit area, as a function of the concentration of the active

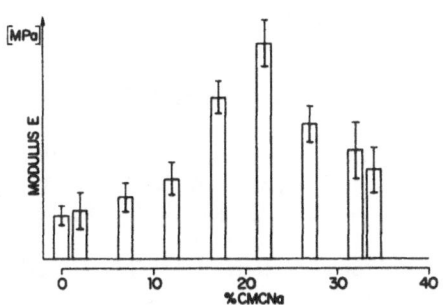

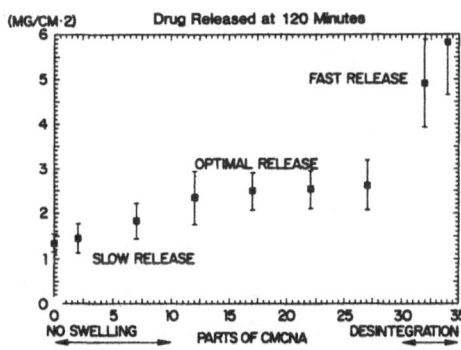

Figure 6.   Initial Modulus of Various Formulations Hydrated for 10 Minutes in Artificial Saliva as a Function of NaCMC Concentration (Expressed as wt % of the Original, Dry System.) The Results are the Average of three Experiments ± s.d.

Figure 7.   Quantity of Febuverine Release after 120 Minutes per Unit Area (in mg/cm^2) from Prehydrated Formulations as a Function of the NaCMC Concentration of the Formulations (wt % of Dry Weight). Average of three Experiments ± s.d.

bioadhesive component. Since the concentration of the other active swellable component, hydrolyzed gelatin, is equal to (34 - x) wt%, where x is the NaCMC concentration, the same plot shows the importance of gelatin in the release process of the drug. The plot may be separated roughly into three regions, of which the middle one, with NaCMC concentrations of 12-25 wt%, gives the optimal amount of released drug. The judicious design of this novel intraoral release system has therefore led to an optimum concentration of NaCMC of 20 wt% where the bioactive bond strength is the maximum and the release drug has the optimum value.

CONCLUSION

Using a careful analysis and evaluation of surface, interfacial and molecular phenomena occurring during bioadhesion of polymers, it is possible to design bioadhesive controlled release devices with desirable bioadhesiveness and controlled release kinetics. This principle has been shown with the design of novel intraoral release systems for delivery of febuverine by adjusting the concentration of the active bioadhesive component.

REFERENCES

1. Gurny, R., Meyer, J.-M. and Peppas, N.A., Biomat., 5:336, 1984.
2. Merill, E.W., Ann. N.Y. Acad. Sci., 283:6, 1977.
3. Huntsberger, J.R., J. Adhesion, 12:3, 1981.
4. Pritchard, W.H., Proc. Conf. Aspects of Adhesion, 6:11, 1971.
5. Bueche, F., Cashin, W.M. and Debye, P., J. Chem. Phys., 20:1956, 1952.
6. Voyutskii, S.S., J. Adhesion, 3:69, 1971.
7. de Gennes, P.G., C.R. Acad. Sci. Paris Ser. II, 292:1505, 1981.
8. Prager, S. and Tirrell, M., J. Chem. Phys., 75:5194, 1981.

9. Gilmore, P.T. and Laurence, R.L., Proc. IUPAC Symp. Macromol., 26:1086, 1979.
10. Huntsberger, J.R., J. Paint. Techn., 39:199, 1967.
11. Rothner, J.T., Cobe, H.M., Rosenthal, S.L. and Bailin, J., J. Dent. Res., 28:544, 1949.
12. Kanig, J.L. and Menago-Ulgado, P., J. Oral Ther. Pharmacol., 1:413, 1965.
13. Kutscher, A.H., Zegarelli, E.V., Beube, F.E., Chilton, N.W., Berman, C., Mercadante, J.L., Stern, I.B. and Roland, N., Oral Surg., Oral Med., Oral Pathol., 12:1080, 1959.
14. Chen, J.L. and Cyr, G.N., In Adhesion in Biological Systems, R.S. Manly, ed., pp. 1, Academic Press, New York and London, 1970.
15. Salter, R. in Aspects of Adhesion, D.J. Alner, ed., pp. 81, University of London Press Ltd., London, 1963.
16. Gross, L. and Hoffman, R. in Adherends and Medical and Biological Bounding Technology Adhesives, p. 818, Academic Press, New York, 1975.
17. Manly, R.S., Adhesion in Biological Systems, Academic Press, New York and London, 1970.
18. Bremecker, K.-D., Strempel, H. and Klein, G., J. Pharm. Sci., 73:548, 1984.

ARTIFICIAL SKIN: A FIFTH ROUTE TO ORGAN REPAIR AND REPLACEMENT

I.V. Yannas and D.P. Orgill

Massachusetts Institute of Technology, Mechanical Engineering Department, Cambridge, Massachusetts, USA

INTRODUCTION

The design of biomaterials has relied extensively, and with considerable success, on the concept of the inert and permanent prosthesis. Ideally, the latter is a device which replaces a diseased or damaged tissue or organ and restores physiological function over the lifetime of the patient without altering the structure and function of tissues adjacent to it and without itself undergoing changes in structure or function. This concept has motivated a great deal of interdisciplinary research, some of it ingenious, which has led to design of several useful prostheses.

An alternative approach to the design of biomaterials, which is much less used, puts aside the twin requirements of biological inertness and engineering permanence. This approach focuses instead on the controlled interaction between the biomaterials device and host tissue. It aims towards regeneration of the damaged or diseased tissue and the simultaneous metabolic disposal of the device. We shall refer to such a device as a biodegradable regeneration template.

We have designed a biodegradable regeneration template and have used it to solve the surgical problem of treating the massively burned patient. Treatment is achieved by providing the patient with a conveniently available biomaterials device, by use of which irreversibly damaged skin can be regenerated in approximately intact form. In the process of developing the solution to this surgical problem we suggest that we have uncovered certain principles by use of which biomaterials science can be applied toward in-vivo regeneration of organs, other than skin, which have become diseased or damaged.

The current surgical treatment of the patient who has suffered deep and extensive burns is prompt closure of wounds, after thorough excision of necrotic tissue, in order to control two life-threatening processes, i.e. extensive fluid loss and massive bacterial infection. A further essential requirement, control of scar formation, is rarely life threatening in a direct way but it frequently leads to phschological devastation of the massively disfigured individual and limits dramatically the individual's ability to function in society.

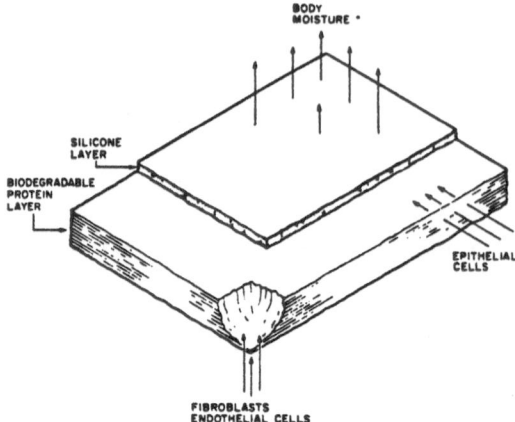

Figure 1. Stage 1 Membranes Comprise a Top Layer of a Silicone Elastomer and a Bottom Layer of a Highly Porous, Covalently Cross-linked Network of Collagen and Glycosaminoglycan. (Reproduced from Science).

Currently, large excised wounds are treated with the split-thickness autograft. Although other approaches have been used (see Discussion), the autograft usually perfoms in a very satisfactory way by adequately controlling fluid loss and infection.

The autograft is often unavailable for prompt use, however, as happens with patients who have suffered deep burns over a substantial fraction of the body surface area. In addition,the process of harvesting it from a previously intact donor site leaves the latter scarred. Furthermore, the surgical operation involved in harvesting the autograft is a serious one, normally requiring support services such as a blood bank.

The biomaterials device described here competes well with the autograft. It is a bilayer polymeric membrane which promptly closes skin wounds in animals and humans and simultaneously serves as a template for the construction of a functional extension of the skin. The top layer of the membrane is a silicone elastomer while the bottom layer is a highly porous, covalently cross-linked network of bovine hide collagen and glycosaminoglycan (GAG) (Fig. 1). We have achieved reproducible conditions under which autologous epidermal cells, seeded onto the membrane before grafting, synthesize mature neoepidermal tissue in-vivo while mesenchymal cells from the wound bed synthesize a neodermal tissue that differs from conventional scar tissue. Whereas the silicone layer is eventually ejected spontaneously or removed nontraumatically and is recovered intact, the collagen-GAG layer is biodegraded within 4 weeks or less and is replaced by neoepidermal and neodermal tissue. These conditions are obtained by controlling several physicochemical and biological parameters of the bottom layer, including the average molecular weight between covalent crosslinks, the ratio of collagen to GAG, the pore structure, the intensity of banding of collagen fibers and the density of autologous epidermal cells seeded before grafting.

Our 11-year design effort has developed in two stages. Stage 1 is a non-cellular, aseptic polymeric membrane capable of being produced in large quantities and of being stored over indefinite periods of time. When grafted on deep wounds without any additional manipulation Stage 1 membranes have been shown to reliably protect animals and humans from fluid loss and infection. Stage 1 membranes do not prevent scar formation unless the silicone layer is eventually replaced with a thin autoepidermal graft. Stage 2 membranes, prepared by seeding Stage 1 membranes prior to

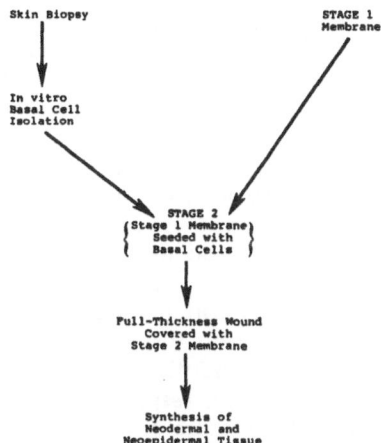

Figure 2.   Flowsheet which Describes the Procedure for Converting Stage 1 Membranes to Stage 2 Membranes.

grafting with a small number of autologous epidermal cells, promptly control fluid loss and infection equally well but, in addition, reduce contraction and scar formation without need for subsequent manipulations, such as harvesting autoepidermal grafts.

In this paper we review briefly the biomaterials design principles which were relied upon in our effort. We then summarize in very condensed form selected experimental results of animal and human studies with Stage 1 and Stage 2 membranes. Emphasis is placed on presentation of recent results obtained with Stage 2 membranes. A detailed presentation of our experimental procedures and results of our ongoing 11-year effort is currently being published in Journal of Biomedical Materials Research (4,6,7).

BRIEF SUMMARY OF DESIGN PRINCIPLES

A detailed discussion of the physicochemical aspects of wounds closure appears elsewhere (1). Briefly it is essential to achieve intimate physicochemical contact between graft and wound bed in order to prevent proliferation of bacteria in microscopic air pockets at the graft-wound bed interface. Achievement of efficient wetting requires use of a membrane with sufficiently low flexural rigidity and critical surface energy. Maintenance of the graft-wound bed bond is achieved by migration of mesenchymal cells from the wound bed into the graft and early synthesis of connective tissue, the latter acting as a "biological adhesive" at the graft-wound interface. Control of moisture flux through the graft is also an indispensable prerequisite for maintenance of a strong bond between graft and wound bed (1).

These essential requirements have been met by iterative design of a non-cellular two-layer polymeric membrane which is referred to here as Stage 1 (Fig. 1). The top layer is a moisture-curing silicone elastomer while the bottom layer is a highly porous covalently crosslinked network of purified bovine hide collagen and chondroitin 6-sulfate (2,3) which may optionally be seeded with autologous epidermal cells (Fig. 2). Functionally, the top layer imparts mechanical strength to the graft, prevents bacterial entry into the wound, and controls the moisture flux; it remains intact and is eventually ejected as a result of neoepidermal tissue synthesis or is peeled off non-traumatically by the surgeon at a time of election. The bottom layer is, however, enzymatically degradable and acts as a tissue support medium utilized by the wound bed to construct neodermal tissue (Stage 1) or neoepidermal as well as neodermal tissue (Stage 2). The rate of enzymatic degradation of the bottom layer must be controlled (4,5) to match approximately the rate of neodermal tissue synthesis (4). The volume fraction of pores is controlled to exceed 96 % while the mean pore size exceeds 50 μm. Failure to meet each of these requirements results in grafts which do not control infection adequately and do not lead to neodermal tissue synthesis.

The limiting dimensions of the graft need to be considered with respect to the migration rate of mesenchymal cells (originating in the wound bed) through the thickness direction and of epithelial cells (originating at the wound edge) along the plane of the membrane. For example, endothelial cells and fibroblasts migrate at rates of about 0.4 mm/day and 0.2 mm/day, respectively. We find that a 0.5-mm thick collagen-GAG layer is populated by these mesenchymal cells within 2 to 5 days following grafting.

At approximate observed speeds of 0.25 mm/day, epidermal cells, advancing from opposite wound edges in the plane of the membrane, between the collagen-GAG and silicone elastomer layers (Fig. 1), typically close a 1.5-cm wound gap in guinea pigs within about 30 days, a period roughly equal to an optimal biodegradation time constant (4). However, the very large wounds which are seen with patients who have suffered extensive burns often exceed 30 cm. Coverage of such large wounds by epidermal cell sheets advancing from the wound edges would require a period of time too long to be clinically acceptable.

We have approached the problem of epithelialization of large wounds in two ways. In one approach (6), which has been used with over 50 patients who had sustained massive third-degree burns, the burned area was originally excised down to viable tissue and grafted with Stage 1 membranes. At a time of election, up to 46 days, the silicone layer was peeled off nontraumatically, exposing a newly synthesized layer of neodermal tissue. The exposed neodermal tissue was then covered with a thin layer of autoepidermal tissue, harvested with a dermatome. The layer of auto-epidermal tissue was sufficiently thin to prevent scar formation at the donor site.

Another approach, which has been used so far only in our work with animals (Stage 2), involves seeding of the porous collagen-GAG layer of the polymeric membrane prior to grafting with a small quantity of uncultured autologous epidermal (basal) cells. Following grafting of the wound with the seeded membrane, these cells have been shown to proliferate at the interface of the two layers of the membrane, forming sheets of mature keratinized neoepidermis within less than 14 days following grafting. Seeding of a properly constructed collagen/GAG layer appears to overcome the limitation of the size of wound which can effectively be treated. This design is a distinct improvement over Stage 1 since it overcomes the current need for eventual harvesting an autoepidermal graft in the treatment of large wounds. Quite importantly, Stage 2 membranes reduce the wound closure time from greater than 20 days to less than 14 days.

ANIMAL SKIN GRAFTING WITH STAGE 1 MEMBRANES

Three major structural parameters of the collagen/GAG layer have been placed under control. The bound GAG content of the collagen/GAG network, determined by hexosamine assay (2), was controlled by adjustment of reaction conditions during the high temperature treatment step under vacuum (following freeze drying), and by adjustment of the conditions during treatment in a glutaraldehyde bath (2). Currently used Stage 1 membranes have a bound GAG content of 8.2 ± 0.8 %-wt. The average molecular weight between crosslinks, M_c, partly controls the biodegradation time constant; the latter can be determined by use of a collagenase assay (7). In-vitro data have been empirically correlated with animal data (5), and a preliminary relation between M_c and fractional weight loss of subcutaneous implants has been obtained (5). Currently, M_c of the collagen-GAG layer, calculated from the tensile modulus measured under conditions of ideal rubber elastic behavior (2), is 13,000 ± 3500. The pore volume fraction of the freeze dried membranes is higher than 0.96 and the mean pore size is 150 ± 30 μm; both values have been determined by application of quantitative stereological procedures to scanning electron photomicrographs of the freeze-dried collagen-GAG layer (3). The pore structure has been controlled by use of a freeze-drying process which was developed following a detailed comparative study of other dehydration procedures (3). Bilayer membranes currently in use have Young's moduli in the range 7-40 x 10^4 N/m^2 while moisture permeability ranges between 1 and 10 mg/cm^2/hr (values obtained in the hydrated state) (8).

Although the above-mentioned physicochemical characteristics have been arrived at after considerable experimentation we wish to emphasize that additional studies, currently ongoing, may dictate modification in the level of these variables.

Full-thickness wounds closed with Stage 1 membranes remained free of infection and exudation. Histological studies showed extensive cellular migration inside the graft. No evidence of inflammation in the area of the wound was observed after about 4 days following excision and grafting. There was no gross indication of rejection, neither was any histological evidence of an immunogenic response detected over more than 30 days of observation following grafting. Lymphocytes were almost never observed. There was also no tissue necrosis nor was there thrombosis or alterations in vascular histological characteristics. By comparison, homografts were usually rejected by the animals between 9 and 14 days after grafting.

Wounds covered with Stage 1 membranes did not begin contracting until 10 ± 3 days in the animals with grafts. Autografts showed much less contraction.

Peeling of Stage 1 membranes at a 90° angle was resisted by forces as high as 4 N/m (4 g/cm) just 6 hrs after grafting with Stage 1 membranes, increasing to about 45 N/m (45 g/cm) after 10 days. Peeling forces of this magnitude compare favorably with the force that peels off conventional adhesive tape from itself. This was followed by a decay to zero peeling strength at the time of confluence by epidermal cell sheets (see below), which occurred between 30 and 40 days with these wounds. Low magnification study of the graft-wound interface following partial peeling showed copious tissue synthesis (8).

Extensive histologic observations show that the neodermis formed when either optimally designed Stage 1 or Stage 2 membranes are used is a well vascularized matrix comprising collagen fibers which appear to possess morphological characteristics similar to those of physiological dermis, rather than of scar tissue. The tissue interface between host and graft is clearly elicited by use of polarized optical microscopy and by electron microscopic study of histological sections. When the design parameters are kept within certain limits the interface comprises loose strands of collagen fibers rather than a layer of well-packed fibers characteristic of fibrous scarring. Extensive control studies (5), suggest that at least 80 % of the original collagen-GAG layer undergoes degradation within 3-4 weeks.

HUMAN SKIN GRAFTING WITH STAGE 1 MEMBRANES

Following primary excision of dead tissue, 49 burn victims received Stage 1 membranes as large as 15 x 25 cm (6). Results with an initial group of ten patients are reported in detail in Ref. 6. After being placed on the wound bed, the grafts were carefully sutured under a slight tension, avoiding wrinkling of the thin membrane. The subjects, 3- to 87 year-old males and females, with total third-degree burn size 50 to 90 % body surface area, received Stage 1 grafts over 15 to 60 % body surface area. No immunosuppression was employed. "Take" of Stage 1 membranes on the excised wound bed was 95 to 100 %, providing continuous physiological closure without infection or rejection. Whenever the graft was next to intact epidermis the epidermal edge migrated between the two layers of the membrane over the distance of a few millimeters. Between 14 and 46 days later the silicone layer was removed from the vascularized neodermal tissue and the wound was closed with a thin auto-epidermal graft (0.1 mm). "Take" of autoepidermis on the neodermis was 85 to 95 %. Neither the donor site nor the grafted area showed significant contraction or scarring following such treatment. By comparison, following removal of split-thickness autografts (0.25 - 0.375 mm), which grafts include a fraction of the dermis in the conventional harvesting procedure, the donor sites are usually significantly scarred. The follow-up in this study ranged from 2 to over 16 months (6).

Histologic findings obtained by light and fluorescent microscopy showed a very favorable response of human host tissue to the collagen-GAG layer. Vascularized connective tissue tufts were shown to have grown into spaces of this layer and in 1-2 weeks the occupation of the lower layer of the graft by newly formed tissue appeared complete. Immunofluorescent microscopic findings confirmed the presence of basement membrane collagen in quantities which were consistent with the presence of high levels of vasculature. The zone of transition from the normal host muscle or fat to the implanted collagen-GAG layer generally consisted only of several fibrous strands and was not characteristic of fibrous scarring. In a few cases thickened zones indicative of scarring were observed. The latter may be attributed to healing in the host bed of a wound partially damaged by burn, in which damaged tissue was imcompletely excised (6).

STAGE 2 MEMBRANES: SKIN REGENERATION IN ANIMALS

After in-vitro seeding with uncultured autologous basal cells, Stage 2 membranes were grafted onto full-thickness skin wounds. In the sterile environment of the wound closure, the basal cells reached confluence within 10-14 days and layers of keratinizing epidermal tissue became evident in the polarizing stage of the optical microscope at about the same time (8,9).

Repeated observations have left no doubt that the neoepidermal sheet nucleates and grows from the basal cell seeds rather than originating at the wound edge. Furthermore, there is no doubt that keratinization of such neoepidermal sheet over the entire wound area has progressed significantly before the 14th day.

Histologic studies of the interface between host tissue and Stage 2 grafts show a close similarity to the findings obtained with Stage 1 grafts. Well-vascularized connective tissue which resembles dermis eventually replaces the collagen-GAG layer in less than about 4 weeks. Collagen fiber bundles posses morphology which resembles that of physiological dermis and does not resemble scar (8,9).

The most striking long-term difference between the performance of Stage 1 and Stage 2 membranes is the gross appearance of the healed wound two months following grafting. The rectangular wound area grafted with a Stage 1 membrane was reduced to a linear scar as a result of strong contraction of wound edges. By contrast, grafting with Stage 2 membranes gave results which were quite similar, though not identical, to those obtained following grafting with unmeshed full-thickness autograft. Four months following grafting with Stage 2 membranes, the wound area was reduced to about 75 % of the original excised area, compared to about 105 % for the autograft. The perimeter of the wounds grafted with Stage 2 membranes consisted of scar tissue as did also the perimeter of wounds covered with autograft. The tissue inside the perimeter was clearly not scar and had almost identical appearance both with Stage 2 grafts and with autografts. Both were soft and extensible, were well vascularized and responded well to touch. Histologically, the tissue inside the wound perimeter was clearly not scar and appeared indistinguishable from intact guinea pig skin except for the absence of hair follicles. (The long-term area value reported for ungrafted wounds and for wounds grafted with Stage 1 membranes is about 25 % (Fig. 2). This value corresponds to the area occupied by scarred tissue between tattoo marks placed at the wound edge prior to inflicting the wounds.)

There seems to be little doubt that two months after being grafted on full-thickness wounds, the collagen/GAG layer of Stage 2 membranes which has been seeded with basal cells has been replaced by new integument comprising both a neoepidermal and a neodermal layer but lacking hair follicles.

The kinetics of contraction of wounds grafted with Stage 2 membranes have reproducibly (10 animals) followed a somewhat complex path. After a significant contraction of the wound area to almost 30 % of the original area by day 30, the grafted wounds increased slowly but unmistakeably in size until, by day 120, the wound area approached 75 % of the original.

Preliminary studies of the effect of viable epidermal cell density (seed cells) on the healing parameters showed that approximately 3×10^6 viable cells could be readily isolated from each cm^2 of skin biopsy. The viable cell density was adjusted so that 5×10^4 to 5×10^5 cells per cm^2 were seeded into the graft by the centrifugation method which we developed (9). An area expansion factor of 6x was thereby obtained when cells were seeded at 5×10^5 /cm^2 and an expansion factor of 60x was obtained at a seed density of 5×10^4 /cm^2. We find, however, that whereas increasing the cell density above 5×10^5 /cm^2 does not significantly affect the time, 10-14 days, normally required for wound closure by formation of a confluent neoepidermis, reduction of cell density to 5×10^4 /cm^2 increases the closure time to approximately 21 days.

A preliminary comparison of properties of newly synthesized (regenerated) skin and intact (normal) skin shows several close similarities. However, differences are also apparent, striking among them being the absence of skin accessory organs, including hair (the guinea pig has no sweat glands).

DISCUSSION

Current treatment of patients who have suffered extensive skin loss emphasizes fluid resuscitation and prompt closure of wounds with autografts, cadaver skin, or pig skin following the excision of dead tissue (10). Failure to achieve closure of massive burn wounds within 3 to 7 days after injury significantly increases the probability that the patient will die (10).

Autografts provide prompt wound closure and leave minimal scarring. However, the patient's intact skin is often in short supply, and the operation to obtain it is undesirable. Homografts, obtained from cadavers and used immediately or after preservation in a skin bank (11) are also in short supply and, unless immunosuppressive agents are used, commonly are rejected early. However, the use of immunosuppressive agents increases the risk of infection. Heterografts, obtained from animals, especially pigs, are available commercially and are widely used to achieve short-term wound closure. Normally they are removed between the third and ninth day following application. A number of natural and synthetic polymer membranes have been employed in the treatment of burns but their use has not reliably prevented infection (1). A temporary skin dressing based on synthetic polymers and peptides derived from collagen has been compared favorably with human homograft and porcine heterograft, especially in covering graft donor sites; however, it requires removal about 7-10 days after application (12). Recently, a culture of autologous epidermal cells was grafted into full thickness skin wounds in humans 5 weeks after harvesting (13). A reconstituted collagen lattice populated by cultured autologous fibroblasts and epidermal cells has been grafted on rats at least 2 weeks after harvesting (14). The latter two procedures require lengthy in-vitro culturing of tissue prior to grafting.

By contrast with temporary dressings, where the obligatory removal exposes the wound bed once more to the risk of infection, Stage 1 membranes provide closure of full-thickness wounds in animals and humans without requiring eventual removal. This is achieved by synthesis of a stable well-vascularized neodermis in the aseptic environment provided by the silicone layer. Although the latter is eventually ejected spontaneously (small wounds) or removed at a time of election (large wounds), the neodermis is not removed, but covered with thin autoepidermal grafts providing continuous physiological wound closure.

Efforts to prepare a long-term wound closure by culturing skin grafts in-vitro (13,14), have shown great promise but they require use of dressings that must be eventually removed to be replaced by the cultured tissue. By contrast, Stage 2 membranes are designed to act as templates for synthesis of skin in-vivo, making prompt and deliberate use of the host's wound tissue as an organ culture medium (9).

Human studies conducted over the past 2 years confirm and extend results from animal studies. They show conclusively that Stage 1 membranes are superior to cadaver and porcine skin grafts. When Stage 1 membranes are eventually covered with thin (0.1 mm) autoepidermal grafts, these membranes equal the split-thickness (0.25-0.4 mm) autograft in clinical performance at the graft site without generating a scarred donor site, as normally occurs after harvesting a split-thickness autograft (6).

Although not yet studied with human subjects, Stage 2 membranes provide a means for closing the largest full-thickness wounds without requiring use of autologous epidermal grafts, as is currently practiced when human subjects are grafted with Stage 1 membranes. This significant simplification in clinical procedure is achieved by seeding the membrane with a small number of cells from a skin biopsy before grafting. A neoepidermis is thereby generated in-vivo inside the sterile environment of the bilayer membrane. In addition, autoepithelial wound closure is reduced from about 20 days, attainable with Stage 1 membranes, to less than 14 days.

An important and reproducible result of the cell-seeding modification which defines Stage 2 membranes is attainment of substantial control of wound contraction

Scar synthesis appears also to be reduced, in the sense that conventional scarring eventually forms only at the perimeter of the wound. Scarring appears to be reduced within the wound perimeter. It appears that Stage 2 membranes induce synthesis of new, nearly physiologic integument within the wound bed.

Preliminary characterization shows that newly synthesized skin is strikinly similar, though not identical, to intact skin (Table I). Ongoing studies are directed towards biochemical characterization of macromolecular components in new skin, detailed morphological analysis and elucidation of the kinetics of synthesis of the new organ mass.

Table I. Comparison of New Skin to Intact Skin in the Guinea Pig.

Property	Intact skin	New skin
Moisture permeability, in-vivo, $g/cm^2/h$[a]	4.5 ± 0.8	4.7 ± 1.0
Mechanical Properties,	31×10^6	14×10^6
In-vitro tensile strength, Pa		
Second derivative of stress-strain curve	+	+
Histological studies[b]		
Multilayered keratinizing epidermis	+	+
Intact dermal-epidermal junction	+	+
Skin accessory organs (eg., hair)	+	—
Dermal vascularization	+	+
Collagen morphology	wavy	less wavy
Epidermal thickness, μm	20 - 40	30 - 40
Dermal thickness, mm	0.8 - 1.3	0.9 - 1.4
Neurological test (pin prick)[c]	+	+
Vascularization test (blanching)[d]	+	+
Color[e]	white	white

[a] Measured value remained invariant, within experimental error, between 1 and 10 months following grafting.

[b] Performed 10 months following grafting.

[c] Positive results obtained by day 21.

[d] Positive results obtained by day 14.

[e] Color changes in the graft were as follows: red, up to about 2 months; pink to off-white about 2-5 months; white, after about 5 months.

230

REFERENCES

1. Yannas, I.V. and Burke, J.F., J. Biomed. Mat. Res. 14:65, 1980.
2. Yannas, I.V., Burke, J.F., Gordon, P.L., Huang, C. and Rubenstein, R.H., J. Biomed. Mat. Res., 14:107, 1980.
3. Dagalakis, N., Flink, J., Stasikelis, P., Burke, J.F. and Yannas, I.V., J. Biomed. Mat. Res., 14:511, 1980.
4. Yannas, I.V., Burke, J.F., Huang, C. and Gordon, P.L., Fed. Proc. Fed. Amer. Soc. Exp. Biol., 38:988, 1979.
5. Yannas, I.V., Burke, J.F., Huang, C. and Gordon, P.L. J. Biomed. Mat. Res., 9:623, 1975.
6. Burke, J.F., Yannas, I.V., Quinby, W.C., Jr., Bondoc, C.C. and Jung, W.K., Ann. Surg., 194:413, 1981.
7. Huang C. and Yannas, I.V., J. Biomed. Mat. Res., Symp. No. 8:137, 1977.
8. Yannas, I.V., Burke, J.F., Warpehoski, M., Stasikelis, P. Skrabut, E.M., Orgill, D. and Giard, D.J., Trans. Am. Soc. Artif. Intern. Organs, 27:19, 1981.
9. Yannas, I.V. and Burke, J.F., Orgill, D.P. and Skrabut, E.M., Science, 215:174, 1982.
10. Shires, G.T. and Black, E.A., eds., Consensus development conferenc, J. Trauma, 19:855, 1979.
11. Bondoc, C.C. and Burke, J.F., Ann. Surg., 158:371, 1971.
12. Woodroof, E.A., Travis, M.J., Grossman, A.R. and Bartlett, R.H., in Advances in Biomaterials 3, Winter, G.D. Gibbons, D.F. and Plenk, H., eds., Wiley, UK (in press).
13. O'Connor, N.E., Mulliken, J.B., Banks-Schlegel, S., Dehinde, O. and Green, H., Lancet, 1981-I:75, 1981.
14. Bell, E., Ehrlich, H.P., Buttle, E.J. and Nakatsuji, T., Science, 211:1052, 1981.

PLASMA POLYMERIZATION AND PLASMA MODIFICATION OF SURFACES FOR BIOMATERIALS APPLICATIONS

A.S. Chawla,

Bureau of Medical Devices, Health and Welfare Canada, Ottawa, Canada

INTRODUCTION

As it is the surface of a biomaterial which comes in direct contact with blood or tissue, it primarily determines the biocompatibility. Therefore, by changing or modifying the surface of a material, it may be possible to improve biocompatibility. Plasma, which may be defined as an ionized gaseous state of matter, can be used for polymerization and the process is known as plasma polymerization. Plasma can also be used for the chemical modification of surfaces. In these processes only the surfaces are modified leaving the bulk material unchanged. Therefore, it may even be more promising than the high energy radiation grafting techniques where materials are affected throughout the bulk.

If a gas, say argon, is passed through an electric discharge, part of it will be ionized as shown in Figure 1. This partially ionized gas is in a non-equilibrium state where electron temperature (T_e) is 10 to 100 times higher than the gas temperature (T_g). The process produces high temperatures and may not be useful for surface modification of polymeric materials. Therefore, for biopolymer applications low pressure plasma, where the pressure is of the order of a few mm Hg, and the temperature of the gas remains close to ambient is used. The free electrons produced in the plasma can react further with gases or other materials present in system. Thus, if organic vapours are introduced in it, they will undergo secondary ionization by reacting with these high energy electrons. The secondary electrons and ions can react further to produce a number of reactive particles and radiation such as cations, anions, free radicals, excited molecules, UV radiations, etc. These particles and radiation are the basis of plasma chemistry and are used for polymerizations, surface modifications and surface chemical reactions. Thus, for our purposes the plasma technology involves the use of these species to produce useful biomedical materials.

Let us now look at how plasma is produced. There are a variety of energy sources such as lasers and ionizing radiations which may be used to produce plasma but for practical purposes, the choice is between microwave and radiofrequency (RF) discharge. For the commercial RF generators, the frequency is dictated by the Federal

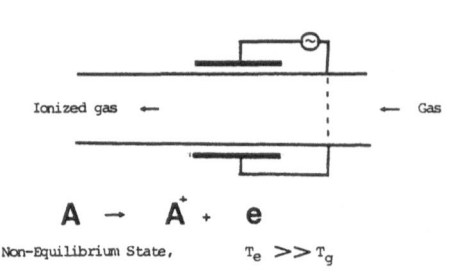

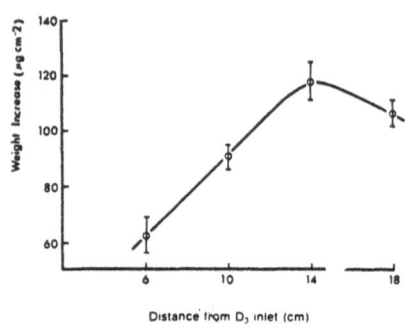

Figure 1.   Schematics of Plasma Generation. A = Argon Gas.

Figure 2.   Plasma Polymerization of Hexamethylcyclotrisiloxane over Celgard Membranes at Various Distances from the Monomer inlet in the Plasma Reactor.

Communication Commission, U.S.A. and is set at 13.45 MHz. The RF can be coupled to a reaction vessel capacitatively or inductively. For example, in our work RF was coupled capacitatively to the reaction vessel by placing copper electrodes outside a glass reactor.

As mentioned above, plasma technology can be used for (a) depositing a layer of a polymer on a substrate or (b) for surface modification by adding new groups. These processes are dependent upon a number of variables. Some of these are described next.

The power from an energy source (say an RF generator) is transmitted to the gas and this is responsible for ionization and other secondary processes. Therefore, it is obvious that the higher the power input, the higher the number of active species produced and the higher the associated temperatures. Also, as in polymerization reaction kinetics, excess of initiator would produce short chain polymers which may not be desirable. Therefore, depending upon other conditions, a moderate amount of power, say less than 100 watts, should suffice for laboratory chambers of about 12 cm in diameter and 30 cm in length. For chambers of different dimensions, the power density can be considered to be a good parameter to scale. In our work, we used about 30 watts.

The gas flow rate and pressure determine the time available for chemical reactions and ionization produced. Thus, at higher gas flow rates, reaction time is reduced and the number of reactive species per unit volume would be less.

Other variables are the reactor configuration and contents and the time a substrate or a biopolymer spends in the reaction vessel. Depending upon the type of monomers, the inert gas and other gases present, we should expect different end products. Like any kinetics the chemical yield is increased with time of reaction.

The position of a substrate in the reaction vessel could affect the rate of reaction. Figure 2 shows the results where the position of the substrate was varied from the organic vapour inlet. As the distance is increased, the amount of polymer deposited goes through a maximum at about 10 cm from the inlet. This should be expected because close to the inlet there has not been enough time for complete polymerization and at the distal end the rates fall off due to the shortage or non-availability of feed or monomer and reduction in number of polymer initiating species due to recombination and consumption in polymerization.

It should be clear from above discussions that there are many factors which affect the plasma polymerization. Therefore, it would not be too much to say that polymerization is system dependent. This lack of portability may be one reason that the technique is not used more often. It will take additional research and development efforts for this technology to reach a state of control suitable for commercial production of biomaterials and medical devices.

PREPARATION OF SILICONE COATED BIOMATERIALS

As silicone polymers are among the most biocompatible materials available (1), it was hoped that depositing plasma polymerized silicone polymer on the surfaces of biomaterials would improve their biocompatibility. Preparation and some of the characterizations of these biomaterials are described. Results of our in-vitro and ex-vivo experiments are also presented.

Materials and Methods

Hexamethylcyclotrisiloxane (D_3) and octamethylcyclotetrasiloxane (D_4) used for the plasma polymerization were purified by fractional distillation. The substrate materials used were : (a) microporous polypropylene membranes (Celgard-2400[R], Celanese Corp., Summit, N.J.) ; (b) Silastic[R] membranes (Dow Corning Corp. Midland, Michigan, Cat. No. 500-1) ; (c) polypropylene film (Eastman Kodak) ; (d) polyurethane film (Tuftane[R], B.F. Goodrich) ; (e) Teflon[R] (du Pont) ; and (f) precleaned glass slides.

All the substrate materials, including the washed Silastic membranes, were washed with 70% ethanol using an ultrasonic cleaner. These were then washed with distilled water and dried overnight in a vacuum oven at about 70°C. These membranes were ready for use except polyurethane which had to be pumped under a vacuum of about 10^{-3} torr overnight. This was done to remove the volatile materials coming out of the polyurethane film.

The plasma polymerization reactor used is shown schematically in Figure 3. The radio-frequency plasma generator (RFG) was capacitatively coupled to the reaction vessel by placing the electrodes outside it. Samples were placed at 10 cm down stream from the D_3 inlet and the reactor was evacuated to about 10^{-3} torr. Argon was fed at a rate so as to stabilize the pressure inside the reactor at 0.4 torr. The pulsed RF power of 30 watts was used in a 2x on and 2x off mode. After 30 sec pretreatment of the substrate materials, the D_3 feed was started, the feed rate being 2.7×10^{-3} gm min^{-1}. The details of these experiments have been described in a previous publication (2). The increase in the weight of the substrate material was determined gravimetrically. From the weight increase, the thickness of the deposited film was calculated.

To find the leachable fractions of the deposited polymer, the glass slides having plasma polymerized film on them were extracted with toluene. The preweighed slides were placed in a large excess of toluene at room temperature for 24 hrs. The slides were then taken out, rinsed with fresh toluene and then dried in a vacuum oven at about 70°C overnight and weighed. From these weights the percentage loss of the deposited polymer was calculated.

234

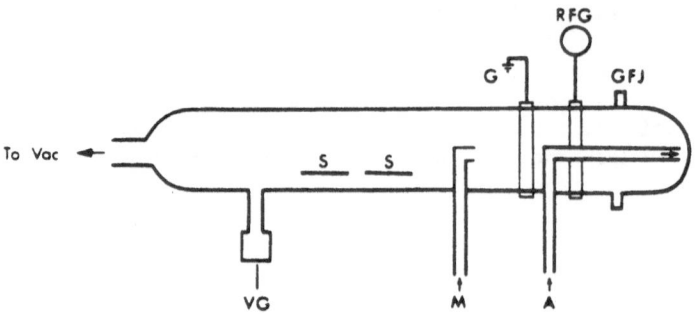

Figure 3.   Plasma Polymerization Reactor. RFG : Radio Frequency Generator, Along with Associated Electronic Setup; GFJ: Glass Flange Joint; G: Ground; A: Argon Inlet; M: Monomer or Other Vapours Inlet; VG: Vacuum Gauge; S: Sample Positions.

To find the nature of the deposited film, a Fourier-transform infrared spectro-photometer was used (Nicolet 7000 Series, FT-IR system). Infrared spectra were obtained using Attenuated Total Reflection (ATR) techniques. For this work high density polyethylene (HDPE) films were coated with plasma polymerized silicone polymer. The film samples were applied on both sides of a KRS-5 reflection plate. To obtain a better signal to noise ratio, 200 scans were performed and then averaged.

To test the biocompatibility of the membranes, in-vitro blood compatibility studies were done. Medical grade 0.005-inch-thick Silastic sheets (Cat. No. 500-1, Dow Corning Corporation, Midland, Michigan, U.S.A) were used as control material. These were washed with Ivory soap flakes, rinsed thoroughly with distilled water and, finally, steam sterilized, a procedure recommended by the manufacturer.

Two flow-through test cells decribed previously (2) were used for these bio-compatibility studies. The cells were made of two Plexiglas[R] plates seperated by an ellipical gasket cut from a 0.12-inch-thick Silastic sheeting (Cat. no. 502-5, Dow Corning Corporation , Midland, Michigan, U.S.A.). The gaskets, which had been cleaned as described in the above paragraph for Silastic sheeting, were equipped with inlet and outlet ports at the apexes. The test membranes were placed on the gasket surface, one on either side, and held in place by the Plexiglas plates. Therefore, when a cell was filled with blood, the two membranes were exposed to it simultaneously. Cell No.1 contained a glass slide (control) and silicone coated Celgard (SCC) and cell No.2 contained the Silastic sheet and SCC. The assembled cells were washed, filled with normal saline, and then incubated at 37°C for one hour. The saline was displaced with citrated canine blood (blood was used within 30 minutes of withdrawal) using a syringe infusion pump. The test cells containing the blood were incubated at 37°C with constant shaking at 110 cycles per minute.

These cells were turned over every five minutes. This was to prevent settling of the blood cells on the lower membrane. At the end of a 30-minute incubation period, the blood was washed off with normal saline at a constant flow rate of 24 ml/min. After disassembling the cells, the samples were rinsed in saline and then fixed with methanol. These were then stained with Wright's stain and examined microscop-ically using oil-immersion techniques. Only central portions of the samples were used for blood cell counts. The blood cell counts were used to compare the biocompatibility of the test materials with control material. A minimum of 25 fields of view were used for each sample.

The silicone coated Celgard (SCC) membranes were also tested in ex-vivo shunts. Uncoated Silastic sheets were used as control material. The ex-vivo shunts were the same flow-through cells described above. Blood at a flow rate of 15 ml/min entered the lower end and left at the apex of the gasket. Anesthetized mongrel dogs were used. Before using them for the blood compatibility studies, their blood was tested to confirm that it was normal. Both femoral vein and artery were cannulated using 8 mm OD siliconized plastic tubing. After taking the blood samples for hematological data, the dog was systemically heparinized (100 U/kg). The flow-through cells were primed with normal saline and then the blood flow was started by manipulating the stopcocks and also switching on the blood pump in the experimental set up shown in Figure 4. After each predetermined time intervals of 1.5 and 10 mins, blood flow was stopped and the membranes were washed with normal saline. The central portions of the membranes were cut for observations. These were fixed by 2 different methods, one for light microscopy and the other for scanning electorn microscopy (SEM). For observations under light microscopy, these were fixed with methanol and then stained with Wright's stain. For SEM observations, a 3 g/dl glutaraldehyde solution was used for fixation (3). These methods have been described in detail in our previous publication (4).

Results and Discussion

The weight increases of the substrate materials Celgard-2400, Silastic, polypropylene, polyurethane, and Teflon, are shown in Figure 5. It is evident that increases in the weights of the substarate materials are linear with time. The weight increases at the end of a 30 min reaction time are shown in Table I. From these weights, the thicknesses of the deposited polymer layers were calculated and shown in Table I. Also from the results of Figure 5, the rates of plasma polymerization were calculated from the slopes of the curves and are shown in the last column of the table. They vary between 2.83 to 4.45 $\mu g\, cm^{-2}\, min^{-1}$.

Table I. Plasma Polymerization of D_3 after 30 Minutes over Various Substrate Materials.

Substrate Material	Amount of Polymer Deposited ($\mu g\, cm^{-2}$)	Thickness of Deposited Layer (μm)	Rate of Polymerization ($\mu g\, cm^{-2} min^{-1}$)
Celgard-2400[R]	120	1.22	3.84
Silastic[R]	105	1.07	3.22
Polypropylene(Tenite[R])	88	0.90	2.83
Polyurethane(Tuftane[R])	122	1.24	4.45
Teflon[R]	118	1.20	3.95

The polymer deposited on the glass slides was scratched with a blade. This polymer was not soluble in toluene, indicating that the material was cross-linked (uncrosslinked silicone polymers are readily soluble in toluene). The glass slides were extracted with toluene. The average weight loss was 4.2 ± 2.8 % (n = 5) indicating that the deposited polymer layer is tightly bound to the glass slides and cannot be washed

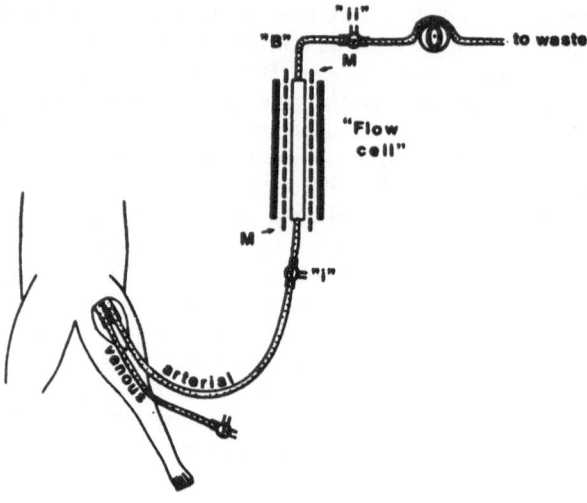

Figure 5. Kinetics of Plasma Polymerization Over Various Substrate Materials. PP: Polypropylene; PU: Polyurethane.

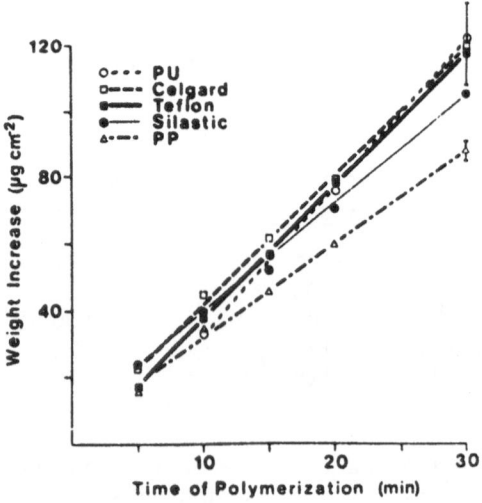

Figure 6. Fourier Transform Infrared Spectra of (a) High Density Polyethylene and (b) Silicone Coated High Density Polyethylene.

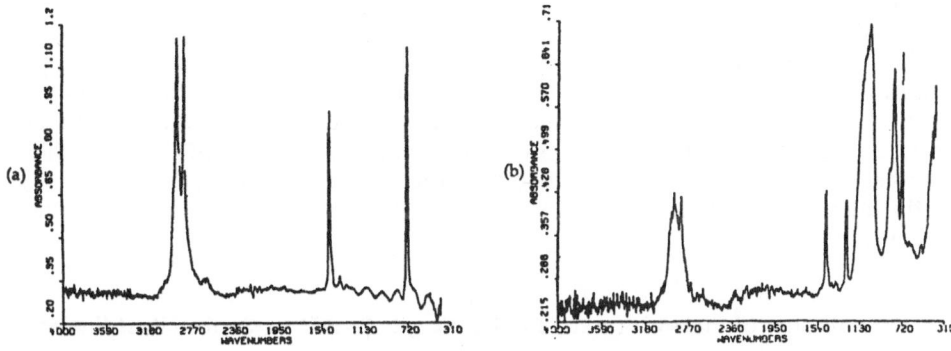

Figure 4.   Ex-Vivo Shunt Arrangement for the Evaluation of the Membranes.

off even by toluene. These results show that the deposited polymer layer was cross-linked and bonded to substrate materials.

Figure 6 shows the Fourier-transform ATR spectra of the uncoated and coated HDPE. The peaks at 1262, 1020, and 801 cm^{-1} are due to Si-CH$_3$ bending, Si-O-Si stretching, and Si-CH$_3$ out of plane bending, respectively. Similar peaks were obtained for other coated materials, and these results are summarized in Table II. There are some variations in the position of these peaks. These variations are to be expected and results from the binding of the silicone polymer to various other groups present in the substrate polymers.

Table II. Infrared Spectral Assignments for Various Polymer Films Coated with Plasma Polymerized Silicone.

	Absorption bands (cm^{-1})		
Polymer film	Si-CH$_3$ Bending in-plane	Si-O-Si Stretching	Si-CH$_3$ Bending out-of-plane
Polyethylene (H.D.)	1262	1020	802
Polypropylene	1270	1000	776
Teflon	1261	1025	802
Polyurethane	1261	1017	804

The test results of in-vitro blood compatibility studies are shown in Table III. It is apparent that there is a wide variation in the number of platelets and leukocytes adhering to a particular surface. These variations, in addition to being due to random errors, are thought to be mainly due to variations in the blood from different animals.

The results for cell No. 1, in which glass and SCC were used, show that the number of platelets on glass was greater than on SCC, except in sample No. CGD-44, in which SCC had 1.4 more platelets per field of view than glass had. Statistical analysis showed that the glass had significantly more platelets than the SCC ($P < 0.05$). Similarly, for cell No. 2, in which the Silastic and the SCC were compared, statistical analysis showed that the Silastic had significantly more platelets than the SCC ($P < 0.025$). From these results it may be concluded that the coated surfaces (SCC) were better than the glass or the Silastic surfaces as far as the platelet-foreign surface interactions were concerned.

Table III. Adhesion of Platelets (Plat.) and Leukocyte (WBC) to Various Test Surfaces.

Sample Code No	Initial Blood Platelet Count, $\times 10^3/\mu l$	Cell No.1				Cell No.2			
		Glass		SCC		Silastic		SCC	
		Plat.	WBC	Plat.	WBC	Plat.	WBC	Plat.	WBC
CGD-41	228	93.6	0.1	19.7	0	167.4	0	0.7	0
-41	256	60.0	0.3	45.0	0	52.1	0	65.1	0
-42	186	18.3	0	16.3	0	94.3	0.3	39.4	0
-44	224	9.1	0.1	10.5	0	45.7	0.3	17.7	0
-45	264	0.1	0	0	0	0.5	1.4	0	0
-46	228	0.2	0.2	0	0	0.9	0	0.1	0.1
-47	224	1.3	0	0.2	0	10.0	0.3	0.5	0
-47	241	0.5	0.1	0.4	0	0.3	0.1	0.1	0
-52	193	3.0	0	3.0	0	0.3	0.1	0	0
-52	285	79.6	0.1	4.8	0	132	0	0.5	0
-54	183	0.8	0	0	0	9.2	1.2	0	0.1
-54	275	66.2	0.5	47.7	1.0	25.6	2.5	40.6	0.8
-55	245	84.4	2.7	23.8	0.3	110.5	0.5	72.1	0.02

It is also evident that there were fewer leukocytes on SCC than on the glass or the Silastic. The exact significance of these leukocytes is uncertain, but they would normally invade a surface after the plasma proteins and the platelets have conditioned the surface.

From the above discussions of the platelets-biomaterials and leukocytes-biomaterials interaction, the SCC surfaces are tentatively judged to be superior than the glass or the Silastic surfaces as far as the blood-surface interactions were concerned.

Table IV shows the hematological data obtained for one of the dogs used. The dog has normal blood cell count and normal whole blood clotting time. The numbers of platelets and leukocytes adhering to the membranes were found by counting them under light microscopy. Either 20 fields of view or 1000 cells, whichever came first were counted. The results are shown in Table V. It is evident that even after 1 min of blood flow, the platelets could be found on the membranes. After 5 min the number of platelets per field on the coated membrane was only 26 compared to 140 on the Silastic membrane. The number of leukocytes on both the membranes were almost the same. After 10 min, the number of platelets per field on the coated Celgard membrane was 148 compared to 234 on the Silastic membrane. In addition

Table IV. Hematological Data for one Experimental Dog's Blood.

Whole Blood Clotting Time	10 mins.
Hematocrit	38 %
Platelet Count	$247 \times 10^3 / \mu l$
WBC Count	$10.1 \times 10^3 / \mu l$

to these platelets, some platelet clumps were also seen on the Silastic membrane. Also, coated Celgard had 2 leukocytes per field of view compared to 3.4 on the Silastic. Furthermore, some leukocytes were in the platelet clumps on the Silastic membranes and could not be counted. From the results of Table V it is evident that after 5 and 10 min of blood flow, the coated Celgard had fewer platelets compared to the Silastic membrane. Similarly, after 10 mins, coated Celgard had fewer leukocytes compared to those on the Silastic membranes.

Table V. Blood Cell Adhesion on Silicone Coated Celgard (SCC) and Silastic (Field of view area = 0.14 mm^2).

Sample	Time of Blood Flow	Avarage Number of Platelets Per Field	Average Number of Leukocytes Per Field
SCC	1 min	15	0
Silastic	1 min	9.7	0
SCC	5 mins	26	1.7
Silastic	5 mins	140	1.3
SCC	10 mins	148	2.0
Silastic	10 mins	234 +Platelet Clumps	3.4 +in Clumps

The SEM of the Silastic and the coated Celgard membrane after 10 mins of blood exposure were observed. Higher number of platelets and leukocytes were found on the Silastic membrane compared to those on the coated Celgard. The platelets and the leukocytes on the Silastic membrane had undergone greater morphological changes then those on the coated Celgard membrane. The platelets on the Silastic membrane had put out pseudopods, and some fibrin strands were visible. Thus, the Silastic membrane not only had a higher number of platelets and leukocytes adhering to it, but these blood cells underwent greater morphological changes compared to those on the coated Celgard.

The number and the morphological changes of the platelets adhering to foreign surfaces have been used to evaluate biomaterials (3-11). It is generally agreed that the lower the number of platelets on a biomaterial and the lesser the morphological changes in these, the better the biomaterial. Thus, from the results presented in Table IV, it may be concluded that the silicone coated Celgard membranes are better then the Silastic membranes as far as platelet biomaterial interactions are concerned.

ATTACHMENT OF ALBUMIN TO POLYPROPYLENE SURFACE

We shall now describe a case where reactive amino groups were added by plasma treatment and, these in turn, were used to bind albumin to the substrate surface. Albumin neither initiates coagulation nor attracts blood platelets. Therefore, it was reasoned that albuminated surfaces prepared would be biocompatible.

Material and Methods

In an ammonia discharge a number of reactive species such as N, H, NH, NH_2 etc. are generated (12). These species can be used to initiate a chemical reaction. Simultaneously, the surface of the polypropylene membrane is activated by irradiation with plasma. The reactive species then react with the activated surface, perhaps, by the following reaction (13) :

$$
\begin{array}{ccc}
\underset{\underset{CH_3}{|}}{\overset{\overset{H}{|}}{-CH_2-C-CH_2-}} & \xrightarrow[\text{bombardment}]{\text{Plasma}} & \underset{\underset{CH_3}{|}}{-CH_2-CH-CH_2-} \quad \xrightarrow{\cdot NH_2} \quad \underset{\underset{CH_3}{|}}{\overset{\overset{NH_2}{|}}{-CH_2-C-CH_2-}}
\end{array}
$$

Similarly, amino groups could have attached to any other carbon atom. The net result is that the polymer surface acquires amino groups and this material will be referred to as Celgard $-NH_2$. These membranes were prepared using various ammonia pressures in the plasma reactor.

The membranes with amino groups prepared as above were soaked in a 5 ml solution of 3 g % human albumin (Sigma Chemical) in phosphate buffer, 0.5 M, pH 7.5, for one hour. These membranes were washed throughly with the phosphate buffer to remove superficially bound albumin. The membranes were then divided into two groups. One group was evaluated without any additional treatment. The second group was further treated with a solution of 1.5% glutaraldehyde in phosphate buffer to cross-link the albumin. After one hour the membranes were removed from the glutaraldehyde solution and washed with the buffer. In order to eliminate any free aldehyde groups, the membranes were immersed in 0.13 M glycine in the phosphate buffer for overnight. Thus, 2 types of albuminated surfaces were prepared: one without cross-linking and the other cross-linked with glutaraldehyde, and were referred to as albuminated Celgard (AC) and cross-linked albuminated Celgard (CAC), respectively. The surfaces of these membranes were characterized by Fourier-transform infrared spectroscopy using ATR techniques.

Once the albuminated membranes had been prepared, it was essential to find out if the albumin would be washed out by flowing saline or plasma. To do this ^{125}I-labelled albumin (New England Nuclear, Boston, Massachusetts) was used.

Results and Discussion

Table VI shows the relative IR absorption of the band at 1660 cm^{-1} and the corresponding pressure of the gaseous plasma used in the preparation. It can be seen that the attachment of the NH_2 group is greatest at a pressure of 400 militorr. This may result from the fact that at lower pressures there is not enough ammonia for reaction whereas at higher pressure, the mean free path for collisions between reactive species decreases, leading to higher consumption of the initiating species in the gaseous phase. Thus, at higher pressures not enough initiating species are available at the membrane surface for attaching NH_2 groups. Therefore, the amino group attached membranes prepared at 400 militorr pressure were used for the albumin binding.

Table VI. Pressure and Gaseous Plasma and The Relative IR Adsorption Band of Amino Group at 1660 cm^{-1}.

Sample Code No.	Pressure (militorr)	Relative Absorption
PP031	160	0.263
PP030	400	0.470
PP033	500	0.330
PP029	900	0.246

Fourier Transform infrared spectra of control Celgard and AC are shown in Figures 7A and 7B, respectively. It can be seen from Figure 7B that the amide I band of albumin occurs at 1658 cm^{-1}, while the absorption band for amide II appears at 1540 cm^{-1}. The appearance of these amide I and amide II absorption bands show that the deposited material is indeed a protein and hence albumin. The characteristic bands for the protein were observed for both types of albuminated Celgard (AC and CAC) even after washing in distilled water for 48 hours. FTIR spectra of control membranes exposed to albumin and then washed with distilled water showed no absorption bands for albumin.

The albuminated membranes were prepared for possible use as biomaterials for fabricating blood-contacting medical devices. For the membrane to be an effective biomaterial, albumin should not be washed off by flowing blood. Therefore, it was important to study the stability of the attached albumin both in saline and in plasma. Both the albuminated (AC) and the cross-linked albuminated Celgard (CAC) were tested. The results of washing AC and CAC membranes with normal saline are shown in Figures 8A and 8B, respectively. The concentration of albumin shown on the ordinate refers to the amount retained per cm^2 of the membrane surface. It is evident from Figure 8 that, after the initial rapid removal of albumin, the level stabilized. The concentrations of albumin retained on AC and the CAC membranes were 275 and 357 µg/cm^2, respectively. It is evident that the cross-linking with glutaraldehyde does improve the stability of the attached albumin. Thus, even after 48 hours of washing, higher concentrations were retained by cross-linking. Even without cross-linking, very high concentrations of 275 µg/cm^2 were retained compared to 28 µg/cm^2 reported in literature (14). Thus, our method of plasma treatment yields much higher albumin concentrations on the polymer surface.

The results obtained by washing with human plasma for AC and CAC are depicted in Figures 9a and 9b, respectively. It can be seen from Figure 9 that the amount of albumin on the membranes tends to stabilize after initial rapid washing of albumin. The concentrations of albumin retained on AC and CAC membranes were 325 and 335 µg/cm^2, respectively. The level of albumin retained on the CAC membrane is somewhat higher than that on the AC membranes. The differences among the concentrations of albumin retained after washing with saline and human plasma are

242

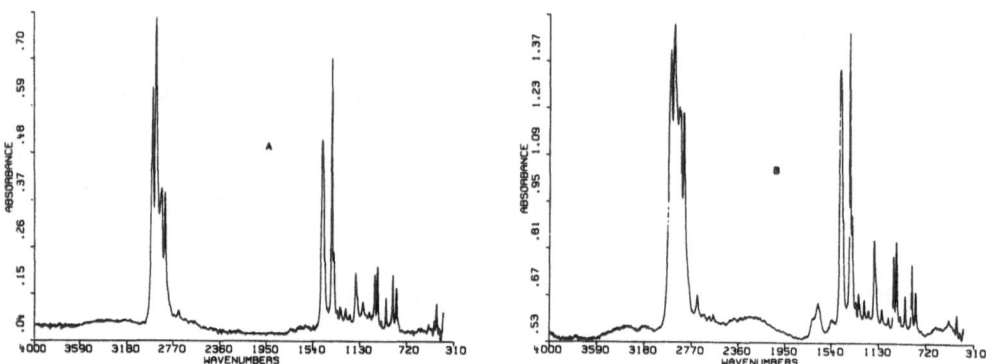

Figure 7.   ATR-IR Spectra of Control Celgard (A) and Albuminated Celgard (B).

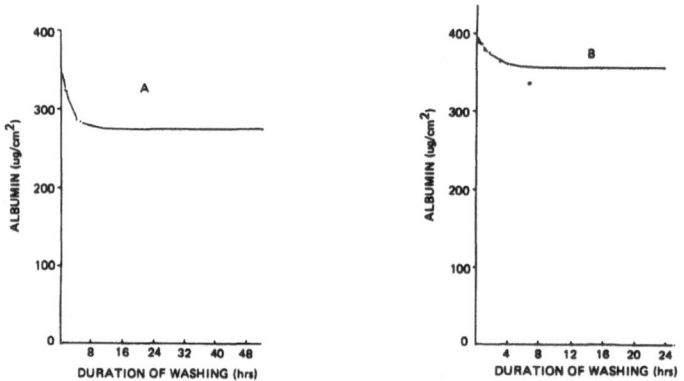

Figure 8.   Washing of Albuminated Celgard Membranes with Saline. 8A: Albuminated Celgard without Cross-Linking. 8B: Albuminated Celgard Cross-Linked by Glutaraldehyde.

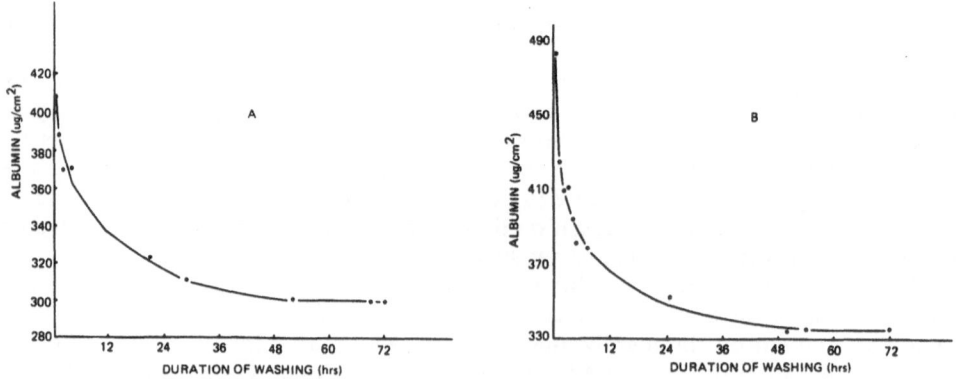

Figure 9.   Washing of Albuminated Celgard Membranes with Human Plasma. 9A: Albuminated Celgard without Crosslinking. 9B: Albuminated Celgard Cross-Linked by Glutaraldehyde.

hard to explain, but these might be due to the fact that human plasma contains about 4 g % albumin. This may be effecting the washing of albumin from the membranes.

The above results show that the albumin can be attached to the polymer surface efficiently by plasma chemistry. It is anticipated that the albuminated biomaterials thus prepared will find applications in medical devices.

ADDITIONAL BIOMEDICAL APPLICATIONS OF PLASMA POLYMERIZATION

This section is presented to bring out the scope of the technology rather than to review the literature.

Silicone rubbers contain about 30% silica as a filler and it appears that part of the silica may reside on the surface. Silica particles act as nuclei for initiating coagulation and the formation of microthrombi (15). To overcome this problem, a number of methods, including plasma polymerization have been used to deposit a layer of filler free silicone polymer over the silicone rubber (2,5,6,16-19). The added layer masks the exposed silica leading to improved biomaterials.

Plasma treatment has been used in controlled drug release devices. For example, the rate of release of progesterone through silicone rubber membrane can be reduced by plasma treatment (20). In another application, the life of an oxygen sensor has been improved by depositing on it a layer of plasma polymerized polypropylene film (21). This prevented the fouling of the electrode by body fluids. Similarly, neurological electrodes were treated with glow discharge to improve their stability (22).

There are a number of additional applications reported in the literature. These may be found in the bibliography provided in the refence section.

REFERENCES

1. Whitford, M.J., Biomaterials, 5:298, 1984.
2. Chawla, A.S., Trans. Amer. Soc. Artif. Intern. Organs, 25:287, 1979.
3. Rembaum, A., Yen, Y.P.S., Ingram, M., Newton, J.F., Hu, C.L., Frasher, W.G., and Barbour, B.H., Biomat., Med., Dev., Artif. Organs, 1:99, 1973.
4. Chawla, A.S., Biomat. Med. Dev., Artif. Organs, 6:89, 1978.
5. Kolobow, T., Stool, E.W., Weathersby, P.K., Pierce, J., Hayano, F., and Suaudeau, J., Trans. Amer. Soc. Artif. Intern. Organs, 20A:269, 1974.
6. Zapol, W.M., Bloom, S., Carvalho, A., Wonders, A., Skoskiewicz, M., Scheider, R., and Snider, M., Trans. Amer. Soc. Artif, Intern. Organs, 21:587,1975.
7. Mason, R.G., Bull, N.Y.Acad. Med, 48:407,1972.
8. Brash, J.L., Brophy, J.M., and Feurerstein, I.A., J.Biomed, Mater. Res., 10:429, 1976.
9. Muzykewicz, K.J., Crowell, E.B., Jr., Hart, A.P., Schultz, M., Hill, C.G.J., Jr., and Cooper, S.L., J.Biomed, Mater. Res., 9:487,1975
10. Salzman, E.W., Lindon, J., Brier, D., and Merrill, E.W. Ann. N.Y. Acad. Sci., 283:114, 1977.
11. Lindsay, R.M., Prentice, C.R.M., Burton, J.A., Ferguson, R., and Kennedy, A.C. Trans. Amer. Soc. Artif. Intern. Organs, 19:487, 1973.
12. Devins, J.C. and Burton, M., J.Amer. Chem. Soc., 76:2618, 1953.
13. Hollahan, J.R., and Stafford, B.M., J. Appl. Poly. Sci., 13:807, 1969.

14. Hoffman, A.S., Schmer, G., Harris, C. and Kraft, W.G. Trans. Amer. Soc. Artif. Intern. Organs, 18:10, 1972.
15. Kolobow, T., Tomlison, T.A. and Pierce, J.E. J. Biomed. Mater. Res., 11:471, 1977.
16. Gifford, G.H., Jr., Merrill, E.W., and Morgan, M.S. J. Biomed. Mater. Res., 10:857, 1976.
17. Chawla, A.S. Artif. Organs, 3:92, 1979.
18. Chawla, A.S. Biomaterials, 2:83, 1981.
19. Chawla, A.S. and Sipehia, R.,J. Biomed. Mater. Res., 18:537, 1984.
20. Colter, K.D., Bell, A.T., and Shen, M.,Biomat., Med. Dev., Artif. Organs, 5:13, 1977.
21. Hahn, A.W., Nichols, M.F., Barr, R.E., Sharma, A., And Hallmuth, E.W., in Biomedical Sciences Instrumentation, Vol. 15, p. 7-10, Proceedings of 16th Ann. Rocky Mountain Bioengineering Symposium, Denver, Co. 1979.
22. Cannon, J.G., Dillon, R.O., Bunshah, R.F., Crandall, P.H. and Dymond, A.M., J.Biomed. Mater. Res., 14:279, 1980.

SURFACE MODIFICATION OF BIOPOLYMER MATERIALS

H.Chmiel and H.Bauser

Fraunhofer—Institut für Grenzflaechen-und Bioverfahrenstechnik Stuttgart, FRG

INTRODUCTION

The interactions between a polymeric material and the surrounding biosystem are more or less a function of the surface of the biomaterial. An example is the adsorption of plasma proteins on surfaces in contact with blood. These adsorptive interactions are directly or indirectly related to more than one of the requirements for blood compatibility (Table I): Plasma protein adsorption may influence the integrity of structure and function of proteins, the adhesion of cells, and finally the development of thrombi or emboli (1). In addition, the function of polymeric membranes in artificial organs is impaired by protein adsorption not only indirectly by clogging with trapped emboli, but also immediatley by the formation of protein deposits at membrane surfaces.

Table I. Conditions for Blood Compatibility.

Biomaterials must not induce
— thrombi or emboli
— impairment of cell function or destruction
— alteration of plasma proteins
— toxic or allergic reactions
— immuno reactions
— cancer
— release of particles or harmful substances

By this token, surface modification of polymeric materials, if applied to minimize the interaction between surface and proteins, may be considered from two angles : improving thromboresistance and reducing membrane fouling. This paper is devoted to the latter aspect.

MATERIALS AND METHODS

Glow-discharge methods allow many substances to be deposited or grafted onto many polymeric substrates. Plasma deposition and plasma polymerisation have been used in order to attach functional groups to surfaces or to form coatings, such as polyacrylonitrile, isotropic carbon, sulfino groups, polysiloxane, etc. Another glow–discharge deposition technique is sputtering, which has mainly been used to prepare isotropic carbon layers (similar to LTI carbon (2)) on polymers. On ultra-filtration membranes, a granular structure of carbon layers (3) allows access of the feed solution to the membrane pores. Layers of below 10 nm suffice for surface modification.

Substrate materials have been polyurethane, polycarbonate, polysulfone, poly-tetrafluoroethylene etc. Membrane materials used were mostly Cuprophane[R] HDF flat membranes (cut-off approximately 10,000 Dalton) and Nuclepore[R] polycarbonate membranes with pore diameters of 0.03 and 0.4 µm.

For filtration experiments with flat membranes, cross-flow test cells were used with 0.3 mm X 0.3 mm straight channels. These experiments were performed under controlled conditions for solution flow, transmembrane pressure, and temperature. Filtrate and retentate flow were recorded continually by weighing. Only feed-solution sides of membranes were surface modified. Filtration tests were made with bovine blood serum or with different protein solutions.

TESTING

Electron and infrared-reflection spectroscopy were applied for chemical surface characterization of native and modifed polymer substrates. ESCA can also be used to detect adsorbed protein layers after a substrate has been exposed to a protein solution (4). The growth of a protein adsorption layer and its decrease upon desorption can be observed as a function of time by a dielectric method described elsewhere (4). A third method is adsorption measurement by radioactive tracers. Results have been reported elsewhere (3).

FILTRATION EXPERIMENTS

As a consequence of the separation process at the membrane, the wall concentration of retained molecules, particles or cells exceeds their bulk concentration (Fig. 1). This concentration polarization of retained species, if high enough, gives rise to the formation of a gel layer. Proteins, because of their attractive interaction with the membrane surface, contribute to gel-layer formation even if their molecular diameter is smaller than the pore diameter. This will be confirmed below. Consequently, (a) the transmembrane flux decays in the course of time, and (b) its pressure dependence is sublinear (Fig. 2).

If the feed-solution side of a membrane is surface-modified for smaller protein interaction, the performance of the membrane may be improved. However, the results of filtration experiments with protein solutions suggest a qualitatively different improvement for the micro- and ultrafiltration membranes tested so far.

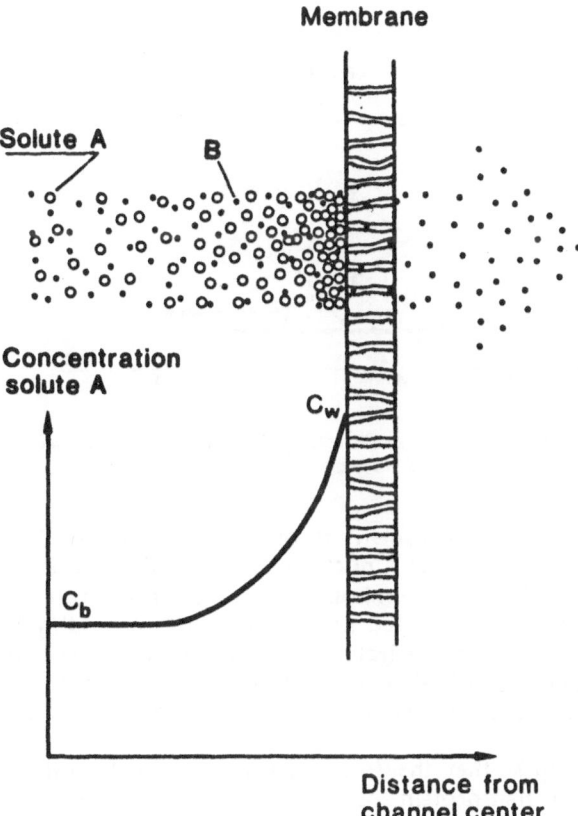

Figure 1.   Concentration Polarisation at a Membrane (Schematic).

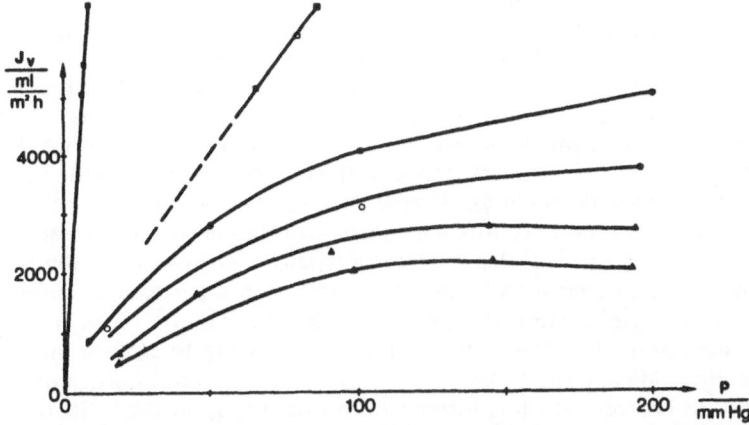

Figure 2.   Plot of Transmembrane Flux I_V Versus Transmembrane Pressure p of Hollow-Fibre Membranes for Plasma Separation. Filtration of NaCl Solution before and after □ Plasma Separation. Plasma with Platelet Counts of 5,000 ● and 40,000 ○. Whole Blood with Hematocrit of 36 % ▲ and 38 % △.

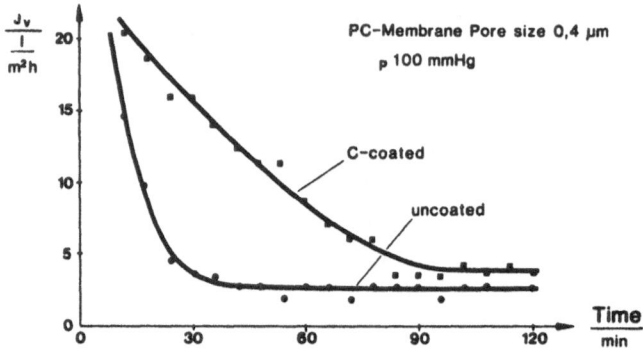

Figure 3.   Transmembrane Flux I_V Versus Filtration Time of Bovine Blood Serum through Uncoated and Isotropic Carbon-Coated Nuclepore[R] Membranes.

An only temporary improvement is obtained for microfiltration membranes. This is illustrated in Figure 3 for a nucleation-track polycarbonate membrane with 0.4 μm pore diameter. The transmembrane flux drops in the course of time both at the uncoated and the carbon coated membrane. Surface modification in this case only retards the flux decay. Such a treatment would therefore be of use only in applications where the duration of filtration would only last one or two hours (e.g. in therapeutic hemofiltration), or where the periods between back washing would be this short.

These results suggest that the formation of protein deposits at the membrane surface is reduced, but that protein adsorption at the pore walls, which have not been modified, finally causes the flux to decay to nearly the same steadystate value as at the uncoated membranes. (The protein molecular diameter in this case is much smaller than the pore size, therefore, the protein molecules in principle should pass the pores).

Qualitatively similar though quantitatively different results were obtained with other carbon coatings (differences due to other deposition parameters), with titanium layers, or with sulfone groups on the same base membranes.

Qualitatively different results, however, have been achieved with ultrafiltration membranes. The representation chosen in Figure 4 for Cuprophane[R] HDF membranes displays the gel-layer resistance $R_{g,t}$ as a function of time. Within the duration of the experiments the gel-layer resistance of the unmodified membrane keeps increasing (i.e. the flux keeps decreasing), whereas the carbon-coated or - with a somewhat more modest success - the polysiloxane-coated membranes reach a steady state after about 30 to 40 minutes. The steady-state resistance remains below the still growing resistance of the uncoated membrane, thus indicating a permanent improvement of the membrane function. Here the protein molecules cannot sneak into the pores. Hence the reduction of protein-deposit formation owing to surface modification at the feed-solution side appears to be sufficient for a permanent improvement.

In order to corroborate this interpretation based upon the influence of protein adsorption and its reduction by surface modification, Figure 5 shows for a protein solution adsorption and desorption measurements at a Cuprophane[R] HDF membrane without and with isotropic carbon coating.

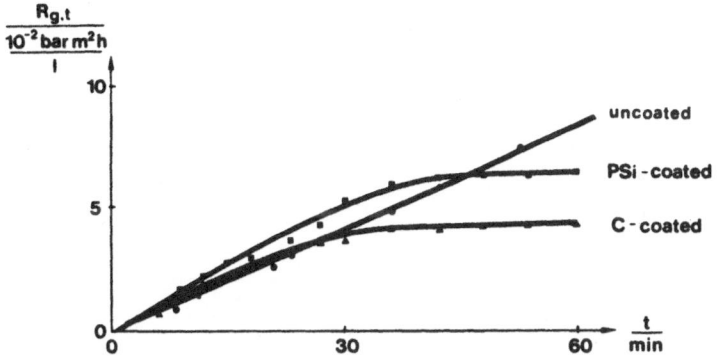

Figure 4. Flow Resistance of Gel Layer on Unmodified, Polysiloxane-Coated and Carbon-Coated Cuprophane(R) HDF Membranes as a Function of Time (Solution with 0.7 % Albumin and 0.2 % Globulins). Transmembrane Pressure 1 Bar.

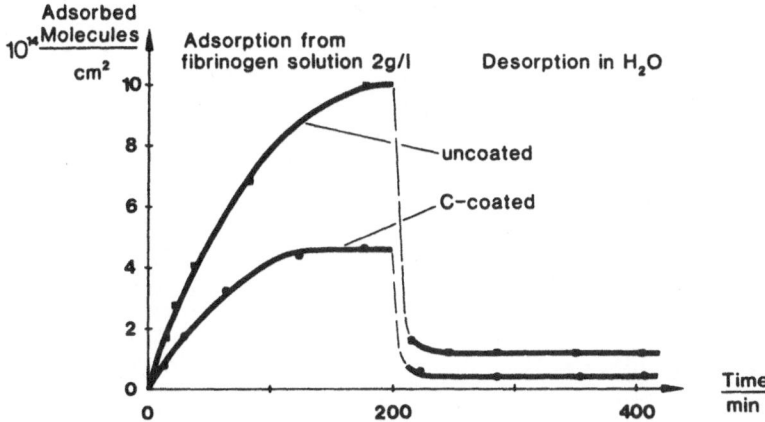

Figure 5. Adsorption of Bovine Fibrinogen from a 0.2 % Solution (0 to 200 min) and Desorption in Water (200 to 400 min) of Uncoated and Isotropic Carbon-Coated Cuprophane(R) HDF Membranes.

REFERENCES

1. Bruck, S.D., Properties of Biomaterials in the Physiological Environment, CRC Press Inc., Boca Raton, Fl., 1980.
2. Bokros, J.C., Carbon, 15:335, 1977.
3. Bauser, H., Chmiel, H., in Polymers in Medicine, E. Chiellini and P. Giusti, eds., pp. 297, Plenum, New York, 1984.
4. Hellwig, G., Chem.-Ing.-Technik, 51:530, 1979.

KEY WORDS FOR SUBJECT INDEX

Polymeric Biomaterials, E. Piskin and A.S. Hoffman

252

CHAPTER 9, *Piskin 3,*
—Biological App—

256